Cardiovascular Disease in Primary Care

RCGP Curriculum for
General Practice Series

Cardiovascular Disease in Primary Care

A guide for GPs

Edited by
F.D. Richard Hobbs,
Richard J. McManus
and Clare J. Taylor

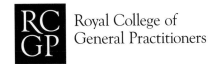

Royal College of
General Practitioners

The Royal College of General Practitioners was founded in 1952 with this object:

'To encourage, foster and maintain the highest possible standards in general practice and for that purpose to take or join with others in taking steps consistent with the charitable nature of that object which may assist towards the same.'

Among its responsibilities under its Royal Charter the College is entitled to:

'Diffuse information on all matters affecting general practice and issue such publications as may assist the object of the College.'

British Library Cataloguing-in-Publication Data
A catalogue record for this book is available from the British Library

© Royal College of General Practitioners
F.D. Richard Hobbs, Richard J. McManus and Clare J. Taylor 2011

Published by the Royal College of General Practitioners 2011
1 Bow Churchyard, London EC4M 9DQ

Disclaimer
This publication is intended for the use of medical practitioners in the UK and not for patients. The authors, editors and publisher have taken care to ensure that the information contained in this book is correct to the best of their knowledge, at the time of publication. Whilst efforts have been made to ensure the accuracy of the information presented, particularly that related to the prescription of drugs, the authors, editors and publisher cannot accept liability for information that is subsequently shown to be wrong. Readers are advised to check that the information, especially that related to drug usage, complies with information contained in the *British National Formulary*, or equivalent, or manufacturers' datasheets, and that it complies with the latest legislation and standards of practice.

Designed and typeset at the Typographic Design Unit
Printed by Hobbs the Printers Ltd
Indexed by Carol Ball

ISBN: 978-0-85084-330-9

Contents

Contributors

Editors

Professor F.D. Richard Hobbs FRCP FRCGP FESC FMedSci is currently Professor and Head of Primary Care Clinical Sciences at the University of Birmingham, UK. He is the Director of the National Institute for Health Research (NIHR) National School for Primary Care Research (2009–) and was co-Director of the Quality and Outcomes Framework (QoF) Review Panel from 2005–9. He sits on several national and international scientific and research funding boards, and currently chairs the Council for Cardiovascular Primary Care, the European Society of Cardiology (ESC), the Prevention and Care Board, the British Heart Foundation, and the European Primary Care Cardiovascular Society (EPCCS). Professor Hobbs's research interests focus on cardiovascular epidemiology and clinical trials, especially relating to vascular and stroke risk, and to heart failure. Overall, his publications comprise twenty-eight book chapters, twelve edited books and over 290 original papers in peer-reviewed journals such as the *Lancet, Annals of Internal Medicine* and the *British Medical Journal*. His research has impacted on international health policies and clinical guidelines. Within the NHS he has consulted on National Service Frameworks for coronary heart disease, atrial fibrillation and heart failure, as well as several National Institute for Health and Clinical Excellence (NICE) reviews. He has provided clinical care in inner-city general practice for nearly 30 years.

Professor Richard J. McManus BSc MSc PhD MBBS FRCGP is a Professor of Primary Care Cardiovascular Disease, Clinical Director of the Midlands Research Practice Consortium (MidReC) and a part-time GP at Greenridge Surgery in Billesley, Birmingham. His research interests lie mainly in cardiovascular disease and he has published work on the management of chest pain in primary care, electronic blood pressure measurement, stroke management in primary care and self-monitoring in hypertension. He holds an NIHR Career Development Fellowship and leads the Stroke Theme of the Birmingham Collaboration for Leadership in Applied Health Research and Care (CLAHRC) as well as several NIHR-funded studies on the primary care management of hypertension and chronic kidney disease. He supervises PhD students undertaking projects in diabetes, hypertension and chronic kidney disease, and is external examiner for the Primary Care MSc at Barts and the London. He is Guardian of RCGP curriculum statement 15.1, *Cardiovascular Problems*, and has provided expert advice to NICE, the Department of Health and the ESC.

Dr Clare J. Taylor MA MB MPH BChir DCH MRCP MRCGP qualified from the University of Cambridge in 2002. She completed a medical rotation at Addenbrooke's Hospital, gaining Membership of the Royal College of Physicians, then did a year of Paediatrics before moving to Birmingham to train in academic General Practice. She now works as a salaried GP in central Birmingham and is an NIHR In-Practice Fellow at the University of Birmingham with an interest in cardiovascular research. Her research has focused on the prognosis of patients with heart failure and the management of atrial fibrillation. She is also Clinical Lead for two cardiovascular disease modules in the Masters in Primary and Community Care at the University of Birmingham and a clinical examiner at the Medical School. Dr Taylor was Chair of the RCGP's Associates-in-Training Committee, 2008–9, and is now the 'First5' Continuing Professional Development Fellow at the College, looking at the learning needs of GPs within the first 5 years of qualification. She is also a member of the Clinical Knowledge Summaries editorial board and the GP Extraction Service project board at Connecting for Health.

Contributing authors

Dr Paul Aveyard is a reader in Behavioural Medicine at the University of Birmingham and a GP in the Blythe Practice, Knowle, Solihull. He has been researching tobacco control, particularly in the area of smoking cessation, for the past 10 years. His current research interests focus on behavioural and pharmacological methods to enhance cessation, particularly in testing the possibility of helping people unwilling to quit smoking to accept treatment, and if this is beneficial.

Professor Matthew Cooke is the National Clinical Director for Urgent and Emergency Care at the Department of Health in England. He is also Professor of Emergency Medicine at Heart of England NHS Foundation Trust and Warwick Medical School. His research interests focus on emergency care systems design, safer clinical systems and clinical trials in soft-tissue injuries and pre-hospital care.

Dr Russell Davis has been a consultant cardiologist at Sandwell and West Birmingham Hospitals NHS Trust since 2002 and is Honorary Senior Lecturer at the University of Birmingham. He trained at King's College, Cambridge, and Cambridge Clinical School, graduating in 1988. He then undertook specialty training in cardiology, including 3 years as Clinical Research Fellow in the Department of Primary Care and General Practice at the University of Birmingham. Here he was involved with the ECHOES study of heart failure prevalence in the community, which was the subject of his MD thesis. His main clinical and research interests are heart failure and cardiac imaging.

Dr Olaolu Erinfolami is a Consultant in Emergency Medicine and Foundation Training Programme Director at the Heart of England NHS Foundation Trust. He has a keen interest in evidence-based medicine, observation emergency medicine (clinical decision units) and medical education. He is a member of the Editorial Panel for NHS Evidence – emergency and urgent care (formerly a Specialist Library of the National Library for Health), the Lead Clinician for the Clinical Decision Units at the Trust and a member of the American College of Emergency Physicians (observation section). He is also a Senior Clinical Examiner for the University of Birmingham.

Professor David Fitzmaurice is a GP and Professor of Primary Care at the University of Birmingham. His primary research interest lies in cardiovascular disease, in particular oral anticoagulation management. He is a board member of the Primary Care Cardiovascular Society (PCCS), for which he chairs the Anticoagulation Working Group, is Primary Care Adviser to several NICE guidelines (including *The Management of Atrial Fibrillation*), author of UK guidelines for patients' self-management of oral anticoagulation and co-author of a recent systematic review of cost-effectiveness of self-management of oral anticoagulation for the Health Technology Assessment programme.

Dr Simon Fynn is a Consultant Cardiologist at Papworth Hospital, Cambridge. He specialises in the investigation and treatment of cardiac arrhythmias and undertakes radiofrequency catheter ablation and cardiac device implantation (e.g. pacemakers and defibrillators). He has a particular interest in atrial fibrillation and has published numerous papers on the mechanisms and treatment of cardiac arrhythmias.

Dr Paramjit Gill is a Clinical Reader in Primary Care Research at the University of Birmingham and works part time as a GP in Birmingham. His research interests include addressing health inequalities, particularly amongst migrant populations, and evidence-based health care and its application to healthcare delivery.

Dr Patrick Heck read medicine as an undergraduate at Caius College, Cambridge, before completing his degree at Brasenose College, Oxford. Having started as a cardiology specialist registrar in 2004, he is currently undertaking an electrophysiology fellowship at the Royal Melbourne Hospital for 18 months before returning to Papworth Hospital in 2011.

Dr Carl Heneghan is Deputy Director of the Centre for Evidence-Based Medicine. He is a GP and Clinical Lecturer in the Department of Primary Health Care at the University of Oxford. He is a principal investigator in the Oxford Centre for Monitoring and Diagnosis in Primary Care (MaDOx), a new research programme funded by the NIHR, and works with the Oxford Vascular Study (OXVASC) on the incidence, prevention and treatment of acute coronary events from a population perspective.

Professor Kamlesh Khunti has been Professor of Primary Care Diabetes and Vascular Medicine, and Head of Division of General Practice and Primary Health Care, University of Leicester, since 2007. He leads a research group in the Department of Health Sciences, undertaking important research into early identification and interventions in people with diabetes and pre-diabetes.

Professor Michael Kirby worked as a GP in Letchworth, Hertfordshire, 1973–2007, and was Director of HertNet (the Hertfordshire Primary Care Research Network), 1998–2007. He is currently a Visiting Professor to the Faculty of Health and Human Sciences and consultant to the Clinical Trials Co-ordinating Centre (CTCC) at the University of Hertfordshire. His clinical work is now at the Prostate Centre in London. He is editor of the *Primary Care Cardiovascular Journal* (PCCJ) and he also holds membership of several NHS advisory boards. He has published more than 200 clinical papers and twenty-three books.

Dr Su May Liew is a Senior Clinical Lecturer and Family Medicine Special-ist at the University of Malaya, Malaysia. She is currently pursuing a DPhil in Primary Health Care at the University of Oxford. Her research area is cardio-vascular disease prevention in primary care, focusing on cardiovascular risk assessment. Dr Liew also works with the AsiaLink programme, funded by the European Commission to establish common, sustainable knowledge and capacities in Asia in evidence-based medicine and clinical epidemiology.

Professor Paul Little is a GP and Professor of Primary Care Research at the University of Southampton. He has a particular interest in self-management of acute and chronic conditions, and in the use of web-based interventions to support behaviour change. He was the GP on the NICE panel for the treat-ment of obesity.

Professor Jonathan Mant is Professor of Primary Care Research at the University of Cambridge, Associate Director for Primary and Social Care of the Stroke Research Network, and Honorary Consultant in Public Health. His research focuses on prevention and treatment of cardiovascular disease, particularly stroke, in community settings.

Dr Edmond Walma qualified as a GP in 1982 in Rotterdam, the Neth-erlands, and he has practised in Schoonhoven since 1984. His thesis was about diuretic therapy in the elderly with hypertension and heart failure. Since then he has been involved in the production of national and Euro-pean guidelines on several cardiovascular disease topics. He is affiliated with the Department of General Practice of Erasmus University, Rotterdam, is a board member of the EPCCS and is also a member of the ESC'S Council on Cardiovascular Primary Care.

Dr Azhar Zafar is a GP in Northampton and an NIHR In-Practice Fellow working at the Division of Diabetes and Cardiovascular Medicine at the University of Leicester. His research interest is Type 2 diabetes in the Southeast Asian community.

Foreword

The important role of GPs in managing cardiovascular disease has always been underestimated. Although the recent development of interventions to limit the tissue damage caused by acute ischaemia has turned stroke and myocardial infarction into 999 events that often bypass primary care, the importance of the GP to cardiovascular health has not diminished. Death and serious disability from vascular disease before old age should not happen – every stroke and heart attack in a younger person should make a practitioner ask him or herself whether everything possible was done to prevent it.

Prevention used to mean simply taking the blood pressure and giving advice on smoking cessation and healthy eating. It now means much more than that. Identifying vascular disease at an early stage often means that the catastrophic event can be postponed or averted by appropriate treatment. Immediate treatment of transient ischaemic attacks prevents strokes. Early treatment of ventricular dysfunction prevents heart failure. Early treatment of unstable angina prevents heart attack. Good management of diabetes minimises the risk of all vascular complications. All these preventive interventions need to be done effectively and efficiently in general practice.

Making an early and accurate cardiovascular diagnosis is therefore the key to much preventive activity. It is also the key to treating effectively the many disabling symptoms caused by vascular pathology. A number of chapters in this book deal with the early recognition of vascular pathology, including stroke and peripheral vascular disease, as well as the common heart problems encountered in general practice such as arrhythmias, murmurs and pump failure. It is essential that GPs are confident and competent at dealing with these issues and have access to the necessary investigative technologies described in these chapters – it is neither efficient nor sustainable for NHS hospital cardiologists to be providing care that does not require their specialist skills.

The fact that the RCGP has commissioned this textbook reflects the commitment of the College to making sure that we apply the latest research evidence in general practice to deliver the highest possible quality of cardiovascular care in the UK. We should be proud that much of the cutting-edge research that underpins this evidence originated in UK general practice. We should also be proud that many UK general practices already apply this evidence base to the highest possible standard. But we have to admit that this is not always the case. The quality of the cardiovascular care we provide in UK primary care remains patchy. This book is a step towards remedying that situation.

Professor David Mant
Emeritus Professor of General Practice, University of Oxford

Professor Roger Boyle CBE
National Director for Heart Disease and Stroke, Department of Health

Preface

Cardiovascular disease is the number one cause of morbidity and mortality both in the UK and worldwide. GPs and other members of the primary healthcare team see a spectrum of patients with cardiovascular disease. Our day-to-day practice includes the identification and treatment of patients with modifiable risk factors, the management of patients presenting with acute stroke or myocardial infarction, and the provision of effective palliative care to patients who are dying.

This book is based on RCGP curriculum statement 15.1, *Cardiovascular Problems*, and covers the key aspects of these issues plus other cardiovascular disease relevant to primary care. Practical tips are combined with evidence-based practice. We have included case-based discussions that put the theory in the text into practice and, in many chapters, have included self-assessment questions. We hope you find the book useful, relevant and enjoyable to read. We would like to thank Dr Rodger Charlton for reviewing the manuscript and for his helpful comments.

F.D. Richard Hobbs, Richard J. McManus and Clare J. Taylor

Abbreviations

ABI	ankle brachial index
ABPI	ankle brachial pressure index
ACC	American College of Cardiology
ACCORD	Action to Control Cardiovascular Risk in Diabetes
ACCP	American College of Chest Physicians
ACE	angiotensin-converting enzyme
ACS	acute coronary syndrome
ADVANCE	Action in Diabetes and Vascular Disease: Preterax and Diamicron Modified Release Controlled Evaluation
AF	atrial fibrillation
AI	aortic incompetence
AMI	acute myocardial infarction
AR	aortic regurgitation
ARB	angiotensin II receptor blocker
ARVD	arrhythmogenic right ventricular dysplasia
AUC	Areas Under the ROC Curve
AVNRT	atrioventricular nodal re-entrant tachycardia
AVRT	atrioventricular re-entry tachycardia
BB	beta-blocker
BHF	British Heart Foundation
BMI	body mass index
BNP	B-type natriuretic peptide
CABG	coronary artery bypass graft
CAD	coronary artery disease
CAST	Cardiac Arrhythmia Suppression Trial
CAST	Chinese Acute Stroke Trial
CCB	calcium channel blocker
CHD	coronary heart disease
CI	confidence interval
CK	creatinine kinase
CKD	chronic kidney disease
CLI	chronic limb ischaemia
CMO	Chief Medical Officer
CNST	Clinical Negligence Scheme for Trusts
COPD	chronic obstructive pulmonary disease
CT	computerised tomography
CTPA	CT pulmonary angiogram
CTT	Cholesterol Treatment Trialists

CVD	cardiovascular disease
CVD	cerebrovascular disease
CXR	chest X-ray
DVLA	Driver and Vehicle Licensing Agency
DVT	deep-vein thrombosis
DWI	diffusion weighted imaging
EBCT	electron beam computerised tomography
ECG	electrocardiogram
ED	emergency department
ED	erectile dysfunction
ESC	European Society of Cardiology
ETT	exercise tolerance test
FAST	Face, Arm, Speech Test
FH	familial hypercholesterolaemia
GTN	glyceryl trinitrate
GTT	glucose tolerance test
GUCH	grown-up congenital heart disease
HCM	hypertrophic cardiomyopathy
HDL	high-density lipoprotein
HOCM	hypertrophic obstructive cardiomyopathy
HOT	Hypertension Optimal Treatment study
HRT	hormone replacement therapy
ICDs	implantable cardioverter defibrillators
ICU	intensive care unit
IE	infective endocarditis
IFG	impaired fasting glucose
IGT	impaired glucose tolerance
IHD	ischaemic heart disease
INR	international normalised ratio
IST	International Stroke Trial
JVP	jugular venous pressure
LBBB	left bundle branch block
LDL	low-density lipoprotein
LFTs	liver function tests
LMWH	low molecular weight heparin
LR	likelihood ratio
LVEF	left ventricular ejection fraction
LVH	left ventricular hypertrophy
LVSD	left ventricular systolic dysfunction
MHRA	Medicines and Healthcare products Regulatory Agency
MMAS	Massachusetts Male Aging Study

MR	modified release
NASCET	North American Symptomatic Carotid Endarterectomy Trial
NICE	National Institute for Health and Clinical Excellence
NRAF	non-rheumatic atrial fibrillation
NRT	nicotine replacement therapy
NSTEMI	non-ST-segment elevation myocardial infarction
NSVT	non-sustained ventricular tachycardia
NYHA	New York Heart Association
PAC	premature atrial complex
PACs	premature atrial contractions
PAD	peripheral arterial disease
PCI	percutaneous coronary intervention
PE	pulmonary embolism
PSA	prostate-specific antigen
PSVT	paroxysmal supraventricular tachycardia
PTT	partial thromboplastin time
PVC	premature ventricular complex
PVCs	premature ventricular contractions
PVD	peripheral vascular disease
RF	radiofrequency
ROC	receiver operator characteristic
ROSIER	Recognition of Stroke in the Emergency Room
RR	rate ratio
RR	relative risk
RVOT	right ventricular outflow tract
QoF	Quality and Outcomes Framework
SHIM	Sexual Health Inventory for Men
SIGN	Scottish Intercollegiate Guidelines Network
SPCs	summary of product characteristics
SSS	sick sinus syndrome
STEMI	ST-segment elevation myocardial infarction
SVT	supraventricular tachycardia
TASC	TransAtlantic Intersociety Consensus
TC	total cholesterol
TG	triglycerides
TIA	transient ischaemic attack
TIMI	Thrombolysis In Myocardial Infarction
T-LOC	transient loss of consciousness
UKPDS	United Kingdom Prospective Diabetes Study
VADT	Veterans Affair Diabetes Trial

VF   ventricular fibrillation
VT   ventricular tachycardia
VTE   venous thromboembolism
WOSCOPS   West of Scotland Coronary Prevention Study

Overview of cardiovascular disease

Clare J. Taylor

Aim

The aim of this chapter is to give an overview of the broad topic of cardiovascular disease (CVD) in relation to the Royal College of General Practitioners (RCGP) curriculum statement 15.1, *Cardiovascular Problems*. The chapter will discuss the epidemiology of cardiovascular disorders, the most common presenting symptoms and how to carry out an appropriate cardiovascular examination within the time limits of a general practice consultation. Also reviewed are the investigations available in primary and secondary care, use of evidence-based treatments and the importance of prognostic information and quality of life for patients with CVD.

Key learning points

▶ CVD is the commonest cause of death in the UK.
▶ Effective management of modifiable risk factors such as hypertension, smoking, hyperlipidaemia and diabetes could reduce the prevalence of CVD.
▶ Common causes of CVD are related to atherosclerosis. However, degenerative conditions of the heart or structural disorders that may be present from birth should not be forgotten.
▶ The main symptoms of CVD are chest pain, shortness of breath, ankle oedema, palpitations, syncope and, in the case of stroke, muscle weakness or difficulty speaking.
▶ An appropriate cardiovascular examination can be completed within the 10-minute consultation.
▶ Investigations such as blood tests, urinalysis and electrocardiograms (ECGs) are available in primary care.
▶ Appropriate and timely referral to secondary care is crucial to allow appropriate intervention and ensure patient safety.
▶ Prognostic information and end-of-life care is important to patients with CVD and their families.

▶ Acute presentations of CVD are amongst the commonest emergencies to present in primary care, and recognition and prompt management of these can be life saving.

Importance of cardiovascular disease

Mortality

CVD is the most common cause of death in the UK, resulting in 198,000 deaths annually.[1] Coronary heart disease is responsible for around 48 per cent of these deaths, and stroke around 28 per cent. CVD is also the commonest cause of premature mortality (death before the age of 75). The healthcare costs of CVD are substantial. The cost of prescriptions for all CVD is around £1.9 billion per annum. The number of cardiac procedures has increased to over 73,000 percutaneous interventions being carried out annually. Recent estimates suggest CVD costs the NHS over £14 billion and costs the UK economy over £30 billion due to loss of productivity and informal care of people with CVD.[1]

The picture is similar in the rest of Europe, where CVD is the main cause of death, accounting for over 4.3 million people each year – 48 per cent of all deaths. Coronary heart disease (CHD) and stroke are again the main causes of CVD associated with death. Despite reductions in incidence in Western European countries, CVD has increased in Central and Eastern Europe in recent years.[2]

CVD is also the leading cause of death globally. According to World Health Organization statistics, 29 per cent of deaths worldwide are caused by CVD. An estimated 17.1 million people around the world die per year from CVD; 7.2 million of these deaths are due to CHD and 5.7 million are due to stroke. Eighty-two per cent of CVD deaths occur in low- or middle-income countries.[3]

Burden of disease

CVD can affect all age groups, from the fetus to the elderly. Advanced surgical techniques have dramatically improved survival from congenital heart disease, resulting in an increasing number of patients reaching adulthood.[4] Cardiac arrhythmias and structural heart disease can affect children and adults, and can be associated with a fatal outcome. The major burden of CVD, however, is due to CHD. Each year in the UK there are around 96,000 new cases of angina and 146,000 patients have a myocardial infarction. The underlying cause is usually atherosclerosis. Lifestyle factors such as smoking, diet and physical activity, as well as diseases such as diabetes and hyperlipidaemia, can predispose to atherosclerotic plaque formation. However, effective prevention and treatment of CHD are available. As the population ages (median age has increased by 2 years in the last decade)[5] and survival from CVD improves, the incidence of heart failure is also increasing.[6] Around 68,000 new cases of heart failure are diagnosed each year in the UK. The prognosis of heart failure is poor and worse than many cancers.[3,4,7]

CVD is an important cause of significant morbidity and mortality, which GPs should feel confident in managing. Accurate and timely diagnosis, appropriate use of effective treatments, and well co-ordinated prevention programmes within primary care are vital to address this huge burden of disease.

RCGP curriculum

The RCGP curriculum has 32 curriculum statements. The generic competences and attributes required to be a GP are described in the core curriculum statement *Being a GP*.[8] Patients with CVD commonly present to GPs. A sound knowledge base and an ability to demonstrate the core competences of a GP in the context of CVD are required to manage these patients effectively.

The six domains of *Being a GP*

Domain 1: Primary care management

▷ The GP is often the first point of contact for patients with CVD. GPs should have the knowledge and skills to safely manage a spectrum of disease.
▷ Urgent and timely referral to secondary care may be necessary for a patient presenting with acute chest pain suggestive of coronary artery disease. However, a patient with end-stage heart failure may require optimal palliative treatment in the community.
▷ GPs are responsible for overall co-ordination of care and should be able to effectively liaise with secondary care colleagues and other primary healthcare professionals to ensure optimal patient care.
▷ Many patients will be unaware of their underlying risk of CVD and may benefit from cardiovascular risk assessment to allow risk factor modification.
▷ Health promotion is important for all patients in general practice to prevent CVD.

Domain 2: Person-centred care

▷ Patients may present with symptoms suggestive of cardiac disease but have their own health beliefs about what may be causing the problem. For example, angina is frequently mistaken for indigestion. It is important for a GP to understand the patient's perspective in order to provide an adequate explanation about the possible diagnosis and negotiate an effective management plan.

▷ Primary prevention is important to reduce the incidence of CVD. However, the asymptomatic patient may not appreciate the importance of risk factor modification. Cardiovascular risk should be communicated in a way that the patient can understand, and his or her autonomy should be respected if he or she chooses not to take medication after adequate discussion.

▷ Many CVDs result in heart failure and GPs should feel able to initiate end-of-life discussions to allow patients to make informed choices about palliative care.[9]

Domain 3: Specific problem-solving skills

▷ Patients with suspected CVD require thorough clinical assessment and appropriate, timely investigation. Prompt action may be required in the emergency situation, and making the distinction between what is or is not an emergency can be key. Chest pain and shortness of breath, for example, are common, potentially serious symptoms of cardiac disease but have multiple other possible causes.

▷ A careful history can help to determine a likely diagnosis.

▷ Cardiovascular examination is important to identify an irregular pulse, heart murmur or signs of heart failure, but may be normal in the presence of some CVDs such as paroxysmal arrhythmias or angina.

▷ Cardiovascular risk factors should be addressed through lifestyle advice and medication, and this requires patient motivation.

▷ Cardiovascular emergencies such as myocardial infarction, stroke and critical ischaemia require urgent intervention.

Domain 4: A comprehensive approach

▷ Patients often present with multiple conditions and co-morbidities. GPs need to prioritise the patient's complaints and deal with them in order of importance. The patient may need to be seen several times to ensure all of their issues have been addressed.

▷ Patients over the age of 40 are more likely to have modifiable cardiovascular risk factors and may benefit from cardiovascular risk assessment and primary prevention treatment.

▷ Lifestyle interventions for all patients can reduce the risk of developing CVD in the longer term.

Domain 5: Community orientation

▷ Cardiovascular investigations can be expensive and healthcare systems only have finite resources. The role of the GP is to correctly identify those patients who require investigation and refer appropriately.

▷ Open-access services in the community, such as echocardiography, can help to improve access and reduce the number of clinicians the patient is required to see for a definitive diagnosis to be made.

▷ Evidence-based treatments should be used for prevention, and generic prescribing can reduce the overall cost of drugs.

▷ Patients with CVD may be at risk of further events. They are recommended not to drive in some circumstances to avoid putting themselves and others in the community at risk.

▷ GPs should advise patients of driving restrictions but it is the patient's responsibility to inform the Driver and Vehicle Licensing Agency (DVLA). A comprehensive and up-to-date guide to driving restrictions according to cardiovascular disorder is available from the DVLA website.[10]

Domain 6: A holistic approach

▷ CVD can affect the psychological wellbeing of patients in addition to their physical health.

▷ Myocardial infarction or malignant arrhythmias can be incredibly frightening for the patient and his or her family. Even after they have been effectively treated and have recovered from the acute event, patients can remain very anxious and become aware of minor physical ailments, which they may attribute to heart problems (so called 'cardiac neurosis').

▷ Cardiac rehabilitation programmes can help to address concerns of patients and their relatives, and help to build confidence to allow a return to normal life.

▷ The wider impact of the disease on other family members may also be seen by GPs. Adequate understanding of their concerns, and explanation and reassurance where needed, are important aspects of holistic care.

5

The three essential features of *Being a GP*

There are three essential features of being a GP, which are described throughout the RCGP curriculum: contextual, attitudinal and scientific aspects.

Contextual aspects

▷ CVD is a major public health problem. GPs should be aware of the population trends in the prevalence of risk factors and CVD in the community where they practise. They should also be aware of the provision of cardiovascular services locally and the implications of journey times for ambulances responding to cardiovascular emergencies, particularly in rural areas.

▷ Government policy can also have an impact on the range of services available and the priorities for the healthcare system. GPs should keep up to date with the latest guidelines and other policy documents that shape the wider context of the healthcare environment.

Attitudinal aspects

▷ There are many factors that will influence risk of CVD and outcome after cardiovascular events, such as smoking, exercise, alcohol, age, ethnicity or gender.

▷ The GP should not allow his or her own opinions about these factors to influence the management of patients.

Scientific aspects

▷ Evidence-based medicine is important to ensure high-quality care for patients in general practice as much as in any other specialty. It is therefore important for all GPs to have a sound understanding of key research and national guidelines.

Psychomotor skills

▷ There are several important psychomotor skills that are needed by all GPs for effective management of CVDs. It is important that an appropriate cardiovascular examination is conducted where indicated. An example of a cardiovascular examination that is feasible within the 10-minute consultation is given later in the chapter.

▷ It is important that GPs are able to perform and interpret an ECG in the surgery.
▷ GPs should also be proficient in basic cardiopulmonary resuscitation for children and adults.

Main causes of cardiovascular disease

The main causes of CVD can be considered in terms of blood vessel blockage (atherosclerosis and clot formation), electrical abnormalities or problems with the structural components of the heart.

Blood vessel blockage

ATHEROSCLEROSIS

A major underlying cause of CVD is atherosclerosis.[11] The process of athero-sclerotic plaque formation can start during childhood and may not become clinically apparent until many decades later. Fatty deposits build up in the intimal layer of the blood vessel wall, prompting an inflammatory response that results in the formation of an atherosclerotic plaque. The resultant nar-rowing compromises the patency of the blood vessel or, if the plaque ruptures, promotes blood clot formation, resulting in complete occlusion.[12] This may result in a compromised blood supply and can lead to ischaemia or infarction of the tissue. Atherosclerosis predominantly affects the proximal portion of large arteries. Blockage of the main blood vessels to the heart, brain and lower limbs results in CHD (see Chapter 3), stroke (see Chapter 4) and peripheral vascular disease (see Chapter 5) respectively.

There are several risk factors associated with plaque development, progres-sion and rupture, such as smoking, cholesterol, diabetes and hypertension. Managing these modifiable risk factors with effective treatments can reduce the progression of atherosclerosis and increase plaque stability.[13]

CLOT FORMATION

Atherosclerotic plaque fissuring or rupture can cause blood clot formation in the main arteries. Occlusion of the venous system can also occur due to a single large blood clot or multiple smaller clots. An imbalance of the coagu-lation cascade due to acquired factors, such as immobility and cancer, or inherited clotting disorders can predispose to venous clot formation.[14] Clot in the venous system, most commonly in the lower limbs, may be asymptomatic, cause local symptoms or may dislodge and enter the pulmonary circulation causing a potentially catastrophic pulmonary embolus. This is discussed further in Chapter 10.

Blood clots may also form in the left atrium of patients with atrial fibrillation (AF) due to uncoordinated left atrial contraction as well as other important thrombogenic factors.[15] Blood clots from the left atrium can enter the cerebral circulation and cause a transient ischaemic attack (TIA) or stroke (see Chapter 4).

Electrical abnormalities

Abnormal electrical activity can be caused by acquired disorders such as fibrosis of the conducting system with age, electrolyte abnormalities and diseased blood vessels, or, less commonly, genetic mutations of ion channels in the cardiac membrane.[16] The clinical consequences of abnormal conduction can range from minor symptoms like occasional palpitations to cardiac arrest. Cardiac arrhythmias are discussed in more detail in Chapters 6 and 7.

Structural abnormalities of the heart

The structure of the heart, including the valves and great vessels, is important to allow optimal function as a pump. Valvular abnormalities may be caused by degenerative or ischaemic disease or, more commonly in developing countries, by infection, which can disrupt the integrity of the valve.[17] Other structural abnormalities of the heart, such as hypertrophic cardiomyopathy, may be caused by genetic abnormalities in key cardiac proteins.[18] Acquired disorders such as infection, toxins or alcohol may damage the structural integrity of the myocardium leading to dilated cardiomyopathy.[19] A detailed description of structural and valvular heart disease can be found in Chapter 8.

Presentation

CVD may present in a variety of ways. Patients without cardiac symptoms may be found to have risk factors for CVD through screening in primary care. Patients may present with a history of gradually worsening central chest pain on exertion and may require an urgent referral to a rapid-access chest pain clinic. An acute presentation with crushing central chest pain that is not relieved by rest may be due to a myocardial infarction and requires emergency admission by ambulance for further management. This may involve thrombolysis or primary angioplasty.

Sudden death may unfortunately be the first presentation for patients with an underlying malignant arrhythmia. Patients with chronic heart failure may require long-term follow-up and ultimately well-planned and co-ordinated palliative care. The symptoms and signs that are used to establish an accurate diagnosis of CVD are discussed in detail below.

Symptoms

Chest pain

CHD is an important diagnosis that should not be missed. However, the cause of chest pain in primary care is not always cardiac.[20] Gastrointestinal, musculoskeletal and respiratory causes of chest pain are also common in general practice. A careful history and physical examination is crucial in establishing an accurate diagnosis.[21] A good understanding of the epidemiology of those diseases in the differential diagnosis and their associated risk factors is also important to determine the most likely cause of chest pain.

CARDIAC

Central crushing chest pain that radiates to the left arm or neck is the classical description of cardiac chest pain, and in a patient over 40 years of age with cardiovascular risk factors is likely to be due to CHD.[22] If the pain is related to exertion and relieved by rest the diagnosis is likely to be stable angina, whereas if the pain is prolonged and is not relieved by rest or glyceryl trinitrate spray then a diagnosis of myocardial infarction should be suspected (see Chapter 3).

Aortic dissection is also a rare but important cause of chest pain. The pain classically starts in the central chest and radiates to the back. Pain is often severe and can be described as a tearing sensation. Dissection can affect branches of the aorta, such as cerebral, renal or iliac vessels, and more than one-third of patients develop symptoms secondary to inadequate blood supply to other organs.[23]

Cardiac chest pain can also be due to pericarditis. The pain is usually sudden onset, sharp, pleuritic, left sided and is made better by leaning forward. There is commonly a prodromal illness of fever, malaise and myalgia.[24]

GASTROINTESTINAL

Dyspepsia and gastro-oesophageal reflux can be difficult to distinguish from cardiac chest pain.[25] Epigastric pain, which radiates to the chest and throat, is worse after food, is associated with belching and relieved by antacids, is more likely to be due to a gastrointestinal cause. Risk factors for gastric irritation such as use of non-steroidal anti-inflammatory drugs or excessive alcohol intake are important factors to consider. However, anginal chest pain may be precipitated by a large meal due to the resultant increased cardiac output.

RESPIRATORY

Lung diseases such as pneumonia, pneumothorax, pulmonary embolism (PE) or lung cancer are also associated with chest pain. Coexistent symptoms such as productive cough, shortness of breath and fever make a diagnosis of pneumonia likely. Pneumothorax can occur spontaneously (more commonly in tall, thin males) or after chest trauma. The patient usually complains of one-sided pleuritic chest pain with increasing breathlessness.

PE is a rare but important cause of chest pain, which can be fatal if undiagnosed and untreated. PE often occurs as a result of deep-vein thrombosis, which may or may not be recognised before an individual presents with chest pain. Risk factors for venous thromboembolism such as immobility, recent surgery, cancer, advanced age, female hormone use and inherited clotting disorders are important to consider in the history.[26] Chest pain due to PE is usually unilateral, worse on inspiration and may be associated with shortness of breath and haemoptysis.

Lung cancer can also cause chest pain but other signs of malignancy such as productive cough, haemoptysis, breathlessness, weight loss, tiredness, bone pain and a history of smoking may be present.

MUSCULOSKELETAL

The most common cause of chest pain in patients presenting to primary care is musculoskeletal.[21] This differs from hospital care, where the commonest diagnosis is CVD. This reflects the different populations seen by GPs compared with hospital physicians, and the role of the GP as gatekeeper to secondary care. Pain is often constant, worse on certain movements and can be precipitated by palpating the chest wall.

PSYCHIATRIC DISORDER

Chest pain can be related to anxiety. If the patient has other symptoms of anxiety, such as palpitations or hyperventilation, or has significant stressors, panic disorder may be a likely diagnosis. Exclusion of a significant underlying cause is important before attributing chest pain to anxiety. An understanding of the patient's psychosocial context is important to establish the diagnosis.

GPs have a longitudinal relationship with the patient and his or her family, and so are often aware of psychological and social factors that may influence the patient's presentation.[27]

Shortness of breath

CARDIAC

Shortness of breath, with or without chest pain, can be a symptom of CHD. Heart failure is a complication of many cardiac disorders including ischaemic heart disease, valvular heart disease, structural heart disease and arrhythmias. Shortness of breath on exertion, ankle swelling and fatigue suggest a diagnosis of heart failure.[28] This is discussed in more detail in Chapter 9.

RESPIRATORY

Pulmonary embolism should be suspected in patients with the risk factors described above who develop shortness of breath. Many lung disorders cause shortness of breath and a list is shown in Box 1.1. Respiratory disorders may coexist with CVD due to common underlying causes such as smoking.

Box 1.1 ○ *Respiratory causes of shortness of breath*

▶ Chronic obstructive pulmonary disease.

▶ Asthma.

▶ Pneumonia.

▶ Pulmonary embolism.

▶ Pleural effusion.

▶ Pneumothorax.

▶ Pulmonary fibrosis.

▶ Muscle disorders.

▶ Chest wall abnormalities.

Swollen ankles

Patients with CVD may have ankle swelling (or oedema). Causes of oedema are multiple and depend on the presence of other symptoms and signs. If the patient has oedema associated with shortness of breath, fatigue and has a history of CHD, valvular disease or other cardiac abnormality the cause is likely to be heart failure (see Chapter 9).

However, the commonest cause of swollen ankles is probably venous stasis with or without varicose veins. Low protein states associated with liver or renal disease can also cause fluid to leak into the tissues causing bilateral oedema. Unilateral oedema may be due to local causes. Redness and swelling of one leg may be caused by deep-vein thrombosis, cellulitis or a ruptured baker's cyst. This is discussed further in Chapter 10.

Syncope

Syncope is a transient loss of consciousness resulting from an insufficient supply of oxygen to the brain.[29] The causes of syncope can be classified as neurally mediated, orthostatic hypotension, cardiac arrhythmia and structural cardiac or cardiopulmonary disease.[30] A study of the aetiology of syncope found that neurally mediated causes such as vasovagal attacks accounted for 66 per cent of syncopal episodes. Orthostatic hypotension due to volume depletion or autonomic disorders such as Parkinson's disease accounted for a further 10 per cent. Cardiac arrhythmias such as sinus node dysfunction, conduction disorders and ventricular arrhythmia accounted for a further 11 per cent and structural cardiac disorders just 5 per cent.

The European Society of Cardiology guidelines on management of syncope suggest all patients presenting with loss of consciousness should be evaluated with a thorough history, physical examination including supine and upright blood pressures, and an ECG.[30]

Palpitations

Palpitations are an awareness or sensation of a rapid or irregular heartbeat. They can be caused by a cardiac arrhythmia, anxiety, drugs, systemic disorders or other cardiac disorders. Extracardiac causes such as anaemia or fever, which may induce sinus tachycardia, can also be felt by the patient. A thorough family history is required to identify high-risk patients.

A history of dizziness or syncope in a child or young adult in the presence of palpitations should raise suspicion of an underlying inherited arrhythmia. A full cardiovascular examination and ECG is required to assess patients adequately. Further assessment of palpitations is discussed in Chapter 6.

Other symptoms

Fatigue is a common symptom in patients with heart failure (discussed further in Chapter 9). Stroke or TIA presents with neurological symptoms such as facial weakness, slurred speech or loss of power on one side of the body. The symptoms and signs of stroke are discussed further in detail in Chapter 4. Pain in the calves on walking and skin changes are important symptoms of peripheral vascular disease and these are further discussed in Chapter 5.

Signs

A 10-minute consultation is a short amount of time to carry out a full clinical assessment, explain the diagnosis to the patient, arrange any follow-up or referrals, and document findings in the medical record. It is, however, possible to do a thorough cardiovascular examination in just a few minutes. Examination is vital to diagnose some cardiovascular disorders such as atrial fibrillation, valvular heart disease or heart failure. It should be remembered, however, that examination may be entirely normal despite the presence of significant CVD such as CHD or paroxysmal arrhythmia.

Some important cardiovascular signs are shown in the picture section at the end of this chapter.

Appearance

The appearance of the patient when he or she walks into the consulting room can be very helpful. A patient who is breathless on walking may have heart failure, angina or an underlying respiratory disorder. If the patient is pale he or she may be anaemic or generally unwell. Cyanosis (blue lips) would suggest inadequate oxygenation, which may be due to underlying cardiovascular or respiratory disease. The smell of smoke may be present in patients who smoke or who live with a smoker.

Pulse

Pulse palpation is a vital aspect of the cardiovascular examination and should be carried out in addition to any automated blood pressure monitor readings:

▷ **rate** ▶ a normal pulse rate is 60–90 beats per minute
▷ **rhythm** ▶ occasional missed beats may be due to ventricular ectopics, while an irregularly irregular pulse is due to atrial fibrillation. An

abnormal pulse should be followed up with an ECG in order to diagnose the arrhythmia
▷ **volume** ▶ a low pulse volume suggests inadequate cardiac output
▷ **symmetry** ▶ asymmetric radial pulses are suggestive of aortic dissection so palpation of both radial arteries should be conducted if this is a possible diagnosis.

Blood pressure

Blood pressure should be measured with the patient in a comfortable sitting position with the arm well supported and after about 5 minutes' rest. An appropriate-size cuff should be used. The patient should not talk during blood pressure measurement. Both mercury and automated sphygmomanometers should be calibrated each year to ensure accuracy.[31]

Blood pressure can vary due to multiple factors, and hypertension is not usually diagnosed until a raised blood pressure has been recorded on three separate occasions (see Blood pressure section, Chapter 2). A low blood pressure can suggest inadequate cardiac output, and in the presence of a brady- or tachycardia can represent significant cardiovascular compromise.

Jugular venous pressure

Jugular venous pressure (JVP) is a measure of central venous pressure and should be assessed with the patient supine at 45°. The anatomical markings of the internal jugular vein are from the earlobe to the medial end of the clavicle; the double pulsations of the column of blood in the vessel may be seen along this path. If the vertical distance between the sternal angle and the level of pulsations is more than 3 cm the JVP is raised. This suggests increased pressure in the venous system, which can be seen in heart failure, tricuspid regurgitation and pericardial disorders. JVP can be difficult to accurately assess but, if raised, may be useful in predicting an adverse outcome in patients with heart failure.[32]

Precordium

Scarring from previous surgery may be evident. Palpation of the chest may reveal a heaving apex (a result of left ventricular enlargement) or thrills (palpable heart murmurs). Heart sounds on auscultation are important. A split-second heart sound is associated with aortic valve disease and added heart sounds are found in the presence of ventricular dysfunction. Murmurs are important in diagnosing valvular disease. The differential diagnosis of murmurs is discussed in detail in Chapter 8.

Lungs

Listening to the lung bases is important to identify crepitations, which may be associated with heart failure. Respiratory disease commonly exists with CVD and so a full respiratory examination may be appropriate if the diagnosis is unclear.

Liver and ascites

The liver may be palpable in patients with right heart failure but other cardiovascular signs are likely to be present. Isolated hepatomegaly may be due to a variety of causes and should be investigated further. Abdominal distension may also be present in patients with severe heart failure due to ascites.

Lower limbs

The appearance of the lower limbs is important in diagnosing peripheral arterial and venous disease. Varicose veins are usually easily seen and may be associated with skin changes such as varicose eczema or lipodermatosclerosis. A cool, pale limb is suggestive of peripheral vascular disease.

Bilateral oedema is common in heart failure but may be present due to other systemic conditions, such as liver disease, nephrotic syndrome or other low-protein states, or due to local disorders such as bilateral varicose veins. The extent of the oedema should be recorded in the notes to ensure any deterioration or improvement can be established at follow-up appointments.

Investigations

There is a limited range of investigations available in primary care. A thorough history and careful examination are crucial in establishing the diagnosis. However, simple tests in the surgery can be helpful in diagnosing and managing CVD.

Blood tests

Blood tests are helpful in identifying modifiable risk factors and for treatment monitoring. A lipid profile (including cholesterol, high-density lipoprotein and triglycerides) and fasting glucose are needed to calculate cardiovascular risk. A renal function test is helpful to identify patients with chronic kidney disease, which frequently coexists with CVD.

Patients with venous thromboembolism may require treatment with oral anticoagulants, which can be monitored through blood testing in primary care. Statins are commonly used in patients with CVD and can rarely cause hepatic damage or myopathy. Liver function tests should be monitored in patients with this complication. Creatine kinase can also be helpful to assess muscle damage in any patients on statins with significant muscle pain.

Urine testing

Urinalysis is carried out to identify any end-organ damage in patients with high blood pressure in the diagnosis of hypertension (described further in the Blood pressure section of Chapter 2). Urine dipstick may also be positive for blood in patients with endocarditis.

Chronic kidney disease (CKD) can commonly coexist with CVD. Albumin–creatinine ratios are recommended for the assessment of patients with CKD to establish the extent of renal damage and to guide referral to specialists. The albumin–creatinine ratio from a urine sample is used to quantify proteinuria, which is related to severity of disease.[33] Optimal management of cardiovascular risk factors is a crucial part of CKD treatment.

Electrocardiogram

Many practices have an ECG machine. GPs should be able to carry out an ECG in an emergency. ECG interpretation can be difficult, but all GPs should be able to recognise important abnormalities such as ischaemic changes (see Chapter 3) or important arrhythmias such as complete heart block or ventricular tachycardia, which require urgent referral (see Chapter 6). Some GPs may not feel confident in routine interpretation of ECGs.[34] Depending on local arrangements, GPs may be able to fax ECGs to GPs with a Special Interest in cardiology or cardiologists for formal interpretation and reporting.

Specialised equipment

Some practices will have facilities to measure ankle brachial pressure index to diagnose peripheral vascular disease or venous Doppler ultrasound machines to diagnose deep-vein thrombosis. In some areas, echocardiography may be offered by appropriately trained GPs in the community. The provision of these types of equipment and services will depend on the local skill mix and healthcare economy.

Secondary care investigations and management

Primary care is well placed to co-ordinate prevention strategies and chronic disease management, and to ensure continuity of care for patients with CVD. However, appropriate and timely referral to secondary care is needed in some circumstances.

Urgent management of patients with chest pain is discussed further in Chapter 3. Further investigation such as troponin measurement or angiography and definitive management can be arranged in the safe environment of hospital, where complications of myocardial ischaemia such as arrhythmias can be effectively treated.

Patients presenting with clinical features of stroke also require urgent management. Admission by ambulance, usually without GP review, is now recommended to allow timely investigation with CT scan and interventions such as thrombolysis where appropriate.[35]

Out-patient referral is also necessary to establish a definitive diagnosis for patients with CVD. Rapid-access chest pain clinics will see patients with a short history of stable cardiac chest pain and arrange further investigation, such as exercise stress testing. The availability of ambulatory blood pressure monitoring, 24-hour tape recording and ECG services vary between regions, and may be directly accessible to primary care or may require referral to a cardiologist.

Treatments

A large amount of research has been carried out in the area of CVD. Evidence-based medicine demands that clinical decisions about individual patients should be made based on appropriate, reliable research findings.[36] However, many of the trials on which GPs base judgements were conducted in highly selected secondary care populations. The study participants may not exactly reflect the patient in the surgery. GPs need to put the research evidence into the context of the patient they are dealing with and take into account any co-morbidities and other medications, as well as the patient's health beliefs and wishes.[37]

The overall goal of management should be considered, and with this in mind the best treatments offered and discussed in a way the patient is able to understand. The management of individual conditions is discussed in detail throughout this book.

Prognosis

CVD covers a spectrum of clinical presentations. Patients may be asymptomatic and require risk factor management in order to reduce the risk of any future cardiovascular events. Patients with angina may be disabled by their symptoms. Ventricular arrhythmias can cause sudden death, but this may be preventable with appropriate treatment. Heart failure can be a consequence of other cardiovascular disorders such as CHD, valvular heart disease and arrhythmia, and carries a prognosis that is comparable to many cancers.[38] It is important that prognosis is discussed with patients where appropriate to allow them to make informed decisions about treatment options, and to plan appropriate end-of-life care.[39,40]

Summary

CVD is a common cause of morbidity and mortality worldwide. Patients presenting with symptoms of CVD require careful clinical assessment and appropriate, timely referral when necessary. GPs should offer evidence-based treatments to improve outcomes in patients with CVD. GPs are also well placed to offer health promotion and assess cardiovascular risk in appropriate patients, in order to reduce the incidence of cardiovascular events. The core principles of patient-centred, comprehensive, holistic care should be applied to CVD management in order to provide effective, safe, high-quality care to patients and their families.

Useful resources

There are many national guidelines and online resources that provide helpful information about CVD:

▷ Department of Health • **www.dh.gov.uk** • The National Service
   Framework for Coronary Heart Disease, published in 2000,
   is a landmark document and is particularly valuable.
▷ National Institute for Health and Clinical Excellence • **www.nice.org.uk**
▷ Scottish Intercollegiate Guidelines Network • **www.sign.ac.uk**
▷ Clinical Knowledge Summaries • **www.cks.nhs.uk**
▷ British Heart Foundation • **www.bhf.org.uk**
▷ European Society of Cardiology • **www.escardio.org**
▷ American Heart Association • **www.americanheart.org**

▷ Primary Care Cardiovascular Society • **www.pccs.org.uk**
▷ British Hypertension Society • **www.bhsoc.org**.

References

1 • Allender S, Peto V, Scarborough, *et al. Coronary Heart Disease Statistics* London: British Heart Foundation, 2008.

2 • European Cardiovascular Disease Statistics, 2008. www.ehnheart.org/cdv. statistics.html [accessed September 2010].

3 • World Health Organization. *Cardiovascular diseases (CVDs)* Geneva: WHO, 2009, www.who.int/mediacentre/factsheets/fs317/en/print.html [accessed September 2010].

4 • British Heart Foundation. www.heartstats.org/datapage.asp?id=3390 [accessed September 2010].

5 • Office of National Statistics. www.statistics.gov.uk/cci/nugget.asp?ID=6 [accessed September 2010].

6 • Barker WH, Mullooly JP, Getchell W. Changing incidence and survival for heart failure in a well-defined older population, 1970–1974 and 1990–1994 *Circulation* 2006; **113(6)**: 799–805.

7 • Tribouilloy C, Buiciuc O, Rusinaru D, *et al.* Long-term outcome after a first episode of heart failure. A prospective 7-year study *International Journal of Cardiology* 2010; **140(3)**: 309–14.

8 • Royal College of General Practitioners. *GP Curriculum and Assessment Website,* www.rcgp-curriculum.org.uk [accessed September 2010].

9 • Shipman C, Gysels M, White P, *et al.* Improving generalist end of life care: national consultation with practitioners, commissioners, academics, and service user groups *British Medical Journal* 2008; **337**: a1720.

10 • Drivers Medical Group, Driver and Vehicle Licensing Agency. *At a Glance Guide to the Current Medical Standards of Fitness to Drive* Swansea: DVLA, 2009, www.dft.gov.uk/dvla/medical/ataglance.aspx [accessed September 2010].

11 • Insull W. The pathology of atherosclerosis: plaque development and plaque responses to medical treatment *American Journal of Medicine* 2009; **122(Suppl 1)**: S3–14.

12 • Rauch U, Osende JI, Fuster V, *et al.* Thrombus formation on atherosclerotic plaques: pathogenesis and clinical consequences *Annals of Internal Medicine* 2001; **134(3)**: 224–38.

13 • Napoli C, Cacciatore F. Novel pathogenic insights in the primary prevention of cardiovascular disease *Progress in Cardiovascular Disease* 2009; **51(6)**: 503–23.

14 • Dahlback B. Blood coagulation *Lancet* 2000; **355(9215)**: 1627–32.

15 • Watson T, Shantsila E, Lip GYH. Mechanisms of thrombogenesis in atrial fibrillation: Virchow's triad revisited *Lancet* 2009; **373(9658)**: 155–66.

16 • Shah M, Akar FG, Tomaselli GF. Molecular basis of arrhythmias *Circulation* 2005; **112(16)**: 2517–29.

19

17 • Enriquez-Sarano M, Akins CW, Vahanian A, *et al.* Mitral regurgitation *Lancet* 2009; **373(9672)**: 1382–94.

18 • Richard P, Charron P, Carrier L, *et al.* Hypertrophic cardiomyopathy: distribution of disease genes, spectrum of mutations, and implications for a molecular diagnosis strategy *Circulation* 2003; **107(17)**: 2227–32.

19 • Gavazzi A, De Maria R, Parolini M, *et al.* Alcohol abuse and dilated cardiomyopathy in men *American Journal of Cardiology* 2000; **85(9)**: 1114–18.

20 • Buntinx F, Knockaert D, Bruyninckx R, *et al.* Chest pain in general practice or in the hospital emergency department: is it the same? *Family Practice* 2001; **18(6)**: 586–9.

21 • Cayley WE. Diagnosing the cause of chest pain *American Family Physician* 2005; **72(10)**: 2012–21.

22 • Diamond GA, Forrester FS. Probability of CAD *Circulation* 1982; **65(3)**: 641–2.

23 • Khan IA, Nair CK. Clinical, diagnostic and management perspectives of aortic dissection *Chest* 2002; **122(1)**: 311–28.

24 • Tingle LE, Molina D, Calvert CW. Acute pericarditis *American Family Physician* 2007; **76(10)**: 1509–14.

25 • Locke GR, Talley NJ, Fett SL, *et al.* Prevalence and clinical spectrum of gastroesophageal reflux: a population-based study in Olmsted County, Minnesota *Gastroenterology* 1997; **112(5)**: 1448–56.

26 • Kyrle PA, Eichinger S. New diagnostic strategies for pulmonary embolism *Lancet* 2008; **371(9621)**: 1312–15.

27 • Bruyninckx R, Van den Bruel A, Hannes K, *et al.* GPs' reasons for referral of patients with chest pain: a qualitative study *BMC Family Practice* 2009; **10**: 55.

28 • European Society of Cardiology, Heart Failure Association of the ESC (HFA), European Society of Intensive Care Medicine (ESICM), Dickstein K, Cohen-Solal A, Filippatos G, *et al.* ESC guidelines for the diagnosis and treatment of acute and chronic heart failure 2008: the Task Force for the diagnosis and treatment of acute and chronic heart failure 2008 of the European Society of Cardiology. Developed in collaboration with the Heart Failure Association of the ESC (HFA) and endorsed by the European Society of Intensive Care Medicine (ESICM) *European Journal of Heart Failure* 2008; **10(10)**: 933–89.

29 • Hainsworth R. Pathophysiology of syncope *Clinical Autonomic Research* 2004; **14(Suppl 1)**: 18–24.

30 • Brignole M, Alboni P, Benditt D, *et al.* Guidelines on management (diagnosis and treatment) of syncope: update 2004 *Europace* 2004; **6(6)**: 467–537.

31 • O'Brien E, Asmar R, Beilin L, *et al.* European Society of Hypertension recommendations for conventional, ambulatory and home blood pressure measurement *Journal of Hypertension* 2003; **21(5)**: 821–48.

32 • Drazner MH, Rame JE, Stevenson LW, *et al.* Prognostic importance of elevated jugular venous pressure and a third heart sound in patients with heart failure *New England Journal of Medicine* 2001; **345(8)**: 574–81.

33 • Crowe E, Halpin D, Stevens P on behalf of the Guideline Development Group. Early identification and management of chronic kidney disease: summary of NICE guidance *British Medical Journal* 2008; **337**: a1530.

34 • Mant J, Fitzmaurice DA, Hobbs FDR, *et al*. Accuracy of diagnosing atrial fibrillation on electrocardiogram by primary care practitioners and interpretative diagnostic software: analysis of data from screening for atrial fibrillation in the elderly (SAFE) trial *British Medical Journal* 2007; **335(7616)**: 335–6.

35 • Stroke Association. www.stroke.org.uk/campaigns/raising_awareness/act_fast.html [accessed May 2010].

36 • Sackett DL, Rosenberg WMC, Gray JAM, *et al*. Evidence-based medicine: what is it and what isn't it *British Medical Journal* 1996; **312(7023)**: 71–2.

37 • Greenhalgh T. Is my practice evidence based? *British Medical Journal* 1996; **313(7063)**: 957–8.

38 • Stewart S, MacIntyre K, Hole DJ, *et al*. More 'malignant' than cancer? Five-year survival following a first admission for heart failure *European Journal of Heart Failure* 2001; **3(3)**: 315–22.

39 • Shipman C, Gysels M, White P, *et al*. Improving generalist end of life care: national consultation with practitioners, commissioners, academics, and service user groups *British Medical Journal* 2008; **337**: a1720.

40 • Zapka JG, Moran WP, Goodlin SJ, *et al*. Advanced heart failure: prognosis, uncertainty, and decision making *Congestive Heart Failure* 2007; **13(5)**: 268–74.

21

Picture section

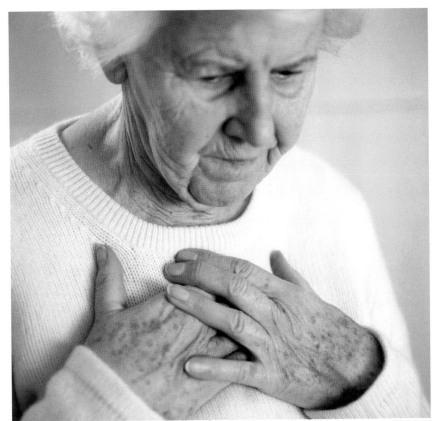

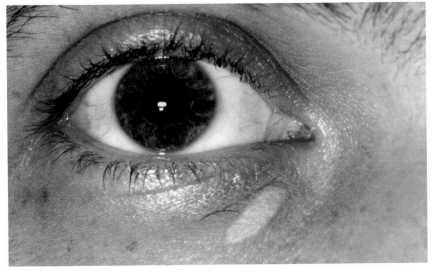

Image © Science Photo Library

Image © Science Photo Library

Top **Figure 1.1** An older patient experiencing the crushing central chest pain of angina (Chapter 3)

Bottom **Figure 1.2** Patients with familial hypercholesterolaemia may have cholesterol deposits (xanthelasma) in the eyelids, as shown here (Chapter 3)

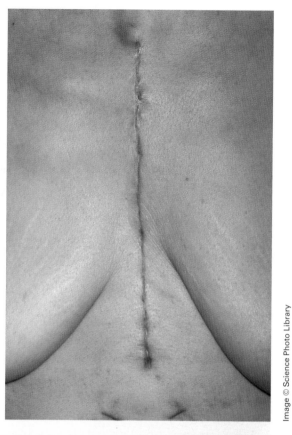

Right **Figure 1.3** This patient has had recent cardiac surgery, as shown by the healing sternotomy scar

Below **Figure 1.4** This patient with heart failure has ascites (Chapter 1)

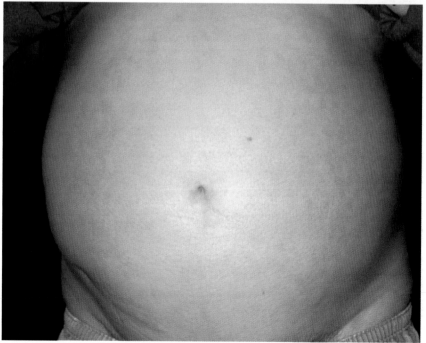

Image © Science Photo Library

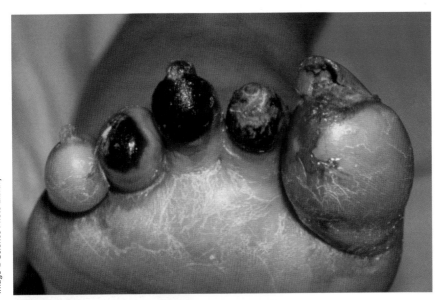

Above **Figure 1.5** Patients with peripheral vascular disease may develop gangrene (Chapter 5)

Left **Figure 1.6** A patient with unilateral swelling of the lower limb due to a deep-vein thrombosis (Chapter 10)

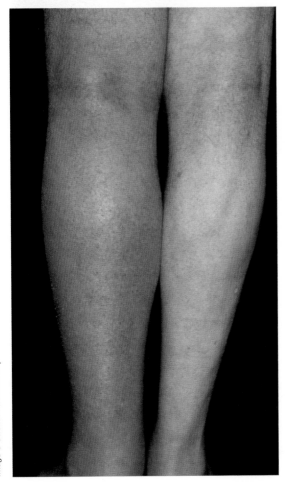

Image © Science Photo Library

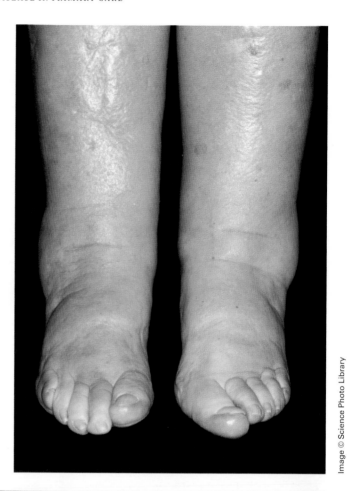

Figures 1.7a and 1.7b This elderly patient has bilateral pitting oedema of the lower limbs due to heart failure

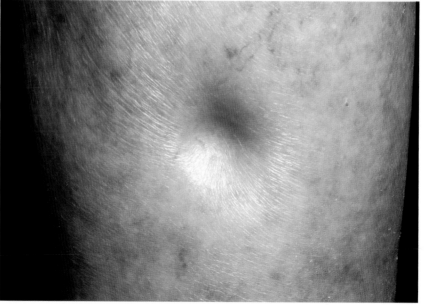

Prevention of cardiovascular disease

2

Richard J. McManus, Paul Aveyard, Paul Little, Paramjit Gill,
F.D. Richard Hobbs, Kamlesh Khunti and Azhar Zafar

Aims

This chapter aims to:

▷ discuss the key risk factors both fixed and modifiable in terms of epidemiology and importance
▷ explain how these can be managed and modified where appropriate
▷ consider how this fits into holistic management in primary care.

Key learning points

▶ Cardiovascular risk calculation can help to target preventive treatment to those who will benefit most.
▶ Blood pressure is a continuous risk factor for cardiovascular disease (CVD), at least above 110 mmHg systolic, which can be reduced by both pharmacological and non-pharmacological means.
▶ Smoking tobacco is highly addictive and is most effectively stopped with a combination of brief behavioural support and pharmacological intervention.
▶ Cholesterol is an independent risk factor for CVD, and primary prevention with a statin is cost-effective.
▶ Type 2 diabetes leads to important increases in cardiovascular risk, and such risk comprises the main target for intervention.
▶ Effective treatment for obesity is now available and has appreciable effects on cardiovascular risk reduction.
▶ In the future, combination treatment of cardiovascular risk factors in a 'polypill' may supersede individual risk factor reduction.

Introduction

CVD is the leading cause of morbidity and mortality worldwide, and hence prevention is a key aspect of medical care in general and primary care in particular.[1] The pathophysiology of CVD involves the development of atherosclerotic plaques within arteries and can be seen to start in childhood.[2] Significantly diseased arteries were seen in post-mortems undertaken on supposedly fit soldiers fighting in Vietnam and Korea, and there seems to be a continuous development of this pathology from fatty streaks in childhood to the full-blown lesions seen in manifest coronary heart disease (CHD).[2]

Cardiovascular risk: calculation and communication

This section discusses methods of calculating cardiovascular risk using the Framingham equations or one of the subsequently developed methods. It will show how such risk calculation can be used in practice.

Learning points

▶ The risk of an individual suffering from a cardiovascular event over a defined time period can guide intervention and has been incorporated into most international primary prevention guidelines.
▶ The Framingham equations were the first developed to calculate such risk and are the most widely cited.
▶ Communicating cardiovascular risk is not straightforward and may be aided by using one of the numerous multimedia tools developed for this purpose.

Definition

Cardiovascular risk is the probability of an individual suffering a cardiovascular event (i.e. stroke, myocardial infarction or cardiovascular cause of death) over a defined period of time, typically 10 years. Risk can be absolute or relative to another group (perhaps someone of the same age with 'average' risk). Cardiovascular risk probabilities can be calculated using combinations of individual risk factors. The concept of such cardiovascular risk calculation first came to the fore with the publication of the Framingham equations, the first almost 20 years ago.[3]

Baseline and event data collected from CVD-free participants in the Framingham epidemiological project were subjected to a series of regression analyses eventually culminating in the publication of the equations. This allowed calculation of a risk 'score' that could be used to attribute risk to an individual. The New Zealand guideline group were the first to widely implement a risk-based approach to cardiovascular risk reduction with their 1993 hypertension guideline and tables, which advocated treatment based on risk as well as blood pressure level.[4] The subsequent publication of the first of the statin trials provided a further rationale for the use of the equations – deciding who best to treat with these expensive new drugs – and the Sheffield tables were developed with this in mind.[5]

Cardiovascular risk calculation

Cardiovascular risk calculated using the Framingham equations has subsequently been included in most major national and international primary prevention guidelines.[6-9] The risk threshold where treatment is recommended has gradually dropped to the current levels of 15 or 20 per cent over 10 years. The major advantage of such thresholds is that they bias treatment towards older, higher-risk individuals for whom treatment will be most effective in terms of numbers needed to treat, and away from younger individuals who have lone raised risk factors such as hypertension. The disadvantage is that, while the latter may be less likely to benefit from treatment, they will live with their risk for much longer, hence accrued benefit may be greater in terms of life years saved.

More recently, newer risk equations have been developed that aim to predict risk more accurately in given populations. In the UK these include QRISK (based on largely English data collected from practices using EMIS) and ASSIGN (developed from the Scottish Heart Health Extended Cohort).[10,11] The latter has been included in the Scottish Intercollegiate guidelines for cardiovascular risk prevention, while the former has yet to be proven in a population with a full dataset and validated outcomes. It is now in its third incarnation following previous updates and corrections.[12]

Cardiovascular risk in practice

Cardiovascular risk equations have been developed into several charts, tables and electronic calculators.[13-15] Use of these in practice may not be straightforward.[16] Several of the primary care clinical systems suppliers including EMIS and VISION have incorporated them into electronic records, allowing use within the consultation. Marshall has proposed the use of the equations, supplemented by epidemiological data for missing values, as a means of prioritising individuals for more accurate risk assessment and subsequent treatment, ensuring that those most likely to benefit from such management are reviewed first.[17] This is important as National Screening Programmes, such as that rolling out from 2009, potentially involve large proportions of the adult population undergoing assessment.

Communication of risk

Communication of risk is an important aspect of primary care management. Experiments have shown that there is a tendency to rank relative risk above absolute risk, with clinical audiences failing to realise that four different presentations of risk were in fact the same but simply presented in different ways. This concept is known as 'framing' and experimental evidence suggests that patients are also affected by the way in which data is presented, preferring positive framing with a graphical presentation.[18]

A large number of decision aids have been developed, ranging from leaflets to interactive DVDs or websites, with the aim of aiding patients and professionals in communicating about risk.[19] A systematic review of this literature found that such aids increased patient participation in decision making, reduced indecision and, importantly, often led to a change from a person's initial position.[19]

Conclusions

In calculating cardiovascular risk in practice some practicalities need to be addressed. The first is the choice of risk calculation tool. The default would be a version of the Framingham equations combining CHD and cerebrovascular diseases, as recommended by the National Institute for Health and Clinical Excellence (NICE) and the Joint British Societies.[7, 14]

In order to calculate risk appropriately one needs to gather the appropriate data by asking about smoking and diabetic status, measuring blood pressure, cholesterol, HDL cholesterol and taking an ECG. These, combined with age and sex, are inputted into the table or programme and a risk generated. This may need to be adjusted in view of ethnicity (or the ETHRISK calculator used), a very strong family history and more controversially the presence of other co-morbidities including erectile dysfunction.[7, 20, 21]

Finally, the result needs to be communicated to the patient, perhaps using one of the decision-making tools described above and then management choices made. Some individuals may make surprising choices when provided with appropriate information.[22]

Smoking: modifiable risk factors

The aims of this section are to:

▷ give a brief overview of why people continue to smoke in the face of good reasons to stop
▷ consider the risks that continuing smoking poses and the benefits to be had from stopping smoking
▷ examine the role and type of brief opportunistic interventions GPs can make to encourage and support their patients to stop
▷ give some information about more intensive intervention that GPs need to manage their patients with tobacco dependence.

31

Key learning points

▶ Understanding why people smoke and express empathy in consultations.
▶ To provide optimum brief interventions respecting patients' autonomy.
▶ To know how to provide safe and effective pharmacotherapy to manage tobacco dependence and where to look for more information.

The hazards of smoking and the benefits of stopping smoking

Smoking will kill half the people who continue with it; half of those deaths will occur before the age of retirement.[23] On average it shortens life by about 10 years.[24] There are three main causes of death from smoking: CVD; cancers (see Figure 2.1 on p.32); and chronic obstructive pulmonary disease (COPD). Almost all smokers know smoking is bad for them, but light smokers often downplay the risks.[25] For cancers and COPD, the risk increases steeply with heaviness of consumption.[23,24] However, for CVD, the biggest killer of smokers, light smokers have nearly the same risk as heavier smokers.[26]

Fortunately, giving up smoking rapidly reverses many of the risks. The risk of CVD declines and within a few years is only marginally elevated from lifelong non-smokers.[27] Even in people with established CVD, stopping smoking reduces the risks of cardiovascular death by a third within 2 years of stop-

Figure 2.1 ○ *Cancer mortality in the UK in 2004*

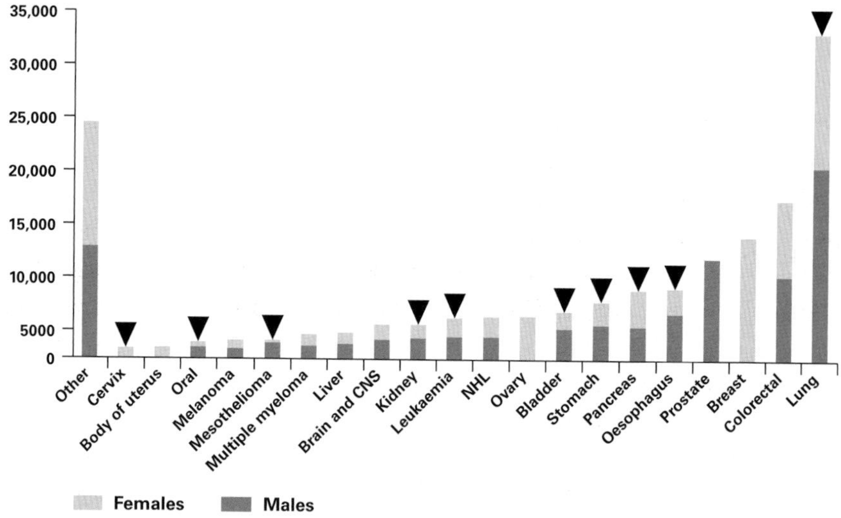

Source: Cancer Research UK. *UK Cancer Mortality Statistics for Common Cancers*, http://info. cancerresearchuk.org/cancerstats/mortality/cancerdeaths/ [accessed September 2010].[28]

Note: Cancers caused by smoking are indicated with a black arrow.

ping.[29] A key statistic to remember relates to stopping at or before the age of 40 years. A smoker who stops before the age of 40 years avoids all or nearly all morbidity and mortality from his or her (usually) 20+ years of smoking (see Table 2.1). A smoker who continues past 40 years loses 3 months of life for every year he or she continues smoking. However, even stopping at age 60 years still brings substantial health benefits to smokers (Table 2.1).

Table 2.1 ○ *Years of life gained relative to continuing smokers – from stopping smoking at various ages*

Age at stopping smoking	Years of life gained
25–34 years	10
35–44 years	9
45–54 years	6
55–64 years	3

Source: Doll R, Peto R, Boreham J, *et al*. Mortality in relation to smoking: 50 years' observations on male British doctors.[24]

Why don't smokers just stop?

Of course there are lots of reasons why smokers do not stop smoking, but the dominant reason that differentiates smoking from other habits is tobacco chemical dependence. Probably the most important factor that drives continued smoking is the presence of urges to smoke.[30] Nicotine binding in the midbrain leads to release of dopamine in the nucleus accumbens[31] and this probably creates urges. These urges are often triggered by cues in the environment, or sometimes mood states act as cues to smoke, triggering urges.[32,33] The urges can be thought of like hunger pangs. You can see food and want to eat it despite not being hungry, but you can want to not eat despite being hungry. Typically, when smokers try to stop smoking, they do not want to smoke (most of the time), but their best intentions are undermined by nicotine hunger pangs or urges to smoke. These come on in situations or moods when smokers have typically smoked and last only a few minutes, but they can be intense.[33] These urges are probably the main reason smokers go back to smoking in the days and weeks following stopping smoking. They diminish after a few weeks without smoking in most smokers.[34] Remember that motivation or wanting not to smoke is fluid. Often in moments of great stress you can feel that 'all bets are off' and ex-smokers often reach for a cigarette. Unfortunately this often reawakens the dormant urges and smokers find themselves trapped again. In addition, smokers suffer tobacco withdrawal symptoms when they go without smoking.[34] A few are physical (mouth ulcers, cough, constipation) but most are psychological (anxiety, depression, restlessness, irritability, insomnia). They probably do not drive return to smoking but they make smokers feel worse when they are trying not to give in to urges and their health declines temporarily and often unexpectedly. Some people become clinically depressed after they stop smoking and most people gain weight, on average 7 kg in the long term.[35] GPs have a role in identifying and managing these problems.

The GP's main role: brief interventions

There is lots of guidance to help doctors give useful interventions to encourage and assist smokers to stop smoking, but much of the guidance is based on extrapolation and expert opinion, and advocates rather lengthy interventions.[36,37] The research evidence indicates that two components are effective in helping smokers stop:

▷ offer help (medication) to smokers to help them stop[38]
▷ advise smokers to stop on medical grounds.[39]

It is important to note that the evidence also suggests that assessing whether smokers want help to stop prior to the offer is probably counter-productive.[40] In trials where smokers were randomised to the offer of treatment and advice to stop smoking or advice to stop smoking only, smokers were 30 per cent more likely to try to stop smoking where treatment was offered.[41–43] Presumably, the offer of treatment increased their motivation to have a go. This is not surprising because nearly all smokers have tried to stop smoking previously and continue because of the failure of previous attempts. Fortunately, offering help to stop smoking and giving some advice on the value of stopping (see above) can be accomplished in only a few seconds and this makes it practical in your surgery. In published studies, somewhere between a quarter and two-thirds of smokers accept help to stop smoking[38] and few people object to offers of help.

A common view of GPs is that they prefer to intervene with smokers when the smoker presents with a smoking-related disease.[44] However, this strategy seems to lead smokers to resist a doctor's advice because they felt this undermined their right to be ill.[45] One benefit of an opportunistic, or 'assistance oriented', intervention strategy is that it fits whenever there is time and not simply when there is a smoking-related disease presented. There is evidence that doctors miss most opportunities to intervene with smokers ready to quit smoking[46] and that the Quality and Outcomes Framework (QoF) has not increased the rate at which doctors assist smokers to stop.[47] The assistance-oriented strategy might change this.

What help to give for the patient who wants to stop smoking?

Some people can stop smoking with little or no help at all, but others require intensive input. There are no characteristics that mean you can easily tell someone who will succeed from someone who will struggle. One thing we do know is that most people, whether heavy or light smokers, fail on any one quit attempt even with the most intensive treatments. However, smokers are four times more likely to succeed with treatment than without.[48] Fortunately, tobacco dependence treatment is cheap and safe, making it 'among the most cost-effective of all healthcare interventions' according to NICE.[49]

The best help a smoker can get is to be referred to the NHS Stop Smoking Service for behavioural support. The service will provide, prescribe, or ask the GP to prescribe medication, which will increase the chance of success by 50–150 per cent.[38,50,51] It will provide regular (usually weekly) advice, support, encouragement, problem solving, and monitoring of smoking status (together termed behavioural support), which increases the chance of success by 50–100 per cent.[52,53] Consequently, the combination of medication and support will quadruple the chance of successful cessation.[48] However, most of these patients will resume smoking, as is the nature of addiction, and they will benefit from re-referral. Patients can lose heart, but a doctor's job is to encourage and re-treat as often as needed.

When patients want to stop smoking but cannot or do not want to use behavioural support, a doctor will need to take over the management of the quit attempt. Supporting quitting well is complicated, but doing so adequately is simple (see Box 2.1). There is good evidence that nicotine replacement therapy is safer than smoking in practically all smokers (there are no absolute contraindications) and that it works to support quitting with no behavioural support.[38] A doctor should become familiar with the use of nicotine replacement therapy (NRT – see resources and Box 2.2 on p. 36). The other medication choices (bupropion[51] and varenicline[50] – see Box 2.3 on p. 36) all have a place, but mainly with behavioural support. GPs will be recommended to prescribe these by the NHS Stop Smoking Service, who will monitor patients using them.

Box 2.1 ○ *Simple advice to patients on how to stop smoking*

▶ Set a day as the last day of smoking.

▶ Review previous quit attempts – what led to relapse and what lessons can be drawn?

▶ Plan ways to deal with the cigarettes that will be hardest to let go. Often this is the one at the start of the day, but can also be ones smoked in the evening. This may involve changing the normal routines to avoid cues to smoke.

▶ Alcohol is a major cause of relapse. Perhaps avoid it altogether for the first week or two. Do not get drunk.

▶ Think of yourself as a non-smoker. Smoking is not even an option. Even one cigarette will seriously reduce your chance of making it.

▶ Many products come with websites or telephone helplines. Encourage use of these or Quitline.

Box 2.2 ○ *Simplified advice for the new prescriber of NRT*

▶ For smokers of ten or more cigarettes per day, use a nicotine patch because adherence to the medication is high. Use the full-strength patches as first choice. The summary of product characteristics (SPC) varies by manufacturer for no good reasons. If smokers have not stopped completely or are getting cravings, *add* a rapid-acting form of NRT as below. This is licensed, evidence-based[16] and not dangerous.

▶ For smokers of fewer than ten cigarettes per day, use gum, lozenge or microtab, with an approximate dose of 1 unit per cigarette. Advise your patients to use more if they have cravings/urges to smoke – it is not dangerous. The patient should practise using these before quit day; it takes time to get used to the unpleasant peppery taste and receive the benefit.

▶ Inhalators or nasal spray are alternatives. Nasal spray is very aversive on first use and is best for heavy smokers. Inhalators are a good choice for those who want something to do with their hands and mouth. Patients should use a new cartridge every 2 hours or so as the nicotine dries up.

Box 2.3 ○ *Simple advice for the new prescriber of varenicline and bupropion for stopping smoking*[54]

Varenicline

▶ Start 1–2 weeks prior to stop date.

▶ Start with 500 mcg once daily for 3 days.

▶ Increase to 500 mcg twice daily for 4 days.

▶ 1 mg twice daily for 11 weeks.

The Medicines and Healthcare products Regulatory Agency (MHRA) guidance currently suggests that varenicline should be used with caution in patients with a history of psychiatric illness, and should be stopped if any patient develops low mood or suicidal ideation.

Bupropion

▶ Start 1–2 weeks prior to stop date.

▶ Start with 150 mg once daily for 6 days.

▶ Increase to 150 mg twice daily and continue for 7–9 weeks.

▶ Stop if no abstinence at 7 weeks.

Bupropion should not be used in patients with a history of seizures, brain tumour or eating disorder, or in patients with acute alcohol or benzodiazepine withdrawal. Use 150 mg once daily in the elderly.

Conclusions

You will put time and effort into helping your patients stop smoking. In the short term, perhaps nine out of ten will fail to quit for good. If you keep going, the large majority will make it, ideally before they develop the complications of tobacco dependence. For many, you need to treat tobacco dependence like other chronic diseases. However, brief encouragement, advice, offers of help and referral to the NHS Stop Smoking Service will help most of your patients to stop.

Smoking cessation resources

▷ A brief guide to clinical management of tobacco dependence can be found at • **www.bmj.com/cgi/content/full/335/7609/37?ijkey= 6mrLxwzzzUXzSrB&keytype=ref** [accessed September 2010].
▷ You can learn more about the treatment of tobacco dependence at • **www.treattobacco.net** [accessed September 2010].
▷ The Cochrane Tobacco Addiction Group publishes its up-to-date evidence-based reviews at • **http://tobacco.cochrane.org/ welcome** [accessed September 2010]. This Cochrane Review argues for the chronic disease model of tobacco dependence.

Obesity

This section aims to put obesity and its management into context in terms of CVD prevention.

Learning points

▶ Deliver intensive lifestyle counselling and follow-up by trained staff.
▶ Target interventions first to those at most risk from obesity (for adults these are those patients with more severe obesity (body mass index (BMI) >35), high waist circumference (>102 cm men, >88 cm women) and/or co-morbidity.
▶ Using local resources, consider referring to local weight management groups that follow best practice.
▶ In adults consider using orlistat if appropriate according to guidelines.
▶ Refer adult patients for bariatric surgery if they have a BMI of 40kg/m^2 or more, or between 35kg/m^2 and 40kg/m^2, and other significant disease and non-surgical measures have been tried and failed.

▶ Refer to specialised multidisciplinary teams for drug or surgical interventions in children (only for older children in exceptional circumstances).

Context

Obesity is a major – and rising – threat to public health. The prevalence of overweight and obese adults in England has trebled in 25 years. In 1980, 8 per cent of adult women and 6 per cent of adult men were classified as obese; by 2004 this had increased to approximately 24 per cent of men and women, with a further 46 per cent of men and 35 per cent of women being overweight.[55] It is associated with a range of secondary co-morbidities (Table 2.2) and significantly impaired quality of life.[56]

Table 2.2 ○ *Relative risk of other diseases in obese adults*

Disease	Relative risk of developing disease	
	Women	Men
Type 2 diabetes	12.7	5.2
Hypertension	4.2	2.6
Heart attack	3.2	1.5
Colon cancer	2.7	3
Angina	1.8	1.8
Gall bladder disease	1.8	1.8
Ovarian cancer	1.7	
Osteoarthritis	1.4	1.9
Stroke	1.3	1.3

Source: National Audit Office. *Tackling Obesity in England.*[57]

The role of primary care

Obesity is not simply a clinical problem. A broad approach to the problem is needed on a number of levels, involving both government and multiple agencies in the health and social sector.[58] Furthermore, the available trial evidence for intervention by primary care teams is limited. Trials are mostly not from typical UK settings,[58-60] mostly had expert lifestyle and behavioural input, and followed up patients intensively (on average 13 times per year). This makes extrapolation of such findings to typical UK primary care settings difficult. Nevertheless, although there is limited evidence from typical UK primary care settings, the risks of obesity are as serious as smoking. As with smoking, GPs can help do something about it – even modest weight loss or stopping weight gain can have considerable health benefits. So for the patients' sakes GPs probably cannot afford to ignore the available trial evidence to date. The systematically reviewed evidence from NICE is as follows:[58]

▷ a 600 kcal per day deficit diet is likely to be effective; a low carbohydrate diet may also be effective, but care is needed with use of lower carbohydrate diets in the medium to longer term since limiting fruit and vegetable consumption is likely to be harmful to health[58,61-63]

▷ a combination of diet and behavioural therapy probably increases weight loss (-7.66 kg; -11.96 to -3.36 kg) compared with diet alone.[58] Important behavioural techniques include:
  □ self-monitoring of behaviour and progress, stimulus control, and goal setting
  □ slowing rate of eating and ensuring social support
  □ problem solving and cognitive restructuring (modifying thoughts)
  □ relapse prevention and strategies for dealing with weight regain

▷ at least 2 to 2.5 hours of moderate-intensity physical activity/week, in addition to diet (600 kcal/deficit or low fat), is likely to be more effective than diet alone (a difference of -1.95 kg; -3.22 to -0.68 kg) at 12 months, which is supported by other systematic reviews[58,64,65]

▷ orlistat with a diet is more effective for weight loss than placebo and diet (-3.3 kg at 12 months), i.e. 5 to 6 kg weight loss in total, which is clinically very important[66]

▷ bariatric surgery for adults if they have a BMI of 40 kg/m² or more.[58]

Putting evidence into practice

Given this evidence, how can the problem be tacked realistically? Raising the issue of obesity with patients is not always easy, and must be done sensitively. Trying to lever reluctant patients into a weight loss scheme will not achieve anything but a deterioration in the doctor–patient relationship. Furthermore, many GPs will have experience of trying but failing with their obese patients. For GPs who decide to intervene, the key issues to address are:

1 ▷ Delivering intensive lifestyle counselling and follow-up by trained staff. The NICE review documented the effectiveness of predominantly intensive lifestyle counselling mostly by highly trained staff[58]

2 ▷ Realistic use of resources: given the prevalence of obesity, even with highly trained staff most general practices are not currently in a position to deliver evidence-based intensive management for all their obese patients (the average intensity of follow-up was more than ten counselling sessions per year in the NICE review).[58] With limited resources, intervention should initially be targeted to those at most risk from their obesity (i.e. in adults with more severe obesity (BMI > 35), high waist circumference (> 102 cm men, > 88 cm women) and/or co-morbidity, e.g. diabetes, hypertension, and who are willing to change their lifestyle[58]

3 ▷ Using local resources: particularly where practice resources are stretched, GPs should consider referral to local weight management groups that follow best practice. Best practice for adults[58] involves:
   □ a realistic healthy target weight (usually 5–10 per cent weight loss), a maximum weekly weight loss of 0.5–1 kg, and long-term lifestyle changes
   □ addressing a long-term healthy-eating approach and advice about physical activity
   □ some behavioural change techniques, such as keeping a diary and advice on how to cope with 'lapses' and 'high-risk' situations
   □ ongoing support

4 ▷ In adults, GPs should consider orlistat – if lifestyle interventions are unsuccessful – for adults who have a BMI of 28 with associated risk factors, or a BMI of 30 kg/m² or more.[58] It is probably not efficient to continue for longer than 3 months if the person has not lost at least 5 per cent of his or her initial body weight since starting drug treatment (but less strict goals for Type 2 diabetes). For orlistat it is worth discussing with patients whether to continue for longer than 12 months for weight maintenance.[58] The dosing schedules used for orlistat are shown in Box 2.4

5 ▷ Refer patients for bariatric surgery for adults if they have a BMI of 40 kg/m² or more, or between 35 kg/m² and 40 kg/m² and other significant disease (for example Type 2 diabetes or high blood pressure), and non-surgical measures have been tried and failed.[3] This will of course depend on the local expertise available, and if specialist teams are not available the local primary care commissioning should make this a priority

6 ▷ Referring to specialised multidisciplinary teams for drug or surgical interventions in children only for older children in exceptional circumstances.[3] Surgery is only indicated if they have achieved or nearly achieved physiological maturity, have a BMI of 40 kg/m^2 or more (or 35–40 and other significant related disease, e.g. Type 2 diabetes, high blood pressure), and all appropriate non-surgical measures have failed to achieve or maintain adequate clinically beneficial weight loss for at least 6 months.

Box 2.4 ○ *Dosing schedules for anti-obesity medication*

Orlistat

▶ For over 18 years; unlicensed in children.

▶ 120 mg before, during or within 1 hour of meal; maximum dose 360 mg daily.

▶ If a meal is missed or the food does not contain any fat, omit dose of orlistat.

Discontinue if:

▶ less than 2 kg weight loss after further 4 weeks at higher dose

▶ weight loss after 3 months less than 5 per cent of initial body weight

▶ weight loss stabilises at less than 5 per cent of initial body weight

▶ individuals regain 3 kg or more after previous weight loss.

Source: British National Formulary. Drugs used in the treatment of obesity.[67]

41

'Lifestyle' risk factors: alcohol, exercise and diet

This section aims to discuss the effect other modifiable risk factors might have on cardiovascular risk. The effects of obesity and smoking have been well described above, but what about other 'lifestyle' factors?

Key learning points

▶ Good evidence exists for the improvement in intermediate end points (for instance blood pressure) in terms of lifestyle factors such as diet, exercise and alcohol.

▶ The evidence that such changes have an effect on long-term cardiovascular risk is less clear, with the best evidence stemming from work evaluating the Mediterranean diet.

What works?

Other so-called 'lifestyle' factors have been shown to be important in the prevention of CVD. The precise effect of these can be difficult to elucidate because – while for instance there is evidence for the reduction of blood pressure with weight loss, increased exercise, reduced alcohol and salt restriction[68] – this evidence is not necessarily converted into benefit in terms of CVD prevention.[69]

This seeming contradiction is probably a factor of both the relatively small effect of these interventions and therefore the problems of detecting such effects: studies designed to detect such effects would need to be large for statistical power. Furthermore, the difficulty of maintaining behaviours is such that experiments over the long periods of time needed for benefit to accrue are likely to produce null benefit. Observational studies that might provide long-term evidence tend to be confounded by the effects of wealth: richer people have better diets and live longer, but it is difficult to tease out the individual factors involved in this. Despite this, good evidence exists regarding the effect of the Mediterranean diet on cardiovascular mortality: pooled relative risk 0.91 (95 per cent CI 0.87–0.95).[70]

Dose response

Increasing amounts of exercise appear to be associated with a dose response in terms of preventing CHD. Those undertaking high and moderate levels of 'leisure time physical activity' gained benefit compared with low-activity individuals: relative risk 0.73 (95 per cent CI 0.66–0.80), $p<0.00001$ and 0.88 (95 per cent CI 0.83–0.93), $p<0.0001$ for high and moderate respectively.[71] Similar effects have been seen for increasing amounts of walking.[72]

No such dose response occurs with salt. For alcohol, a J-shaped curve exists with benefit seen for mild-to-moderate consumption (up to 150 ml wine per day in one meta-analysis) but not at higher intakes.[73]

What advice should I give?

▷ Exercise daily, at least 30 minutes of walking or more intensive physical activity.
▷ Eat a 'Mediterranean diet' consisting of a diet rich in fruits, vegetables, legumes, and cereals, with olive oil as the only source of fat, moderate consumption of red wine especially during meals, and low consumption of red meat.

▷ Reduce salt intake by not adding salt to food. Educate patients about the high amount of salt found in processed foods and encourage them to check labelling. Discuss the availability of low sodium salt options but these may contain potassium so ensure not at risk of hyperkalaemia.

Fixed risk factors: ethnicity

The aim of this section is to provide a brief overview of ethnicity and migration, and effect of the former on CVD. Ethnicity is a non-modifiable risk factor for CVD and ethnic variations in disease rates are closely tied to geographical patterns of disease. For example, there is marked regional variation across Europe in mortality rates with higher CVD rates in the northeast and lower rates in the southwest.[74]

43

Learning points

▶ Ultimately everyone is a migrant.
▶ 8 per cent of the UK population are from a minority ethnic group.
▶ South Asians living in the UK (i.e. Indians, Bangladeshis, Pakistanis) have a 50 per cent greater risk of dying prematurely from CHD than the general population, whereas Caribbeans and West Africans are around half (despite higher rates of hypertension).
▶ Aggressive treatment of cardiovascular risk factors is therefore indicated.

What do we mean by ethnicity?

There has been considerable debate on defining ethnicity and the current consensus is that it is a multidimensional social construct embodying one or more of the following: 'shared origins or social background; shared culture and traditions that are distinctive, maintained between generations, and lead to a sense of identity and group; and a common language or religious tradition'.[75] This definition also reflects self-identification with cultural traditions and social identity, and boundaries between groups. It is also important to remember that *everyone* belongs to an ethnic group and not just those who have migrated to the UK.[76]

Migration to the UK

Since the dawn of humanity people have migrated over vast distances in the search for a better or safer life.[77] Migration to the British Isles has been occurring for the past 40,000 years from all over the world so that everyone living in UK today is either an immigrant or descended from one![78]

Operationalising ethnicity

Given the importance of ethnicity on health, there are pragmatic grounds for assigning people into ethnic groups. The benefit of collecting data on ethnic groups is to help reduce inequalities in health and healthcare delivery.[79] Many have used proxy measures to define ethnic group, such as skin colour, country of birth and name. Each of these has disadvantages and the general consensus is that self-identified ethnicity is the way forward using, for example, the 2001 Census Ethnic Group question.[76] It is also worth noting the Census 2001 question was significant as it asked questions on people of Irish descent and mixed parentage for the first time.

Demographic profile

The UK is a diverse society with 7.9 per cent (4.6 million) of the population from black and minority ethnic groups. The latter is a heterogeneous group residing in all parts of the UK but clustering in the major metropolitan areas.[76]

The largest minority ethnic group is the Asian or Asian British category (50.2 per cent) followed by the black or black British (24.8 per cent). For the first time, the 2001 census also recorded that there were 677,117 (1.2 per cent) people belonging to the 'mixed' ethnic group category – and this is nearly as big as the Pakistani category. It is worth noting that the average age of minority ethnic communities is younger than the white population.

Cardiovascular epidemiology in minority ethnic groups

Cardiovascular morbidity and mortality are higher amongst certain ethnic groups than the white population.[76,80] South Asians living in the UK, as mentioned earlier, have a 50 per cent greater risk of dying prematurely from CHD than the general population.[76] However, premature death rates from CHD for Caribbeans and West Africans are much lower than average –

around half the rate found in the general population for men and two-thirds of the rate found in women – but hypertension is much commoner amongst these groups. Of note, the poorest groups, particularly Pakistanis and Bangladeshis, have the highest mortality rates.

Importantly, the difference in the death rates between South Asians and the rest of the population is increasing. This is because the death rate from CHD is not falling as fast in South Asians as it is in the rest of the population. From 1971 to 1991, the mortality rate for 20–69-year-olds for the whole population fell by 29 per cent for men and 17 per cent for women, whereas in South Asians it fell by 20 per cent for men and 7 per cent for women.[80]

However, a more recent analysis of secular trends in the past 15 years indicates that death from acute myocardial infarction (AMI) among South Asians appears to have declined at a rate similar to that seen in white patients. This is largely caused by reductions in indices of infarct severity (segment on the ECG (ST) elevation, peak creatine kinase, Q wave development on the ECG and treatment with thrombolytic therapy).[81]

The two main ethnic groups within the UK, the black and South Asian groups, are at particularly high risk of CVD, although there are ethnic differences in the prevalence of CVD conditions and cardiovascular mortality.[76] It is also important to note that mortality and morbidity from end-stage renal disease vary by ethnic group, with a much greater burden in both people of African origin and of people from the Indian subcontinent, even among those living in the UK. The prevalence of cardiovascular risk factors and CHD in the UK Chinese population has been reported to be low.[82]

With respect to gender, note that the patterns for cardiovascular morbidity and mortality in men and women differ, with Bangladeshi and Pakistani men being top of the league whereas, in women, the Indian and Irish predominate.

In relation to cerebrovascular disease, this is highest among the African Caribbean populations and high rates are also seen in Chinese and South Asian groups. The major known risk factor for stroke, hypertension, is common in African Caribbeans but not in the Chinese or South Asian populations.

Causes of CVD

The causes of the excess CVD and stroke morbidity and mortality in black and minority ethnic groups (BMEGs) are incompletely understood, though recent work[82–85] indicates that socioeconomic factors are important. However, the role of classical cardiovascular risk factors is clearly important despite the patterns of these risk factors varying significantly by ethnic group.[76,86] Irrespective of these inter-ethnic differences in vascular diseases, cardiovascular morbidity and mortality are still much higher among these BMEGs when compared with the white population.[76]

Implications for clinical practice

As the minority ethnic groups have been under-represented in research, a multitude of guidelines exist for the 'general population'. Risk factor cut-offs such as waist circumference and BMI may need to be varied by ethnicity to accurately reflect the associated cardiovascular risk. However, specific reference and recommendation on primary and secondary prevention guidelines in relation to ethnic groups is extremely limited. Given this, it is still very important to identify and manage those minority ethnic groups at higher CVD risk than the general population.

Other fixed risk factors: age, sex and family history

The section considers other fixed risk factors for CVD, namely age, sex and family history. These are not modifiable but have important consequences for the management of risk.

Learning points

▶ Cardiovascular risk increases with age, male sex, and the presence of a family history of premature CVD.
▶ While absolute risk will be highest at the extremes of age, potential benefit in terms of life years gained may be greatest in younger individuals. This is judged by high relative risks compared with those of similar age.

Age

As a person gets older, the risk of having a cardiac event gradually increases until he or she has a 40 per cent chance of dying from ischaemic heart disease.[87] This increase in absolute risk means that interventions are often more effective in real terms in older people. An example of this is the success in treating systolic hypertension in the elderly where significant reductions in both stroke and death rates have been found.[88,89] Similarly, relative ben-

46

efit from lowering blood pressure in the very elderly is equivalent to younger individuals, although absolute benefit is higher.[90] However, concentrating on the absolute benefit from risk interventions may mask the fact that a younger person at high relative risk may gain more in terms of life years than a patient who is older.

Sex

Men are at higher risk from ischaemic heart disease than women.[91] This differential is highest in younger age groups (3:1) but decreases, to 1.5:1, in the elderly. Female hormones are thought to provide a cardioprotective effect. Interestingly, women smokers are more at risk of CVD than their (smoking) male counterparts and it has been postulated that this is due to a direct effect of smoking on hormonal factors.[92]

Family history

This is another fixed risk factor that cannot be influenced by a patient.[93] At the most extreme, the inheritance of genes for familial hypercholesterolaemia (FH) can lead to a hundred-fold increase in the risk of death from CHD in affected individuals in their twenties and thirties.[93] It is an autosomal dominant inherited disorder, most commonly due to a mutation in the low-density lipoprotein receptor gene. FH only affects around 2:1000 individuals. However, about 30 per cent of all those with CHD fulfil the criteria for a positive family history, leading to around a 30 per cent increase in risk.[94,95] Other genetic disorders such as familial combined hyperlipidaemia, familial high-density lipoprotein deficiency and some coagulation disorders such as Factor V Leiden can also increase risk of coronary events. A detailed account of these disorders can be found in the 'European Guidelines on Cardiovascular Disease Prevention in Clinical Practice' 2007.[96]

Asking about family history in the consultation is therefore an important part of history taking and should include relatives affected under the age of 55 (men) or 65 (women). The Joint British Societies guidelines suggest that the estimated cardiovascular risk should be multiplied by 1.5 in patients with a positive family history. This multiplication factor is pragmatic rather than truly evidence based.[97]

Blood pressure

Aims

This section discusses the importance of blood pressure as a component of cardiovascular risk, the concept of hypertension, and how blood pressure can be lowered in practice.

Key learning points

▶ The relationship between blood pressure and cardiovascular risk is continuous from at least 110 mmHg systolic.
▶ NICE recommends treatment of hypertension where blood pressure is sustained above 160/100 mmHg or above 140/90 mmHg in the presence of additional risk factors, or based on increased cardiovascular risk estimation of >20 per cent 10-year risk.
▶ Accurate blood pressure measurement is a prerequisite for appropriate management.
▶ Non-pharmacological interventions can lower blood pressure and should be recommended for all.
▶ The key to pharmacological management of hypertension is blood pressure lowering. Little difference exists between the efficacy of blood pressure lowering between the major antihypertensive drug classes. Choice of drug is probably best guided by a combination of tolerability, cost and the presence of co-morbidities.

Definition and thresholds

Blood pressure is a key modifiable risk factor for both coronary heart and cerebrovascular disease.[16] The relationship between pressure and risk is a continuous one above approximately 110 mmHg systolic, but it is conventional to assign the label of 'hypertension' to those with a blood pressure above a threshold pressure.[98, 99] In the UK, the level of this threshold has been set by NICE and the British Hypertension Society at an absolute of 160/100 mmHg (sustained) or 140/90 mmHg in the presence of additional risk factors (history of CVD, diabetes, end organ damage) or based on increased cardiovascular risk estimation of >20 per cent 10-year risk of a cardiovascular event.[100, 101] Even lower thresholds have been suggested in those at particularly high risk.[101, 102] Around one-third of the UK population is estimated to have or be treated for raised blood pressure. Prevalence rises with age, meaning that the majority of those over 65 are affected.[103]

Blood pressure measurement

Identifying risk associated with blood pressure depends on accurate measurement.[100] This depends on accurate equipment, appropriate use of it, and careful preparation of the subject.[104] Traditionally, measurement was undertaken using a mercury sphygmomanometer but more recently many primary care practitioners (and indeed patients themselves) have moved towards using automated electronic monitors.[105] Any sphygmomanometer must be validated and calibrated to ensure accuracy. The British Hypertension Society website provides a list of accurate automated models.[106] The same website gives detailed information regarding the appropriate technique for measurement, which includes using an appropriately sized cuff, ensuring that the subject is rested and comfortable, and taking multiple measurements.

Hypertension diagnosis

Diagnosis of hypertension requires measurements on at least three occasions over a time period of 2 weeks to 6 months dependent on the initial level of pressure (see Table 2.3 on p. 50 for thresholds).[100] Repeated measurement over time can lead to surprising drops in blood pressure.[107] Baseline investigations include tests for end organ damage (renal function, urinalysis, ECG), to assess risk (cholesterol, blood glucose) and possible secondary causes (electrolytes, urinalysis, more specialised investigations should a secondary cause be suspected, particularly in the young (<30) or with very high pressure or where control is difficult). Referral may be needed in those where a secondary cause is suspected or to rule out 'white coat hypertension', where 'usual blood pressure' is much lower that office pressure. Secondary causes of hypertension are important as the management of these typically requires specialist input (see Table 2.4 on p. 50). Most cases of raised blood pressure in the UK are of essential hypertension and it is this which is covered in detail in this section. Standard UK criteria for the diagnosis of hypertension as described above are a sustained blood pressure over 160/100 mmHg without other risk factors or over 140/90 mmHg in the presence of end organ damage, additional risk factors or co-morbidity.

Table 2.3 ○ **Diagnostic and treatment thresholds plus treatment choice (NICE guideline)**

Offer treatment (mmHg)	Treatment choice	Target for treatment (mmHg)
All ≥ 160/100 (sustained)	Under 55: ACE inhibitor first line (A)	≤ 140/90 (means both systolic and diastolic below target)
≥ 140/90 plus additional risk: 10-year CHD risk ≥ 15%* 10-year CVD risk ≥ 20%* Existing CVD or target organ damage	55 and older or black patients of any age: calcium channel blocker (C) or thiazide diuretic (D) first line Subsequent choices: <55: A + (C or D) + (C or D) ≥55: (C or D) + A + (C or D)	

Note: * a CHD risk of 15% is equivalent to a CVD risk of 20%; the latter includes stroke risk.

Table 2.4 ○ **Proportion of patients with secondary hypertension – summary of studies**

	Proportion in each category (range %)
Essential hypertension	72.6–95.3
Renal hypertension	2.4–17.2
Renovascular hypertension	0.6–6.1
Primary hypokalaemic aldosteronism	0.1–0.4
Primary normokalaemic aldosteronism	3–18
Phaeochromocytoma	0.2–0.7
Cushing's syndrome	0.1–0.3
Endocrine, other	0.1–0.4
Oral contraceptives	1.5–5.0
Coarctation of the aorta	0.2–0.6
Other	1.0–3.7

Source: adapted from Danielson M, Dammstrom B. The prevalence of secondary and curable hypertension.[108]

Hypertension management

Initial treatment in hypertension should include guidance regarding non-pharmacological measures to lower blood pressure. Interventions that are recommended by NICE and that have been shown to reduce blood pressure include healthy diets, exercise (or a combination of both), reducing alcohol intake, reducing excessive caffeine ingestion and reducing salt (sodium) intake.[100] A systematic review found that blood pressure could be lowered by improved diet, aerobic exercise, alcohol and sodium restriction, and fish oil supplements with reductions in systolic blood pressure of 5.0 mmHg (95 per cent confidence interval (CI) 3.1–7.0), 4.6 mmHg (95 per cent CI 2.0–7.1), 3.8 mmHg (95 per cent CI 1.4–6.1), 3.6 mmHg (95 per cent CI 2.5–4.6) and 2.3 mmHg (95 per cent CI 0.2–4.3), respectively, with corresponding reductions in diastolic blood pressure.[109] Such behaviours may reduce, delay or remove the need for pharmacological treatment of hypertension. Smokers should receive advice to quit in view of the effect on cardiovascular risk, although this will have no effect on blood pressure.

Recommendations for the pharmacological treatment for hypertension are dependent on age and ethnicity, and have been labelled the 'ACD rule'.[100] Those under 55 at diagnosis should be offered initial treatment with an ACE inhibitor (angiotensin II receptor blocker (ARB) only if intolerant) followed by a thiazide diuretic or calcium channel blocker (CCB). The converse is true for those over 55 (diuretic or CCB then ACEI/ARB). People of African Caribbean origin are treated as per over-55s in view of the relative lack of benefit from ACE inhibition in this group because of lower renin levels. Third-line treatment is with the agent not used previously, followed by a beta-blocker, alpha-blocker or additional diuretic as fourth line. Individuals with a particular indication for a class of antihypertensive (for instance beta-blocker post-myocardial infarction) should not have such treatment withheld. Many individuals will be intolerant of, or have a contraindication to, one or more of these recommended classes of agent, hence individualisation is often required. Within classes there is little evidence for differential benefit and the bottom line for treatment is reducing blood pressure in a cost-effective manner.[110] In people with diabetes the treatment choices suggested are largely equivalent to those under 55.[111]

Once treatment has been commenced then targets to aim for again depend on risk and co-morbidities. For essential hypertension the target is below 140/90 mmHg.[100] This is based on evidence from the Hypertension Optimal Treatment (HOT) study, which randomised participants to one of the three diastolic BP targets (90, 85 and 80 mmHg) but found no difference between them in terms of cardiovascular events.[112] This result was probably influenced by the fact that achieved blood pressures were much closer than anticipated (85, 83 and 81 mmHg respectively), which was probably due to participating physicians not being in equipoise and so treating the lesser target groups more aggressively. The targets in diabetes (140/80 or 130/80 mmHg in higher-risk groups) and other co-morbidities such as stroke and renal disease are more aggressive.[100]

People with hypertension need to be followed up to ensure that they are receiving optimum treatment. Such follow-up is typically nurse led and there is evidence that systematic methods with recall and review lead to better outcomes.[113] Current recommendations are for annual review, although a recent paper suggests that blood pressure probably changes very slowly once controlled and that too frequent measurement may lead to false positive raised readings.[114] In the UK, the Quality and Outcomes Framework of the general practice contract (QoF, a pay for performance scheme) requires at least annual follow-up with control below 150/90 mmHg as an audit standard.[115] Slightly oddly, the QoF only rewards review in the last 9 months of the financial year, which is a throwback to the 6-monthly guidance in the British Hypertension Society guidelines. This may change now that NICE is overseeing the development of the QoF.

Conclusions

In conclusion, blood pressure is a key risk factor for CVD that requires careful measurement, increases with age and can be reduced by both non-pharmacological and pharmacological means.

Lipids

The aims of this section are to put the management of lipids into the context of prevention of CVD. There is a special emphasis on CHD, for which intervention is most effective.

Learning points

▶ Dyslipidaemia conveys the greatest risk of the modifiable cardiovascular risk factors.
▶ Reduction of low-density lipoprotein cholesterol is a focus of most international guidelines for cardiovascular prevention.

▶ Statins are the main therapeutic class used with standard dose for primary prevention and higher dose for secondary prevention.

▶ Relative risk reduction for a given dose of statin is similar whatever the underlying risk, but absolute risk reductions are greatest for those at the greatest risk.

Lipids as risk factors for CHD

Abnormal plasma lipid levels (high levels of low-density lipoprotein choles-terol [LDL] and triglycerides [TG], and low levels of high-density lipopro-tein cholesterol [HDL]) are important modifiable risk factors for CVD.[116–119] Studies have shown that 80–90 per cent of CHD patients have at least one modifiable risk factor,[120, 121] and that each risk factor has a continuous, dose-dependent impact on CHD risk,[122, 123] with dyslipidaemia conveying the greatest risk.

A primary focus of most clinical guidelines, such as the US National Choles-terol Education Program Adult Treatment Panel III (NCEP ATP III)[122] and the European Task Force guidelines,[124] is LDL reduction. Therapeutic target levels for LDL are set largely on the basis of observed mean LDL achieved in the intervention arms of the numerous landmark statin studies.[117, 125–129] In most guidelines this is set as a minimum target for LDL below 3 mmol/L (130 mg/dl). There has been considerable debate that this target LDL is too high, with the European guidelines recommending LDL below 2.5 mmol/L in all and 2 mmol/L in those with established CVD. The US ATP guidelines go a step further in the highest-risk patients (those with diabetes and established CVD), recommending an optional target of 70 mg/dl.[122] These reduced target levels are based on four treat-to-differential-target trials, which showed significantly improved cardiovascular outcomes in those treated to around 70 mg/dl com-pared with those treated to around 100 mg/dl.[130] However, these studies were confined to patients with established CHD, and only in those with unstable CHD (acute coronary syndromes) were the additional reductions estimated to be cost-effective. These low targets are also much more difficult to achieve, and require high-dose, potent, long-acting statin (atorvastatin 80 mg).

The NICE and QoF currently maintain an LDL target of below 3 but may change to a lower target in those with established CVD.[131] In Europe, many GPs unfortunately still rely on total cholesterol (TC) targets rather than LDL because they are not provided with full lipid estimations. For these practical reasons, the value of other lipid measurements, such as TC or LDL to HDL ratios or apo-lipoproteins A or B, are not relevant to routine clinical care, though these measures may confer slightly better predictive power than LDL alone.

While LDL remains the most important lipid fraction to control, other lipid parameters such as HDL and TG are important. Strong epidemiological, but limited, clinical trial data suggest a 2–4 per cent decrease in CHD risk for each 0.025 mmol/L (1 mg/dl) increase in HDL.[119, 132–135] Importantly, this relationship is independent of LDL level. The evidence for raised TG levels as an independent risk factor for CHD is less conclusive. Some clinical trials have shown that elevated TG levels are an independent risk factor for CHD, but after adjustment for covariates the relationship was often weakened or abolished.[136–138] In contrast, the 8-year follow-up of PROCAM,[139] the Copenhagen Male Study[140] and a meta-analysis of 17 prospective trials[141] found a raised TG level remained an independent predictor of major coronary events after adjustment for LDL, HDL and diabetes.

Lipids and stroke

The effect of interventions to lower lipids on stroke and transient ischaemic attack (TIA) is not as great as that seen in CHD; subgroup analysis of the Heart Protection Study found that although 40 mg of simvastatin lowered risk of CHD events in people who had had a previous stroke or TIA, it did not lower risk of cerebrovascular events (though cerebrovascular events were lowered in the Heart Protection Study population as a whole).[142] However, the SPARCL study found that high-dose (80 mg) atorvastatin reduced the risk of stroke in people who had had a previous stroke or TIA compared with placebo (5-year absolute reduction in stroke risk, 2.2 per cent; adjusted hazard ratio, 0.84; 95 per cent CI 0.71–0.99; $p=0.03$).[143] The 5-year absolute reduction in the risk of major cardiovascular events was 3.5 per cent (hazard ratio 0.80; 95 per cent CI 0.69–0.92; $p=0.002$). However, no difference was found in overall mortality.

Do statins have differential effects dependent on risk?

The Cholesterol Treatment Trialists' (CTT) Collaborators meta-analysis reviewed the evidence for cholesterol lowering with statins and found a 12 per cent proportional reduction in all-cause mortality per mmol/L reduction in LDL cholesterol (rate ratio [RR] 0.88; 95 per cent CI 0.84–0.91; $p<0.0001$).[144] The major effect was 19 per cent reduction in coronary mortality (0.81; 0.76–0.85; $p<0.0001$), with non-significant reductions in non-coronary vascular mortality (0.93; 0.83–1.03; $p=0.2$) and non-vascular mortality (0.95; 0.90–1.01; $p=0.1$). Further analysis showed that these effects became statistically significant within a year of starting a statin and that the relative reduction in cardiovascular risk was similar whatever the absolute risk at baseline. However, absolute risk reduction and therefore benefit in terms of number needed to treat was greatest at highest risk.[144]

In view of the increase in absolute benefit with increasing risk, NICE in the UK has differentiated between primary and secondary prevention of CVD in their recommendations.[131] This is due to differences in cost-effectiveness seen in the mathematical modelling used to make its decisions. Thus, for most primary prevention, treatment with simvastatin 40 mg in a 'fire and forget' fashion is recommended, whereas secondary prevention with a 4 mmol/L target is suggested.[131]

Table 2.5 ○ *Benefit of LDL-C reduction on coronary events*

Trial	Statin	n	Follow-up	LDL-C reduction from baseline	Reduction in major coronary event
Primary prevention					
AFCAPS/TexCAPS	Lovastatin	6605	5.2 yrs	−25%	−37%
ASCOT-LLA	Atorvastatin	10,305	3.3 yrs*	−35%†	−37%
WOSCOPS	Pravastatin	6595	4.9 yrs	−26%	−31%
Secondary prevention					
4S	Simvastatin	4444	5.4 yrs	−35%	−34%
CARE	Pravastatin	4159	5 yrs	−32%	−24%
HPS	Simvastatin	20,536	5.5 yrs	−38%	−27%
LIPID	Pravastatin	9014	6.1 yrs	−25%†	−24%
PROVE-IT	Pravastatin Atorvastatin	4162	2 yrs	−10% −42%	−16% vs prava
TNT	Atorvastatin	10,001	4.9 yrs	−35%	−22% vs atorva 10 mg
Ischaemia					
AVERT	Atorvastatin	341	18 mths	−46%	−36%‡
LIPS	Fluvastatin	1677	3.9 yrs	−27%	−20%
MIRACL	Atorvastatin	3086	16 wks	−40%	−16%‡

* Stopped early; † vs placebo; ‡ AVERT and MIRACL did not show significant reductions in hard CHD end points; both were short-term trials and were not powered to show such a difference.

Table 2.6 ○ *Lipid goals in global guidelines*

Guideline	Cutpoint for initiating lipid-modifying drugs	Risk level	Goal[a] (mmol/L)			
			LDL-C	TC	TC: HDL-C ratio	Non-HDL-C
Australia	TC: 3.5/5.0 mmol/L[b]	High	—	<3.5/5.0	—	—
		Intermediate	—	—	—	—
		Low	—	<6.5/7.5	—	—
Canada	Treatment recommended in all patients	High	<2.5	—	<4.0	—
		Intermediate	<3.5	—	<5.0	—
		Low	<4.5	—	<6.0	—
Europe	LDL-C: 3.0 mmol/L	High	<2.5	<4.5	used to estimate risk	—
		Intermediate	<3.0	<5.0		—
		Low	<3.0	<5.0		—
New Zealand	TC: 8.0 mmol/L TC: HDL-C: 8.0	High	<2.5[d]	<4.0[d]	<4.5[d]	—
		Intermediate	<2.5[d]	<4.0[d]	<4.0[d]	—
		Low	<2.5[d]	<4.0[d]	<4.0[d]	—
USA	LDL-C: 2.6 mmol/L (optional if LDL-C <2.6 mmol/L)	High	<1.8/2.6	—	—	<3.4[c]
		Intermediate	<3.4	—	—	<3.4[c]
		Low	<4.1	—	—	<3.4[c]
International	LDL-C: 2.6 mmol/L (optional if LDL-C <2.6 mmol/L)	High	<2.6	—	—	<3.4[c]
		Intermediate	<3.4	—	—	<3.4[c]
		Low	<4.1	—	—	<3.4[c]

Notes: **a** Attempts should also be made to increase HDL-C and lower TG levels in appropriate patients; **b** Optional if LDL-C <2.6 mmol/L; **c** If TG ≥3.4 mmol/L; **d** Targets should be individualised to each patient and the calculated risk.

Side effects of statin therapy

Statins, like all drugs, have known side effects.[145] Muscle aches and mild derangement of liver enzymes may occur. More rare complications include rhabdomyolysis and liver toxicity. Liver function tests (LFTs) should be checked at baseline prior to initiation of statin therapy, again 3 months after starting treatment, and then at 12 months. If serum transaminases are more than three times the usual level, the statin should be stopped and LFTs monitored. If significant muscle aches are reported by the patient, checking the creatinine kinase (CK) level can be helpful. A level of CK that is more than

Figure 2.2 ○ *Achieving lower LDL-C reduces coronary events*

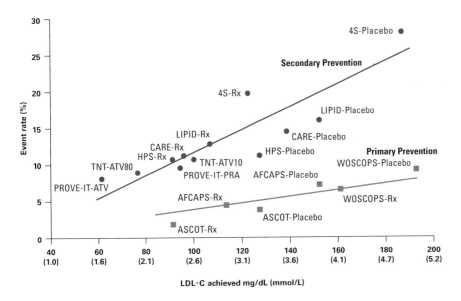

Rx = statin therapy   PRA = pravastatin   ATV = atorvastatin

Source: Cannon CP, Steinberg BA, Murphy SA, *et al*. Meta-analysis of cardiovascular outcomes trials comparing intensive versus moderate statin therapy.[130] Copyright Elsevier (2006). Adapted with permission.

Note: The data show that lower LDL-C levels reduce cardiovascular risk further, therefore supporting the concept that the lower you can get your LDL-C, the better.

five times the normal range may indicate significant muscle problems and the statin should be stopped. Patients at high risk of rhabdomyolysis should have a baseline CK level prior to starting statin therapy.

Conclusions

Lipid lowering is crucial in reducing overall cardiovascular risk. There is a strong evidence base that shows the effectiveness of lipid-lowering drugs, mainly statins, for both primary and secondary prevention of cardiovascular events. Clinical history and blood tests (LFT, CK) are important to identify rare complications of statin use.

Acknowledgement

Some of this section was previously published in Hobbs R, Arroll B. *Cardiovascular Risk Management* Oxford: Wiley-Blackwell, 2009.

Type 2 diabetes mellitus

This section considers the effect of Type 2 diabetes on cardiovascular risk and how this risk should be managed in terms of both pharmacological and non-pharmacological factors.

Learning points

▶ Patient education for healthy diet, increased physical activity, weight management and smoking cessation are key factors in the management of CVD risk in people with Type 2 diabetes.

▶ Intensive management of risk factors reduces cardiovascular risk in people with Type 2 diabetes.

▶ Risk factor targets to prevent CVD include aiming for an HbA1c <7 per cent, BP < 140/80 mmHg, total cholesterol < 4.0 mmol/L and LDL-C < 2.0 mmol/L.

Epidemiology

Type 2 diabetes mellitus is a common chronic and debilitating condition. The global prevalence of Type 2 diabetes mellitus is currently estimated to be 5.1 per cent and is expected to rise to 6.3 per cent by 2025.[146] There are 180 million people with diabetes worldwide [147] and currently 2.5 million people have diagnosed diabetes in the UK.[148] This rising prevalence has been associated with increased life expectancy, higher rates of obesity and a decrease in healthy lifestyle habits. The prevalence of Type 2 diabetes mellitus in certain ethnic groups such as people of South Asian origin is up to four times higher compared with white Europeans.[149] Furthermore, South Asian people develop Type 2 diabetes mellitus at an earlier age compared with white Europeans.[150]

Cardiovascular disease and diabetes

CVD is the most common cause of death in people with diabetes.[151] CVD death rates are either high or appear to be increasing in countries where Type 2 diabetes mellitus rates are high.[152, 153] In addition, advances in glycaemic management have improved the life expectancy of people with Type 2 diabetes mellitus but each year of prolonged life increases the likelihood of cardiovascular complications. CVD is responsible for between 50 per cent and 80 per cent of deaths, as well as for substantial morbidity and loss of quality of life.[154, 155] The risk of cardiovascular events in people with Type 2 diabetes mellitus is two to four times greater than in those people without diabetes.[155, 156]

The risks of mortality are even higher in people with Type 2 diabetes mellitus and established CHD.[157, 158] Although one cross-sectional study suggested that mortality risk from CHD in people with Type 2 diabetes mellitus is as high as in people who have had a myocardial infarction,[155] a more recent UK study showed that the people with Type 2 diabetes mellitus were at lower risk of CVD mortality compared with people with established CHD.[159] Furthermore, these complications are three and half times higher in the lower socioeconomic class[162] and two to three times higher in people with Type 2 diabetes mellitus of South Asian origin.[161] Deprivation is strongly associated with higher levels of obesity, physical inactivity, unhealthy diet and smoking. All these factors are inextricably linked to the risk of diabetes or the risk of serious complications amongst those already diagnosed.

Management of people with Type 2 diabetes mellitus

Intensive management of risk factors in people with Type 2 diabetes mellitus has been shown to be particularly effective, and implementation of these findings into practice should result in improved outcomes. Indeed, the strategy of intensive management of high-risk individuals with Type 2 diabetes mellitus with multiple drug combinations and lifestyle modification showed sustained beneficial effects with respect to vascular complications, and on rates of death from any cause and from cardiovascular causes.[162]

Recently, there have been a number of publications addressing tight glucose control on CVD risk in people with Type 2 diabetes mellitus.[165–166] The Action to Control Cardiovascular Risk in Diabetes (ACCORD) trial suggested that targeting intensive control of HbA1c levels to 6 per cent led to increased mortality as compared with targeting HbA1c levels from 7.0 to 7.9 per cent in people with established Type 2 diabetes mellitus.[164] In contrast to the ACCORD trial, the Action in Diabetes and Vascular Disease: Pre-

59

terax and Diamicron Modified Release Controlled Evaluation (ADVANCE)[21] and the Veterans Affair Diabetes Trial (VADT)[166] trials found no evidence that intensive treatment strategy to control glucose increases mortality. The ADVANCE trial showed that intensive glucose control reduced microvascular events, mainly as a result of a reduction in nephropathy; however, the VADT trial failed to show any microvascular benefits.[167] The speculated possibilities for the excess mortality rate found with intensive glucose control in the ACCORD trial could be the initial level of HbA1c and the rapidity with which intensive glucose control was achieved, as well as combinations of treatments used and the greater weight gain.[167] Unlike these trials of people with established Type 2 diabetes mellitus, the 10-year follow-up of the United Kingdom Prospective Diabetes Study (UKPDS, newly diagnosed people with Type 2 diabetes mellitus) showed that intensive glucose control (HbA1c < 7 per cent) led to significant improvements in CVD, total mortality and microvascular complications.[163] These new trials have therefore suggested that goals of HbA1c should be < 7 per cent rather than 6 per cent, and avoiding hypoglycaemia.[167]

Management of people with Type 2 diabetes mellitus includes comprehensive management of other risk factors including blood pressure and lipids, as well as glucose control. NICE suggests a blood pressure target of < 130/80 mmHg for people with renal or eye disease or CVD and < 140/80 mmHg for people without target organ damage.[168] Current evidence suggests low-dose aspirin should be used for people with established CVD; however, evidence for its use in people without established CVD is lacking.[169] The NICE guideline for Type 2 diabetes mellitus suggests that, when assessing people for premature CVD risk, they should be considered as a high risk unless they are not overweight, their BP is less than 140/80 mmHg without any treatment, there is no evidence of microalbuminuria, they do not smoke, have low-risk lipid profile, have no previous history of CVD and there is no family history of CVD. The guideline recommends estimating risk every 12 months using the UKPDS risk engine[170] if patients are at low CVD risk. NICE recommends targets of total cholesterol of < 4.0 mmol/L and LDL cholesterol of < 2.0 mmol/L.[168] For those at low risk, the NICE guideline suggests managing aggressively all people with Type 2 diabetes mellitus with a 10-year cardiovascular risk greater than 20 per cent using the UKPDS risk engine.[168]

Treating people with Type 2 diabetes mellitus with established CHD for dyslipidaemia, hypertension and hypercoagulability, as well as percutaneous interventions and cardiovascular surgery for acute coronary syndrome, improves event-free survival.[171] To reduce the CVD risk further in people with Type 2 diabetes mellitus, attention should be given to weight management, smoking cessation, patient education for healthy diet and increased physical activity.[172] While patient education has a key role in management of Type 2 diabetes mellitus, the Audit Commission Patient Survey highlighted significant gaps in knowledge, understanding and confidence in managing diabetes in various ethnic groups, which were substantially more pronounced in ethnic minorities.[173] Research carried out by MORI also showed awareness of diabetes and its complications to be extremely low among people in black and minority ethnic groups in the UK.[174] After introduction of pay for performance as part of the QoF, management of CVD risk factors in Type 2 diabetes mellitus has significantly improved.[175, 176] However, there is further scope for improvement through special attention to certain ethnic minority groups and people from low socioeconomic groups, to further reduce inequalities in health.

Management of prediabetes

Prediabetes is found in patients with blood glucose levels that are elevated but not sufficiently high for a diagnosis of diabetes.[177] It encompasses the terms impaired fasting glucose (IFG) and impaired glucose tolerance (IGT). IFG is defined by the World Health Organization as a fasting glucose level of greater or equal to 6.1 mmol/L but less than 7.0 mmol/L and 2-hour post-glucose tolerance test (GTT) of < 7.8 mmol/L. IGT is fasting glucose of greater than 7.0 mmol/L and 2-hour post-GTT ≥ 7.8 mmol/L but < 11.1 mmol/L.[178] Prediabetes is associated with an increased risk of CVD so all cardiovascular risk factors should be aggressively managed in these patients. Five to 10 per cent of patients with prediabetes develop diabetes within one year and most will progress to diabetes within their lifetime without intervention.[179]

Patients presenting to primary care with a blood glucose level of 6.1 mmol/L or above but less than 7.0 mmol/L should be referred for a GTT. The results of a GTT will distinguish between IFG, IGT and Type 2 diabetes. In all cases, the patient should receive diet and lifestyle advice to reduce cardiovascular risk. Other modifiable risk factors such as lipids, blood pressure and smoking should also be addressed to ensure optimal risk factor modification and reduce cardiovascular risk. Patients with prediabetes should have a fasting blood glucose measured annually. Effective lifestyle intervention at an early stage is key to reducing the number of these patients who progress to diabetes.[180]

The polypill: towards combined prevention of cardiovascular disease?

The aim of this section is to consider the potential benefits for cardiovascular prevention from a combined pharmacological intervention, comprising multiple elements known to reduce CVD development.

Learning points

▶ Combined moderate-dose antihypertensive, lipid-lowering and antiplatelet medication has the potential to reduce CVD while minimising side effects.
▶ Such an intervention might be appropriate for large sections of society (say everyone over 55) and has been seen as medicalising ageing, although distribution might conceivably be independent of the medical profession.
▶ No evidence from studies with a clinical outcome yet exists, although the first results of studies with intermediate outcomes (blood pressure and cholesterol) are beginning to appear.

Theoretical considerations

The concept of a polypill was first proposed by Wald and Law in 2003 where, accompanying meta-analyses of the effect of blood pressure and cholesterol lowering, they proposed that a preparation combining three antihypertensives at half normal dose combined with a statin, folic acid and aspirin might reduce CVD 'by more than 80 per cent' if taken by all aged over 55 or with pre-existing CVD.[181] They suggested that a third of individuals might receive a benefit (11 years of life free from a cardiovascular event), with up to 1 in 6 affected by side effects. In a subsequent article they confirm that the effects of major classes of blood pressure-lowering medication in primary prevention are equivalent, albeit that beta-blockers are less effective at lowering blood pressure.[182] Extrapolation of these results to epidemiological studies suggests that the benefit from blood pressure reduction may extend beyond conventionally labelled hypertension, hence the ongoing interest in a 'polypill' for all.

The emergence of evidence

To date only one trial comparing a polypill formulation, 'polycaps', to individual risk factor reduction has been published.[183] This study suggested that similar blood pressure lowering was achieved from a combination formulation as expected from combining individual effects, but that cholesterol lowering from a statin in combination with antihypertensives and aspirin was a little lower than the individual preparation. The clinical consequences of such findings are currently unknown but should become clearer over time.

Case-based discussion

> Box 2.5 ○ *Case scenario*
>
> A 55-year-old man attends surgery. He read in the newspaper that a drug to lower the fat in his blood could prevent him from having a heart attack. He had some blood tests last week and attends for the results. In light of these test results and other factors you need to discuss whether or not he should take a statin to lower his cardiovascular risk. From your records you know his last blood pressure reading was 150/85 mmHg, cholesterol 4.8 mmol/L, HDL cholesterol 1.2 mmol/L and he smokes. He is otherwise fit and well, and does not take any regular medications. He lives with his wife and works as a lorry driver.
>
> 1 What is his cardiovascular risk based on this information?
>
> 2 What primary preventive interventions should you offer him?
>
> 3 Are lifelong prescription medications indicated for him?
>
> 4 Experiment with the risk calculator to see the effect of the development of Type 2 diabetes and/or left ventricular hypertrophy on underlying risk.
>
> 5 He has central obesity. What advice would you give to him?
>
> You will need to use a risk calculation tool that uses the Framingham equations, such as that found at www.patient.co.uk/showdoc/40000133/.
>
> The answers to these questions are considered in the form of a case-based discussion, below.

Practising holistically

This patient has several risk factors for CVD and it is important to address each of these in addition to considering the patient's main query about lipid modification therapy. He attends because of an article he read in the newspaper; however, many patients read medical news stories without it prompting a visit to their GP. His reasons for attending should be further explored. Does he have a reason why he is concerned about having a heart attack? Is he frightened he may lose his job as a lorry driver if he did have heart problems? What does he think statins can do? Is he aware of the other aspects of his lifestyle that may be influencing his risk of heart disease?

Data gathering

A full history to explore all relevant risk factors would be helpful. Ethnicity and family history are important fixed risk factors. The patient is a smoker so a full smoking history including previous attempts to stop may also be helpful. Lifestyle factors such as diet, including salt and alcohol intake, and exercise are also important to explore. He should also have a height and weight measurement in order to calculate BMI. A fasting blood glucose level should also be taken to exclude diabetes.

Making a diagnosis

This patient has a 22 per cent risk of having a cardiovascular event in the next 10 years. He has raised cholesterol, high blood pressure and is a smoker. Further blood pressure readings are needed to establish a definite diagnosis of hypertension.

Clinical management

A risk score above 20 per cent for a cardiovascular event over the next 10 years is the threshold most commonly used in the UK to start cardiovascular preventive therapy, which might include blood pressure-lowering treatment (following confirmation of blood pressure persistently raised above 140/90 mmHg) and/or a statin. In addition his smoking is another key risk factor.

The risk score should be explained in terms that the patient can clearly understand. Diagrammatical aids on some risk score programmes can help. Many patients find the words 'heart attack' and 'stroke' very frightening, so the explanation must be given in a sensitive manner that does not cause undue alarm but still conveys the risk in a truthful way. The patient should be involved in the management decision.

In terms of the options for reducing risk the three main issues are smoking, cholesterol and blood pressure. The order in which these are tackled will vary between patients and is a matter for clinical judgement.

He has read about statins so may have his own thoughts and concerns. If this option is to be taken, the common side effects and regime for a statin should be explained. Baseline LFTs should be checked prior to commencing the statin. For primary prevention, NICE recommends a 'fire and forget' strategy, hence follow-up cholesterol monitoring is not necessarily indicated.

The patient also has raised blood pressure. Lifestyle advice should be given (reduce alcohol and salt intake, increase exercise, lose weight if BMI raised) and arrangements made for a repeat BP check and review.

He is also a smoker. His thoughts and ideas on quitting should be explored. He should be encouraged to attend the smoking cessation clinic to improve his chances of quitting. Simple advice as in Box 2.1 of the smoking section of this chapter should be given (see p. 35).

Managing medical complexity

There are a number of factors that are influencing this patient's cardiovascular risk. Smoking and blood pressure are important in addition to his cholesterol level. He does not have any significant past history of note but may have a family history that requires further exploration. All risk factors will not be adequately addressed within a single 10-minute consultation, so follow-up should be arranged to ensure optimal risk factor management over time.

65

Primary care administration

Primary care records contain large amounts of information on cardiovascular risk factors, which will allow accurate risk calculation.

Working with colleagues

The nurse in the primary healthcare team can contribute to risk factor management. It will be important for other GPs to encourage this patient to stop smoking as success rates at first quit attempt are likely to be low. However, there is considerable potential benefit to the patient if he is encouraged to repeat quit attempts and is eventually able to stop.

Community orientation

It is in the benefit of the wider community to prevent this patient suffering a cardiovascular event. The patient contributes to the healthcare system through paying taxes on income generated from his job as a lorry driver. If he were unable to work due to CVD this would reduce his ability to contribute. There are also high healthcare costs associated with hospital admission following myocardial infarction or stroke. Optimal primary prevention would reduce the risk of these events.

Maintaining an ethical approach

The four medical ethical principles of beneficence, non-maleficence, autonomy and justice should be addressed when considering primary prevention for an individual patient. Primary prevention strategies would reduce the risk of cardiovascular events and therefore benefit the patient. However, treatments such as statins are not without side effects and the risks as well as benefits should be discussed with the patient. Arguably stopping smoking is a more appropriate first intervention than potentially lifelong expensive drug treatment for blood pressure or cholesterol. Once wholly informed, the patient should be fully involved in decision making to ensure his autonomy is respected. Society is likely to benefit from this patient having a reduced risk of cardiovascular events, which will enable him to continue to work and to contribute to the healthcare economy.

Fitness to practise

GPs have a role in health promotion and should encourage patients to adopt a healthy lifestyle. The patient should, however, be the primary concern and he should be fully informed about his individual cardiovascular risk and the options for treatment. The doctor should work within the primary healthcare team to ensure that optimal risk factor management is achieved for this patient over time.

References

1 • Mathers CD, Bernard C, Iburg CM, *et al*. *Global Burden of Disease in 2002: data sources, methods and results* Geneva: WHO, 2003.

2 • McGill HC Jnr, McMahan CA, Gidding SS. Preventing heart disease in the 21st century: implications of the Pathobiological Determinants of Atherosclerosis in Youth (PDAY) study *Circulation* 2008; **117(9)**: 1216–27.

3 • Anderson KM, Odell PM, Wilson PW, *et al*. Cardiovascular disease risk profiles *American Heart Journal* 1991; **121(1 pt 2)**: 293–8.

4 • Jackson R, Barham P, Bills J, *et al*. Management of raised blood pressure in New Zealand: a discussion document *British Medical Journal* 1993; **307(6896)**: 107–10.

5 • Haq IU, Jackson PR, Yeo WW, *et al*. Sheffield risk and treatment table for cholesterol-lowering for primary prevention of coronary heart-disease *Lancet* 1995; **346(8988)**: 1467–71.

6 • National Collaborating Centre for Chronic Conditions. *Hypertension: management in adults in primary care: pharmacological update* London: Royal College of Physicians, 2006, www.nice.org.uk/guidance/index.jsp?action=byID&o=10986 [accessed September 2010].

7 • Cooper A, O'Flynn N. Risk assessment and lipid modification for primary and secondary prevention of cardiovascular disease: summary of NICE guidance *British Medical Journal* 2008; **336(7655)**: 1246–8.

8 • Mancia G, Grassi G. Joint National Committee VII and European Society of Hypertension/European Society of Cardiology guidelines for evaluating and treating hypertension: a two-way road? *Journal of the American Society of Nephrology* 2005; **16(Suppl 1)**: S74–7.

9 • Bhopal R, Unwin N, White M, *et al*. Heterogeneity of coronary heart disease risk factors in Indian, Pakistani, Bangladeshi, and European origin populations: cross sectional study *British Medical Journal* 1999; **319(7204)**: 215–20.

10 • Hippisley-Cox J, Coupland C, Vinogradova Y, *et al*. Derivation and validation of QRISK, a new cardiovascular disease risk score for the United Kingdom: prospective open cohort study *British Medical Journal* 2007; **335(7611)**: 136.

11 • Woodward M, Brindle P, Tunstall-Pedoe H. Adding social deprivation and family history to cardiovascular risk assessment: the ASSIGN score from the Scottish Heart Health Extended Cohort (SHHEC) *Heart* 2007; **93(2)**: 172–6.

12 • Hippisley-Cox J, Coupland C, Vinogradova Y, *et al*. Predicting cardiovascular risk in England and Wales: prospective derivation and validation of QRISK2 *British Medical Journal* 2008; **336(7659)**: 1475–82.

13 • Joshi P, Islam S, Pais P, *et al*. Risk factors for early myocardial infarction in South Asians compared with individuals in other countries *Journal of the American Medical Association* 2007; **297(3)**: 286–94.

14 • British Cardiac Society, British Hypertension Society, Diabetes UK, Heart UK, Primary Care Cardiovascular Society, Stroke Association. JBS 2: Joint British Societies' guidelines on prevention of cardiovascular disease in clinical practice *Heart* 2005; **91(Suppl 5)**: v1–52.

15 • Law MR, Morris JK, Wald NJ. Use of blood pressure lowering drugs in the prevention of cardiovascular disease: meta-analysis of 147 randomised trials in the context of expectations from prospective epidemiological studies *British Medical Journal* 2009; **338**: b1665.

16 • McManus RJ, Mant J, Meulendijks CF, *et al*. Comparison of estimates and calculations of risk of coronary heart disease by doctors and nurses using different calculation tools in general practice: cross sectional study *British Medical Journal* 2002; **324(7347)**: 459–64.

17 • Marshall T, Rouse A. Resource implications and health benefits of primary prevention strategies for cardiovascular disease in people aged 30 to 74: mathematical modelling study *British Medical Journal* 2002; **325(7357)**: 197.

18 • Goodyear-Smith F, Arroll B, Chan L, *et al*. Patients prefer pictures to numbers to express cardiovascular benefit from treatment *Annals of Family Medicine* 2008; **6(3)**: 213–17.

19 • O'Connor AM, Stacey D, Entwistle V, *et al*. Decision aids for people facing health treatment or screening decisions *Cochrane Database of Systematic Reviews* 2003; **2**: CD001431.

20 • Brindle P, May M, Gill P, *et al*. Primary prevention of cardiovascular disease: a web-based risk score for seven British black and minority ethnic groups *Heart* 2006; **92(11)**: 1595–602.

21 • Patel A, MacMahon S, Chalmers J, *et al*.; ADVANCE Collaborative Group. Intensive blood glucose control and vascular outcomes in patients with type 2 diabetes *New England Journal of Medicine* 2008; **358(24)**: 2560–72.

22 • Montgomery AA, Harding J, Fahey T. Shared decision making in hypertension: the impact of patient preferences on treatment choice *Family Practice* 2001; **18(3)**: 309–13.

23 • Peto R, Doll R. The hazards of smoking and the benefits of stopping. In: G Bock, J Goode (eds). *Understanding Nicotine and Tobacco Addiction* Chichester: John Wiley & Sons, 2006, pp. 3–28.

24 • Doll R, Peto R, Boreham J, *et al*. Mortality in relation to smoking: 50 years' observations on male British doctors *British Medical Journal* 2004; **328(7455)**: 1519.

25 • Taylor T, Lader D, Bryant A, *et al*. *Smoking-Related Behaviour and Attitudes, 2005* London: Office for National Statistics, 2006.

26. Bjartveit K, Tverdal A. Health consequences of smoking 1–4 cigarettes per day *Tobacco Control* 2005; **14(5)**: 315–20.

27 • Kawachi I, Colditz GA, Stampfer MJ, *et al*. Smoking cessation and time course of decreased risks of coronary heart disease in middle-aged women *Archives of Internal Medicine* 1994; **154(2)**: 169–75.

28 • Cancer Research UK. *UK Cancer Mortality Statistics for Common Cancers*, http://info. cancerresearchuk.org/cancerstats/mortality/cancerdeaths/ [accessed September 2010].

29 • Critchley J, Capewell S. Smoking cessation for the secondary prevention of coronary heart disease *Cochrane Database of Systematic Reviews* 2003; **4**: CD003041.

30 • West R. Defining and assessing nicotine dependence in humans. In: WA Corrigall (ed.). *Understanding Nicotine and Tobacco Addiction* London: John Wiley & Sons Ltd, 2006, pp. 36–63.

31 • Foulds J. The neurobiological basis for partial agonist treatment of nicotine dependence: varenicline *International Journal of Clinical Practice* 2006; **60(5)**: 571–6.

32 • Shiffman S, Hickcox M, Paty JA, *et al*. Individual differences in the context of smoking lapse episodes *Addictive Behaviors* 1997; **22(6)**: 797–811.

33 • Shiffman S. Reflections on smoking relapse research *Drug and Alcohol Review* 2006; **25(1)**: 15–20.

34 • Hughes JR. Effects of abstinence from tobacco: valid symptoms and time course *Nicotine & Tobacco Research* 2007; **9(3)**: 315–27.

35 • O'Hara P, Connett JE, Lee WW, *et al*. Early and late weight gain following smoking cessation in the Lung Health Study *American Journal of Epidemiology* 1998; **148(9)**: 821–30.

36 • Fiore MC, Jaén CR, Baker TB, *et al. Treating Tobacco Use and Dependence: 2008 update* Rockville, MD: US Department of Health and Human Services, 2009.

37 • National Institute for Health and Clinical Excellence. *Brief Interventions and Referral for Smoking Cessation in Primary Care and Other Settings* London: NICE, 2006, http://guidance.nice.org.uk/PH1/Guidance/pdf/English [accessed September 2010].

38 • Stead LF, Perera R, Bullen C, *et al*. Nicotine replacement therapy for smoking cessation *Cochrane Database of Systematic Reviews* 2008; **1**: CD000146.

39 • Stead LF, Bergson G, Lancaster T. Physician advice for smoking cessation *Cochrane Database of Systematic Reviews* 2008; **2**: CD000165.

40 • Pisinger C, Vestbo J, Borch-Johnsen K, *et al*. It is possible to help smokers in early motivational stages to quit. The Inter99 study *Preventive Medicine* 2005; **40(3)**: 278–84.

41 • Ockene JK, Kristeller J, Pbert L, *et al*. The physician-delivered smoking intervention project: can short-term interventions produce long-term effects for a general out-patient population? *Health Psychology* 2008; **13(3)**: 278–81.

42 • Page AR, Walters DJ, Schlegel RP, *et al*. Smoking cessation in family practice: the effects of advice and nicotine chewing gum prescription *Addictive Behaviors* 1986; **11(4)**: 443–6.

43 • Russell MA, Merriman R, Stapleton J, *et al*. Effect of nicotine chewing gum as an adjunct to general practitioner's advice against smoking *British Medical Journal* (Clinical Research Ed.) 1983; **287(6407)**: 1782–5.

44 • Coleman T, Wilson A. Anti-smoking advice in general practice consultations: general practitioners' attitudes, reported practice and perceived problems *British Journal of General Practice* 1996; **46(403)**: 87–91.

45 • Pilnick A, Coleman T. 'I'll give up smoking when you get me better': patients' resistance to attempts to problematise smoking in general practice (GP) consultations *Social Science & Medicine* 2003; **57(1)**: 135–45.

46 • Coleman T, Wynn A, Barrett S, *et al*. Discussion of NRT and other antismoking interventions in UK general practitioners' routine consultations *Nicotine & Tobacco Research* 2003; **5(2)**: 163–8.

47 • Coleman T, Lewis S, Hubbard R, *et al*. Impact of contractual financial incentives on the ascertainment and management of smoking in primary care *Addiction* 2007; **102(5)**: 803–8.

48 • Aveyard P, West R. Managing smoking cessation *British Medical Journal* 2007; **335(7609)**: 37–41.

49 • National Institute for Health and Clinical Excellence. *Smoking Cessation Services in Primary Care, Pharmacies, Local Authorities and Workplaces, Particularly for Manual Working Groups, Pregnant Women and Hard to Reach Communities* London: NICE, 2008, www.nice.org.uk/guidance/index.jsp?action=byID&o=11925 [accessed September 2010].

50 • Cahill K, Stead LF, Lancaster T. Nicotine receptor partial agonists for smoking cessation *Cochrane Database of Systematic Reviews* 2007; **1**: CD006103.

51 • Hughes JR, Stead LF, Lancaster T. Antidepressants for smoking cessation *Cochrane Database of Systematic Reviews* 2007; **1**: CD000031.

52 • Lancaster T, Stead LF. Individual behavioural counselling for smoking cessation *Cochrane Database of Systematic Reviews* 2005; **2**: CD001292.

53 • Stead LF, Lancaster T. Group behaviour therapy programmes for smoking cessation *Cochrane Database of Systematic Reviews* 2005; **2**: CD001007.

54 • British National Formulary section 4.10 Drugs used in substance dependence>cigarette smoking *British National Formulary* 2010; **59**.

55 • Department of Health. *Health Survey for England: trends* London: Stationery Office, 2005.

56 • Jia H, Lubetkin E. The impact of obesity on health-related quality-of-life in the general adult US population *Journal of Public Health* 2005; **27(2)**: 156–64.

57 • National Audit Office. *Tackling Obesity in England* London: The Stationery Office, 2001.

58 • National Institute for Health and Clinical Excellence. *Obesity: the prevention, identification, assessment and management of overweight and obesity in adults and children* London: NICE, 2006, http://guidance.nice.org.uk/CG43/guidance [accessed September 2010].

59 • Glanville J, Glenny A-M, Melville A, *et al*. The prevention and treatment of obesity *Effective Health Care* 1997; **3(2)**: 1–11.

60 • Thorogood M, Hillsdon M, Summerbell C. Changing behaviour. In: S Barton (ed.). *Clinical Evidence* London: BMJ Publishing Group, 2001, pp. 16–33.

61 • John J, Ziebland S, Yudkin P, *et al*. Effects of fruit and vegetable consumption on plasma antioxidant concentrations and blood pressure: a randomised controlled trial *Lancet* 2002; **359(9322)**: 1969–74.

62 • Liu S, Manson J, Lee I-M, *et al*. Fruit and vegetable intake and risk of cardiovascular disease: the Women's Health Study *American Journal of Clinical Nutrition* 2000; **72(4)**: 922–8.

63 • Bazzano L, He J, Ogden L, *et al*. Fruit and vegetable intake and risk of cardiovascular disease in US adults: the first National Health and Nutrition Examination Survey Epidemiologic Follow-up Study *American Journal of Clinical Nutrition* 2002; **76(1)**: 93–9.

64 • Curioni C, Lourenço P. Long-term weight loss after diet and exercise: a systematic review *International Journal of Obesity* 2005; **29(10)**: 1168–74.

65 • Fogelholm M, Kukkonen-Harjula K. Does physical activity prevent weight gain: a systematic review *Obesity Reviews* 2000; **1(2)**: 95–111.

66 • Tuomilehto J, Lindstrom J, Eriksson J, *et al*. Prevention of type 2 diabetes mellitus by changes in lifestyle among subjects with impaired glucose tolerance *New England Journal of Medicine* 2001; **344(18)**: 1343–50.

67 • British National Formulary, section 4.5, Drugs used in the treatment of obesity *British National Formulary* 2010; **59**.

68 • Dickinson HO, Mason JM, Nicolson DJ, *et al*. Lifestyle interventions to reduce raised blood pressure: a systematic review of randomized controlled trials *Journal of Hypertension* 2006; **24(2)**: 215–33.

69 • Ebrahim S, Beswick A, Burke M, *et al*. Multiple risk factor interventions for primary prevention of coronary heart disease *Cochrane Database of Systematic Reviews* 2006; **4**: CD001561.

70 • Sofi F, Cesari F, Abbate R, *et al*. Adherence to Mediterranean diet and health status: meta-analysis *British Medical Journal* 2008; **337**: a1344.

71 • Sofi F, Capalbo A, Cesari F, *et al*. Physical activity during leisure time and primary prevention of coronary heart disease: an updated meta-analysis of cohort studies *European Journal of Cardiovascular Prevention and Rehabilitation* 2008; **15(3)**: 247–57.

72 • Zheng H, Orsini N, Amin J, *et al*. Quantifying the dose–response of walking in reducing coronary heart disease risk: meta-analysis *European Journal of Epidemiology* 2009; **24(4)**: 181–92.

73 • Di Castelnuovo A, Rotondo S, Iacoviello L, *et al*. Meta-analysis of wine and beer consumption in relation to vascular risk *Circulation* 2002; **105(24)**: 2836–44.

74 • Muller-Nordhorn J, Binting S, Roll S, *et al*. An update on regional variation in cardiovascular mortality within Europe *European Heart Journal* 2008; **29(10)**: 1316–26.

75 • Senior PA, Bhopal R. Ethnicity as a variable in epidemiological research *British Medical Journal* 1994; **309(6950)**: 327–30.

76 • Gill PS, Kai J, Bhopal RS, *et al*. Health care needs assessment: black and minority ethnic groups. In: J Raftery, A Stevens, J Mant (eds). *Health Care Needs Assessment: the epidemiologically based needs assessment reviews* Abingdon: Radcliffe Publishing Ltd, 2007, pp. 227–399.

77 • Gamble C. *Timewalkers: the prehistory of global colonisation* Stroud: Allen Sutton, 1993.

78 • Commission for Racial Equality. *Roots of the Future: ethnic diversity in the making of Britain* London: Commission for Racial Equality, 1996.

79 • Gill PS, Johnson M. Ethnic monitoring and equity *British Medical Journal* 1995; **310(6984)**: 890.

80 • Wild S, McKeigue P. Cross sectional analysis of mortality by country of birth in England and Wales, 1970–92 *British Medical Journal* 1997; **314(7082)**: 705–10.

81 • Liew R, Sulfi S, Ranjadayalan K, *et al*. Declining case fatality rates for acute myocardial infarction in South Asian and white patients in the past 15 years *Heart* 2006; **92(8)**: 1030–4.

82 • Harland JO, Unwin N, Bhopal RS, *et al*. Low levels of cardiovascular risk factors and coronary heart disease in a UK Chinese population *Journal of Epidemiology and Community Health* 1997; **51(6)**: 636–42.

83 • Bhopal R, Unwin N, White M, *et al*. Heterogeneity of coronary heart disease risk factors in Indian, Pakistani, Bangladeshi, and European origin populations: cross sectional study *British Medical Journal* 1999; **319(7204)**: 215–20.

84 • Cappuccio FP, Cook DG, Atkinson RW, *et al*. The Wandsworth Heart and Stroke Study: a population-based survey of cardiovascular risk factors in different ethnic groups. Methods and baseline findings *Nutrition, Metabolism & Cardiovascular Diseases* 1998; **8**: 371–85.

85 • Nazroo JY. *The Health of Britain's Ethnic Minorities* London: Policy Studies Institute, 1997.

86 • Joshi P, Islam S, Pais P, *et al*. Risk factors for early myocardial infarction in South Asians compared with individuals in other countries *Journal of the American Medical Association* 2007; **297(3)**: 286–94.

87 • Prescott E, Hippe M, Schnohr P, *et al*. Smoking and the risk of myocardial infarction in women and men: longitudinal population study *British Medical Journal* 1998; **316(7137)**: 1043–7.

88 • Staessen J, Fagard R, Amery A. Isolated systolic hypertension in the elderly: implications of Systolic Hypertension in the Elderly Program (SHEP) for clinical practice and for the ongoing trials *Journal of Human Hypertension* 1991; **5(6)**: 469–74.

89 • Prevention of stroke by antihypertensive drug treatment in older persons with isolated systolic hypertension. Final results of the Systolic Hypertension in the Elderly Program (SHEP). SHEP Cooperative Research Group *Journal of the American Medical Association* 1991; **265(24)**: 3255–64.

90 • Beckett NS, Peters R, Fletcher AE, *et al*. Treatment of hypertension in patients 80 years of age or older *New England Journal of Medicine* 2008; **358(18)**: 1887–98.

91 • Janghorbani M, Hedley AJ, Jones RB, *et al*. Gender differential in all-cause and cardiovascular disease mortality *International Journal of Epidemiology* 1993; **22(6)**: 1056–63.

92 • Robson J. Information needed to decide about cardiovascular treatment in primary care *British Medical Journal* 1997; **314(7076)**: 277–80.

93 • Risk of fatal coronary heart disease in familial hypercholesterolaemia. Scientific Steering Committee on behalf of the Simon Broome Register Group *British Medical Journal* 1991; **303(6807)**: 893–6.

94 • Hawe E, Talmud PJ, Miller GJ, *et al*. Family history is a coronary heart disease risk factor in the Second Northwick Park Heart Study *Annals of Human Genetics* 2003; **67(Pt 2)**: 97–106.

95 • Myers RH, Kiely DK, Cupples LA, *et al*. Parental history is an independent risk factor for coronary artery disease: the Framingham Study *American Heart Journal* 1990; **120(4)**: 963–9.

96 • Graham I, Atar D, Borch-Johnsen K, *et al*. European guidelines on cardiovascular disease prevention in clinical practice. Fourth Joint Task Force *European Journal of Cardiovascular Prevention and Rehabilitation* 2007; **14(Suppl 2)**: E1–40.

97 • British Heart Foundation. *Joint British Societies' Guidelines on the Prevention of Cardiovascular Disease in Clinical Practice: risk assessment* London: BHF, 2006, www.bhsoc.org/bhf_factfiles/bhf_factfile_jan_2006.pdf [accessed September 2010].

98 • Ball SG. Clinical assessment of the hypertensive patients. In: JD Swales (ed.). *Textbook of Hypertension* Oxford: Blackwell Scientific Publications, 1994, pp. 1009–14.

99 • Law MR, Morris JK, Wald NJ. Use of blood pressure lowering drugs in the prevention of cardiovascular disease: meta-analysis of 147 randomised trials in the context of expectations from prospective epidemiological studies *British Medical Journal* 2009; **338**: b1665.

100 • National Collaborating Centre for Chronic Conditions. *Hypertension: management in adults in primary care: pharmacological update* London: Royal College of Physicians, 2006, www.nice.org.uk/guidance/index.jsp?action=byID&o=10986 [accessed September 2010].

101 • Williams B, Poulter NR, Brown MJ, *et al*. Guidelines for management of hypertension: report of the fourth working party of the British Hypertension Society, 2004-BHS IV *Journal of Human Hypertension* 2004; **18(3)**: 139–85.

102 • Crowe E, Halpin D, Stevens P. Early identification and management of chronic kidney disease: summary of NICE guidance *British Medical Journal* 2008; **337**: a1530.

103 • Joint Health Surveys Unit. *Health Survey for England*, www.ic.nhs.uk/ statistics-and-data-collections/health-and-lifestyles-related-surveys/health-survey-for-england [accessed September 2010].

104 • McAlister FA, Straus SE. Evidence based treatment of hypertension. Measurement of blood pressure: an evidence based review *British Medical Journal* 2001; **322(7291)**: 908–11.

105 • O'Brien E. Ave atque vale: the centenary of clinical sphygmomanometry *Lancet* 1996; **348(9041)**: 1569–70.

106 • British Hypertension Society. Validated blood pressure monitors, www.bhsoc.org/blood_pressure_list.stm [accessed September 2010].

107 • Brueren MM, Petri H, van Weel C, *et al*. How many measurements are necessary in diagnosing mild to moderate hypertension? *Family Practice* 1997; **14(2)**: 130–5.

108 • Danielson M, Dammstrom B. The prevalence of secondary and curable hypertension *Acta Medica Scandinavica* 1981; **209(6)**: 451–5.

109 • Dickinson HO, Mason JM, Nicolson DJ, *et al*. Lifestyle interventions to reduce raised blood pressure: a systematic review of randomized controlled trials *Journal of Hypertension* 2006; **24(2)**: 215–33.

110 • Neal B, MacMahon S, Chapman N. Effects of ACE inhibitors, calcium antagonists, and other blood-pressure-lowering drugs: results of prospectively designed overviews of randomised trials. Blood Pressure Lowering Treatment Trialists' Collaboration *Lancet* 2000; **356(9246)**: 1955–64.

111 • National Collaborating Centre for Chronic Conditions. *Clinical Gudieline 66, Type 2 Diabetes: national clinical guideline for management in primary and secondary care (update)* London: Royal College of Physicians, 2008, http://guidance.nice.org.uk/CG66/Guidance/pdf/English [accessed September 2010].

112 • Hansson L, Zanchetti A, Carruthers SG, *et al*. Effects of intensive blood-pressure lowering and low-dose aspirin in patients with hypertension: principal results of the Hypertension Optimal Treatment (HOT) randomised trial. HOT Study Group *Lancet* 1998; **351(9118)**: 1755–62.

113 • Fahey T, Schroeder K, Ebrahim S. Interventions used to improve control of blood pressure in patients with hypertension *Cochrane Database of Systematic Reviews* 2006; **4**: CD005182.

114 • Keenan K, Hayen A, Neal BC, *et al*. Long term monitoring in patients receiving treatment to lower blood pressure: analysis of data from placebo controlled randomised controlled trial *British Medical Journal* 2009; **338**: b1492.

115 • NHS Information Centre. *Quality and Outcomes Framework: online GP practice results database*, www.qof.ic.nhs.uk/ [accessed September 2010].

116 • Multiple Risk Factor Intervention Trial Research Group. Multiple risk factor intervention trial: risk factor changes and mortality results *Journal of the American Medical Association* 1982; **248(12)**: 1465–77.

117 • Heart Protection Study Collaborative Group. MRC/BHF Heart Protection Study of cholesterol lowering with simvastatin in 20,536 high-risk individuals: a randomised placebo-controlled trial *Lancet* 2002; **360(9326)**: 7–22.

73

118 • Anderson KM, Castelli WP, Levy D. Cholesterol and mortality. 30 years of follow-up from the Framingham study *Journal of the American Medical Association* 1987; **257(16)**: 2176–80.

119 • Assmann G, Schulte H. Relation of high-density lipoprotein cholesterol and triglycerides to incidence of atherosclerotic coronary artery disease (the PROCAM experience). Prospective Cardiovascular Münster study *American Journal of Cardiology* 1992; **70(7)**: 733–7.

120 • Greenland P, Knoll MD, Stamler J, *et al.* Major risk factors as antecedents of fatal and nonfatal coronary heart disease events *Journal of the American Medical Association* 2003; **290(7)**: 891–7.

121 • Khot UN, Khot MB, Bajzer CT, *et al.* Prevalence of conventional risk factors in patients with coronary heart disease *Journal of the American Medical Association* 2003; **290(7)**: 898–904.

122 • Executive Summary of the Third Report of the National Cholesterol Education Program (NCEP) Expert Panel on Detection, Evaluation, and Treatment of High Blood Cholesterol in Adults (Adult Treatment Panel III) *Journal of the American Medical Association* 2001; **285(19)**: 2486–97.

123 • Wilson PW, D'Agostino RB, Levy D, *et al.* Prediction of coronary heart disease using risk factor categories *Circulation* 1998; **97(18)**: 1837–47.

124 • De Backer G, Ambrosioni E, Borch-Johnsen K, *et al.* European guidelines on cardiovascular disease prevention in clinical practice. Third Joint Task Force of European and Other Societies on Cardiovascular Disease Prevention in Clinical Practice *European Heart Journal* 2003; **24(17)**: 1601–10.

125 • Randomised trial of cholesterol lowering in 4444 patients with coronary heart disease: the Scandinavian Simvastatin Survival Study (4S) *Lancet* 1994; **344(8934)**: 1383–9.

126 • Prevention of cardiovascular events and death with pravastatin in patients with coronary heart disease and a broad range of initial cholesterol levels. The Long-Term Intervention with Pravastatin in Ischaemic Disease (LIPID) Study Group *New England Journal of Medicine* 1998; **339(19)**: 1349–57.

127 • Downs JR, Clearfield M, Weis S, *et al.* Primary prevention of acute coronary events with lovastatin in men and women with average cholesterol levels: results of AFCAPS/ TexCAPS. Air Force/Texas Coronary Atherosclerosis Prevention Study *Journal of the American Medical Association* 1998; **279(20)**: 1615–22.

128 • Sacks FM, Pfeffer MA, Moye LA, *et al.* The effect of pravastatin on coronary events after myocardial infarction in patients with average cholesterol levels. Cholesterol and Recurrent Events Trial investigators *New England Journal of Medicine* 1996; **335(14)**: 1001–9.

129 • Shepherd J, Blauw GJ, Murphy MB, *et al.* Pravastatin in elderly individuals at risk of vascular disease (PROSPER): a randomised controlled trial *Lancet* 2002; **360(9346)**: 1623–30.

130 • Cannon CP, Steinberg BA, Murphy SA, *et al.* Meta-analysis of cardiovascular outcomes trials comparing intensive versus moderate statin therapy *Journal of the American College of Cardiology* 2006; **48(3)**: 438–45.

131 • Cooper A, O'Flynn N. Risk assessment and lipid modification for primary and secondary prevention of cardiovascular disease: summary of NICE guidance *British Medical Journal* 2008; **336(7655)**: 1246–8.

132 • Frick MH, Manninen V, Huttunen JK, *et al*. HDL-cholesterol as a risk factor in coronary heart disease: an update of the Helsinki Heart Study *Drugs* 1990; **40 (Suppl 1)**: 7–12.

133 • Jacobs DR Jnr, Mebane IL, Bangdiwala SI, *et al*. High density lipoprotein cholesterol as a predictor of cardiovascular disease mortality in men and women: the follow-up study of the Lipid Research Clinics Prevalence Study *American Journal of Epidemiology* 1990; **131(1)**: 32–47.

134 • Wilson PW, Abbott RD, Castelli WP. High density lipoprotein cholesterol and mortality: the Framingham Heart Study *Arteriosclerosis* 1988; **8(6)**: 737–41.

135 • Abbott RD, Wilson PW, Kannel WB, *et al*. High density lipoprotein cholesterol, total cholesterol screening, and myocardial infarction: the Framingham Study *Arteriosclerosis* 1988; **8(3)**: 207–11.

136 • Assmann G, Schulte H, von Eckardstein A. Hypertriglyceridemia and elevated lipoprotein(a) are risk factors for major coronary events in middle-aged men *American Journal of Cardiology* 1996; **77(14)**: 1179–84.

137 • Criqui MH, Langer RD, Fronek A, *et al*. Mortality over a period of 10 years in patients with peripheral arterial disease *New England Journal of Medicine* 1992; **326(6)**: 381–6.

138 • Jeppesen J, Hein HO, Suadicani P, *et al*. Triglyceride concentration and ischemic heart disease: an eight-year follow-up in the Copenhagen Male Study *Circulation* 1998; **97(11)**: 1029–36.

139 • Assmann G, Schulte H, von EA, *et al*. High-density lipoprotein cholesterol as a predictor of coronary heart disease risk. The PROCAM experience and pathophysiological implications for reverse cholesterol transport *Atherosclerosis* 1996; **124(Suppl)**: S11–20.

140 • Cullen P. Evidence that triglycerides are an independent coronary heart disease risk factor *American Journal of Cardiology* 2000; **86(9)**: 943–9.

141 • Hokanson JE, Austin MA. Plasma triglyceride level is a risk factor for cardiovascular disease independent of high-density lipoprotein cholesterol level: a meta-analysis of population-based prospective studies *Journal of Cardiovascular Risk* 1996; **3(2)**: 213–19.

142 • Collins R, Armitage J, Parish S, *et al*. Effects of cholesterol-lowering with simvastatin on stroke and other major vascular events in 20536 people with cerebrovascular disease or other high-risk conditions *Lancet* 2004; **363(9411)**: 757–67.

143 • Amarenco P, Bogousslavsky J, Callahan A III, *et al*. High-dose atorvastatin after stroke or transient ischemic attack *New England Journal of Medicine* 2006; **355(6)**: 549–59.

144 • Baigent C, Keech A, Kearney PM, *et al*. Efficacy and safety of cholesterol-lowering treatment: prospective meta-analysis of data from 90,056 participants in 14 randomised trials of statins *Lancet* 2005; **366(9493)**: 1267–78.

145 • British National Formulary. Cardiovascular system>lipid-regulating drugs>statins *British National Formulary* 2010; **59**.

146 • International Diabetes Federation. *The Global Burden* Brussels: IDF, 2008, www.diabetesatlas.org/content/global-burden [accessed September 2010].

147 • Wild S, Roglic G, Green A, *et al*. Global prevalence of diabetes: estimates for the year 2000 and projections for 2030 *Diabetes Care* 2004; **27(5)**: 1047–53.

148 • Diabetes UK. www.diabetes.org.uk [accessed September 2010].

149 • Simmons D, Williams DR, Powell MJ. The Coventry Diabetes Study: prevalence of diabetes and impaired glucose tolerance in Europids and Asians *Quarterly Journal of Medicine* 1991; **81(296)**: 1021–30.

150 • Mather HM, Keen H. The Southall Diabetes Survey: prevalence of known diabetes in Asians and Europeans *British Medical Journal (Clinical Research Ed.)* 1985; **291(6502)**: 1081–4.

151 • Murray CJ, Lopez AD. Mortality by cause for eight regions of the world: Global Burden of Disease Study *Lancet* 1997; **349(9061)**: 1269–76.

152 • Thomas RJ, Palumbo PJ, Melton LJ III, *et al.* Trends in the mortality burden associated with diabetes mellitus: a population-based study in Rochester, Minn, 1970–1994 *Archives of Internal Medicine* 2003; **163(4)**: 445–51.

153 • Booth GL, Kapral MK, Fung K, *et al.* Recent trends in cardiovascular complications among men and women with and without diabetes *Diabetes Care* 2006; **29(1)**: 32–7.

154 • Gu K, Cowie CC, Harris MI. Mortality in adults with and without diabetes in a national cohort of the US population, 1971–1993 *Diabetes Care* 1998; **21(7)**: 1138–45.

155 • Haffner SM, Lehto S, Ronnemaa T, *et al.* Mortality from coronary heart disease in subjects with type 2 diabetes and in nondiabetic subjects with and without prior myocardial infarction *New England Journal of Medicine* 1998; **339(4)**: 229–34.

156 • Kannel WB, McGee DL. Diabetes and cardiovascular disease: the Framingham study *Journal of the American Medical Association* 1979; **241(19)**: 2035–8.

157 • Behar S, Boyko V, Reicher-Reiss H, *et al.* Ten-year survival after acute myocardial infarction: comparison of patients with and without diabetes. SPRINT Study Group. Secondary Prevention Reinfarction Israeli Nifedipine Trial *American Heart Journal* 1997; **133(3)**: 290–6.

158 • Mak KH, Moliterno DJ, Granger CB, *et al.* Influence of diabetes mellitus on clinical outcome in the thrombolytic era of acute myocardial infarction: GUSTO-I Investigators. Global Utilization of Streptokinase and Tissue Plasminogen Activator for Occluded Coronary Arteries *Journal of the American College of Cardiology* 1997; **30(1)**: 171–9.

159 • Evans JM, Wang J, Morris AD. Comparison of cardiovascular risk between patients with type 2 diabetes and those who had had a myocardial infarction: cross sectional and cohort studies *British Medical Journal* 2002; **324(7343)**: 939–42.

160 • Weng C, Coppini DV, Sonksen PH. Geographic and social factors are related to increased morbidity and mortality rates in diabetic patients *Diabetic Medicine* 2000; **17(8)**: 612–17.

161 • British Heart Foundation. *Coronary Heart Disease Statistics: 2008 edition* London: BHF, 2009, www.heartstats.org/publications.asp?id=7 [accessed September 2010].

162 • Gaede P, Lund-Andersen H, Parving HH, *et al.* Effect of a multifactorial intervention on mortality in type 2 diabetes *New England Journal of Medicine* 2008; **358(6)**: 580–91.

163 • Holman RR, Paul SK, Bethel MA, *et al.* 10-year follow-up of intensive glucose control in type 2 diabetes *New England Journal of Medicine* 2008; **359(15)**: 1577–89.

164 • Gerstein HC, Miller ME, Byington RP, *et al.* Action to Control Cardiovascular Risk in Diabetes Study Group (ACCORD): effects of intensive glucose lowering in type 2 diabetes *New England Journal of Medicine* 2008; **358(24)**: 2545–59.

165 • Patel A, MacMahon S, Chalmers J, *et al.* ADVANCE Collaborative Group: intensive blood glucose control and vascular outcomes in patients with type 2 diabetes *New England Journal of Medicine* 2008; **358(24)**: 2560–72.

166 • Duckworth W, Abraira C, Moritz T, *et al.* Glucose control and vascular complications in veterans with type 2 diabetes *New England Journal of Medicine* 2009; **360(2)**: 129–39.

167 • Skyler JS, Bergenstal R, Bonow RO, *et al.* Intensive glycemic control and the prevention of cardiovascular events: implications of the ACCORD, ADVANCE, and VA diabetes trials: a position statement of the American Diabetes Association and a scientific statement of the American College of Cardiology Foundation and the American Heart Association *Circulation* 2009; **119(2)**: 351–7.

168 • National Collaborating Centre for Chronic Conditions. *Type 2 Diabetes: national clinical guideline for management in primary and secondary care (update),* London: Royal College of Physicians, www.nice.org.uk/CG66 [accessed September 2010].

169 • Ogawa H, Nakayama M, Morimoto T, *et al.* Low-dose aspirin for primary prevention of atherosclerotic events in patients with type 2 diabetes: a randomized controlled trial *Journal of the American Medical Association* 2008; **300(18)**: 2134–41.

170 • Stevens RJ, Kothari V, Adler AI, *et al.* The UKPDS risk engine: a model for the risk of coronary heart disease in Type II diabetes (UKPDS 56) *Clinical Science* (London) 2001; **101(6)**: 671–9.

171 • Buse JB, Ginsberg HN, Bakris GL, *et al.* Primary prevention of cardiovascular diseases in people with diabetes mellitus: a scientific statement from the American Heart Association and the American Diabetes Association *Diabetes Care* 2007; **30(1)**: 162–72.

172 • British Cardiac Society, British Hypertension Society, Diabetes UK, Heart UK, Primary Care Cardiovascular Society, the Stroke Association. JBS 2: Joint British Societies' guidelines on prevention of cardiovascular disease in clinical practice *Heart* 2005; **91(Suppl 5)**: v1–52.

173 • Healthcare Commission. *Audit Commission Patient Survey Report* London: Healthcare Commission, 2004.

174 • Ipsos MORI. *Public Knowledge of Diabetes,* 2005, www.ipsos-mori.com/ researchpublications/researcharchive/poll.aspx?oItemId=442 [accessed September 2010].

175 • Millett C, Gray J, Saxena S, *et al.* Ethnic disparities in diabetes management and pay-for-performance in the UK: the Wandsworth Prospective Diabetes Study *PLoS Medicine* 2007; **4(6)**: e191.

176 • Khunti K, Gadsby R, Millett C, *et al.* Quality of diabetes care in the UK: comparison of published quality-of-care reports with results of the Quality and Outcomes Framework for Diabetes *Diabetic Medicine* 2007; **24(12)**: 1436–41.

177 • European Society of Cardiology. Guidelines on diabetes, prediabetes and cardiovascular disease *European Heart Journal* 2007; **28(1)**: 88–136.

178 • World Health Organization. *Definition and Diagnosis of Diabetes Mellitus and Intermediate Hyperglycaemia* Geneva: WHO, www.who.int/diabetes/publications/ Definition%20and%20diagnosis%20of%20diabetes_new.pdf [accessed September 2010].

179 • Gerstein HC, Santaguida P, Raina P, *et al.* Annual incidence and relative risk of diabetes in people with various categories of dysglycemia: a systematic overview and meta-analysis of prospective studies *Diabetes Research and Clinical Practice* 2007; **78(3)**: 305–12.

180 • Aroda VR, Ratner R. Approach to the patient with prediabetes *Journal of Clinical Endocrinology and Metabolism* 2008; **93(9)**: 3259–65.

181 • Wald NJ, Law MR. A strategy to reduce cardiovascular disease by more than 80% *British Medical Journal* 2003; **326(7404)**: 1419.

182 • Law MR, Morris JK, Wald NJ. Use of blood pressure lowering drugs in the prevention of cardiovascular disease: meta-analysis of 147 randomised trials in the context of expectations from prospective epidemiological studies *British Medical Journal* 2009; **338**: b1665.

183 • Yusuf S, Pais P, Afzal R, *et al.* Effects of a polypill (Polycap) on risk factors in middle-aged individuals without cardiovascular disease (TIPS): a phase II, double-blind, randomised trial *Lancet* 2009; **373(9672)**: 1341–51.

Coronary heart disease

3

Su May Liew and Carl Heneghan

Aims and key learning points

▶ To enable GPs to recognise and diagnose coronary heart disease (CHD) by means of utilising skills in history, physical examination and investigation.
▶ To prioritise treatment and administer timely management of urgent as well as non-urgent cases.
▶ To institute evidence-based management following the onset of angina/ acute coronary syndrome/myocardial infarction.
▶ To achieve these aims in a primary care setting and in line with primary care principles.

Epidemiology of coronary heart disease

Cardiovascular disease (CVD), which includes both stroke and CHD, continues to be the leading cause of mortality worldwide.[1] Due to increasing rates of diabetes and obesity in developing countries, the burden of disease in these regions will overtake those of developed nations over the next 25 years.[1–2]

More people die from CHD (12.2 per cent of all deaths) compared with cerebrovascular conditions (9.7 per cent of all deaths), although the latter are responsible for greater subsequent disability. CHD is the top reason for premature death (age <75 years) in the UK, causing 1 in 5 premature deaths in men and 1 in 10 in women.[3]

Table 3.1 on p. 80 lists potentially modifiable risk factors for CVD.[4] Non-modifiable risk factors include age, sex and family history. There are also other risk factors for which the evidence is less strong, such as triglycerides, lipoprotein(a), homocysteine, etc. It is important to recognise that the relative impact of risk factors differs for different conditions. For example, cholesterol levels incur greater risk in CHD relative to that for stroke and congestive heart failure.[5] These factors are discussed in more detail in Chapter 2.

Table 3.1 ○ *Established cardiovascular risk factors*

Risk factor	Relative risk
Hypertension	2–3
Cholesterol	1.01 for each 1% increase in total or low-density lipoprotein (LDL) cholesterol or 1% reduction in high-density lipoprotein (HDL) cholesterol
Smoking	1.4 (men) to 2.2 (women)
Diabetes mellitus	2.2 (men) to 3.7 (women)
Obesity	1.2 (men over 50) to 2.1 (women under 50)
Sedentary lifestyle	2.4 (men)
Left ventricular hypertrophy (LVH) on electrocardiogram (ECG)	2.0 (women) to 2.7 (men)
LVH with strain on ECG	2.5 (women) to 5.8 (men)

Source: modified from Padwal R, Straus SE, McAlister FA. Evidence based management of hypertension. Cardiovascular risk factors and their effects on the decision to treat hypertension.[4]

Spectrum of coronary heart disease

CHD can be considered as a spectrum of disorders (see Figure 3.1).

Figure 3.1 ○ *CHD disorders*

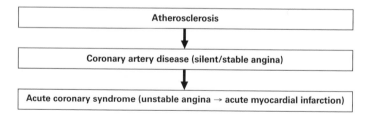

Atherosclerosis of the coronary arteries is a gradual process that builds up over years, as discussed in Chapter 1. There are no symptoms until the narrowing of the arteries results in relative ischaemia during exertion, where the myocardium requires increased blood flow. This causes ischaemic pain and presents as *angina pectoris*, which is now more commonly referred to as stable angina. In the worst-case scenario, rupture of the atherosclerotic plaque causes a clot to form. This prevents blood flow to the cardiac muscles resulting in *acute myocardial infarction* (AMI). An unstable clot may occur at times, creating interrupted blood flow even at rest.[6] This is known as *unstable angina*. The term *acute coronary syndrome* is used for the acute presentation of CHD. This encompasses unstable angina, non-ST-segment elevation myocardial infarction (NSTEMI) and ST-segment elevation myocardial infarction (STEMI).

Angina

Chest pain or *angina pectoris* is the characteristic presentation of CHD, yet only half of the patients that present to hospital with an AMI have preceding angina.[7] Angina is the second most frequently seen complaint in the emergency department.[8] In primary care, chest pain as the presenting complaint is less common but still represents a significant clinical burden with a reported range of frequency from 0.7 to 7 per cent.[9] Despite men having higher rates of myocardial infarction, there is a slightly higher prevalence of angina pectoris in women, with a sex ratio of 1.2. The reason for this is unknown. This finding was consistent despite differences in sex ratio for mortality due to myocardial infarction between populations, so is not purely a consequence of more females surviving cardiovascular events.[10]

Symptoms

The most important step in the evaluation of a patient with chest pain is history taking.[11] A careful history allows the determination of important red flags such as the association of pain with exertion, a significant family history of premature CVD and the presence of important risk factors. Red flags that necessitate urgent referral are listed in Box 3.1.

Box 3.1 ○ *Red flags for chest pain requiring urgent referral*

▶ Chest pain at rest:
- lasting for more than 15–20 minutes
- unresponsive to glyceryl trinitrate.

▶ Recent-onset crescendo angina symptoms.

▶ Associated autonomic symptoms (sweating, vomiting, nausea).

Source: Epstein O, Perkin GD, Cookson J, *et al. Clinical Examination.*[12]

The typical presentation of angina pectoris is a gripping, deep substernal chest pain radiating to the left arm and is associated with sweating and breathlessness.[7] Pain is triggered by increases in cardiac output such as that caused by exertion. It is not related to arm movement. The pain classically reduces within 15 minutes and with rest or use of nitrates.[7,11]

Angina may also present atypically. The pain may radiate upwards and extend towards the jaw. In people with diabetes there may be no pain at all, with sweating or breathlessness the only symptoms. Patients experiencing angina may mistake it for other less serious conditions such as gastrointestinal reflux or musculoskeletal pain. Therefore, the evaluation of chest pain should be treated with caution in patients with high cardiovascular risk, and even atypical presentations such as chest wall tenderness should be evaluated carefully.

Table 3.2 ○ *Clinical classification of chest pain*

Typical angina	1 Substernal chest discomfort with a characteristic quality and duration 2 Provoked by exertion or emotional stress 3 Relieved by rest or nitroglycerin
Atypical angina	Meets two of the typical anginal characteristics
Non-cardiac chest pain	Meets one or none of the typical anginal characteristics

Source: Diamond GA, Staniloff HM, Forrester JS, *et al*. Computer-assisted diagnosis in the noninvasive evaluation of patients with suspected coronary disease.[13]

Signs

Signs are usually absent in patients presenting with angina.[7] There may be tachycardia and increased respiratory rate. There is usually diaphoresis. Doctors should take note that these signs occur during the time when the patient is experiencing angina, which has normally settled by the time the patient is seen in clinic. Examination is therefore largely undertaken to evaluate risk factors such as hypertension, the presence of non-coronary atherosclerosis, e.g. carotid or abdominal bruits, xanthelasma for hypercholesterolaemia, and associated conditions such as valvular heart disease.

Investigations

Doctors frequently feel anxious when patients present with chest pain. There is a tendency to over-investigate because of the fear of missing a serious diagnosis.[14,15] A study involving primary care physicians [16] showed that a multifaceted strategy, which included educational efforts such as improved doctor–patient communication and skills in evidence-based medicine, as well as institutional efforts such as feedback on the use of tests, was effective in decreasing the number of inappropriate tests ordered.

Investigations specific to the determination as to whether or not the chest pain is due to coronary artery disease are as follows:

Table 3.3 ○ *Sensitivity and specificity of diagnostic tests for stable angina*

Investigation	Sensitivity % (mean)	Specificity % (mean)	*LR+	*LR−
ECG stress testing	23–100 (68)	17–100 (77)	3.0	0.4
Exercise testing with echocardiogram	80–85	84–86	5.5	0.2
Exercise myocardial perfusion	85–90	70–75	3.2	0.2
Dobutamine stress echocardiogram	40–100	62–100	3.7	0.4
Vasodilator stress echocardiogram	56–92	87–100	11.4	0.3
Vasodilator stress myocardial perfusion	83–94	64–90	3.8	0.1
Computerised tomography (CT) angiography (with 16-slice CT scanners)	95	98	47.5	0.1
64 detector scanners	90–94	95–97	23	0.1
Electron beam computerised tomography (EBCT) detection of calcium	85–100	41–76	2.2	0.1

Source: modified from Fox K, Garcia MA, Ardissino D, *et al*. Guidelines on the management of stable angina pectoris: executive summary.[11]

* LR = likelihood ratio. This is a measure of how many times more (or less) likely patients with the disease are to have an abnormal test result than patients without the disease.

Investigations in primary care

Resting 12-lead ECG

This is of limited use as the resting ECG is normal in more than 50 per cent of patients with stable angina.[7] ST-segment depression is the characteristic ECG abnormality indicating ischaemia. A resting ECG may be useful in detecting previous cardiovascular events such as a myocardial infarction, as indicated by a Q-wave, or assisting in diagnosing differential diagnoses such as pericarditis.[11]

Stress ECG or exercise tolerance test (ETT)

Exercise can be used to stress the myocardium in order to detect changes in the electrocardiogram. Because the effectiveness of an exercise test at detecting CHD differs with the likelihood that an individual has CHD on the basis of his or her history, it is helpful to think of the pre-test probability when interpreting the results of the stress test to generate the post-test probability for a given patient (Table 3.4).

Table 3.4 ○ *Determining post-test probability for stress ECG*

	Likelihood ratio for a positive result (LR+) = 3	Likelihood ratio for a negative result (LR–) = 0.4
Low probability In a patient with a 5% chance of CHD	Pre-test odds = 5/95 = 0.05 Post-test odds = 0.05 × 3 = 0.15 Post-test probability of having CHD with a positive result = 0.13 or 13%	Pre-test odds = 5/95 = 0.05 Post-test odds = 0.05 × 0.4 = 0.02 Post-test probability of having CHD with a negative result = 0.02 or 2%
Moderate probability In a patient with a 50% chance of CHD	Pre-test odds = 50/50 = 1 Post-test odds = 1 × LR = 1 × 3 = 3 Post-test probability of having CHD with a positive result = 3/(3 + 1) = 0.75 or 75%	Pre-test odds = 50/50 = 1 Post-test odds = 1 × 0.4 = 0.4 Post-test probability of having CHD with a negative result = 0.29 = 29%
High probability In a patient with a 90% chance of CHD	Pre-test odds = 90/10 = 9 Post-test odds = 9 × LR = 9 × 3 = 27 Post-test probability of having CHD with a positive result = 27/(27 + 1) = 0.96 or 96%	Pre-test odds = 90/10 = 9 Post-test odds = 9 × 0.4 = 3.6 Post-test probability of having CHD with a negative result = 0.78 or 78%

As can be seen from Table 3.4, the value of both a positive and negative stress ECG result differs according to the pre-test probability. If the pre-test probability is 5 per cent, then a positive stress test only increases the likelihood of the patient having CHD to 13 per cent. Therefore, even if the patient has a positive stress test, the patient is still more likely not to have CHD. When the probability is very high, as in the patient with a 90 per cent chance of CHD, a negative test will only lower the probability of having CHD from 90 per cent to 78 per cent and so is not able to rule out the disease. It is in patients with moderate probability that the stress ECG has the most value as it allows patients to be differentiated into two distinct groups, where one of the subgroups has a high probability and the other has a low probability of CHD. In the patient with a 50 per cent probability of having CHD, a positive stress test increases the likelihood of the patient having CHD to 75 per cent and a negative stress test decreases the likelihood of the patient having CHD to 29 per cent.

Investigation of risk factors

Once CHD has been diagnosed, investigation for cardiovascular risk factors such as lipid levels and diabetes should be undertaken as soon as possible, and treatment commenced if risk factors are present (see Table 3.5).[11] The use of novel biomarkers for risk stratification has been a subject of interest in the current medical literature. C-reactive protein and apolipoproteins B100 and A-1 as well as lipoprotein(a) have been incorporated into 10-year risk calculators for CVD in men [17] and women.[18]

Table 3.5 ○ *Investigation of other risk factors*

Risk factor	Diagnosis	Target of treatment
Diabetes mellitus [19,20]	Fasting plasma glucose ≥7.0 mmol/L or 2 hour plasma glucose ≥11.1 mmol/L	HbA1c <7.0%
Dyslipidaemia [21]	LDL ≥2.6 mmol/L HDL <1.04 mmol/L TG ≥1.7 mmol/L	LDL cholesterol reduction of 30% to 40%. Once this goal is achieved, HDL and TG levels should be targeted

Investigations in secondary care

Stress imaging studies: echocardiographic and nuclear

Exercise or pharmacological agents may also be used to stress the myocardium in combination with imaging techniques such as echocardiogram and nuclear imaging. Pharmacological stress testing with the use of drugs such as dobutamine is useful in patients with mobility difficulties. Stress imaging should not be used in patients with low or high pre-test probability of coronary artery disease for reasons similar to that for stress ECG.[7] The costs and availability of stress imaging studies limit its use as a first-line investigation.[11]

Coronary calcium scans

Coronary calcium scores can be measured by EBCT or multi-detector slice computerised tomography. Patients with increased coronary calcium scores are at higher risk of coronary artery disease. A systematic review found that calcium scores correlated with risk of coronary artery disease, but the authors could not recommend the routine use of EBCT due to the non-uniformity of studies and lack of individual-level data.[22] There is also significant radiation exposure associated with CT scanning.

Computerised tomography and MRI angiography

Improvements in imaging technology now allow the non-invasive visualisation of the coronary arteries via CT and MRI angiography. However, data are still required with regards to the clinical utility and cost-effectiveness of these investigations in the assessment of patients with suspected coronary artery disease.[23]

Angiography

This is considered the gold standard. The procedure can be immediately followed with a therapeutic intervention such as angioplasty. However, it is the most invasive of all the investigations and is not without risk: the composite rate of death, MI or stroke as a complication of the procedure is 0.1–0.2 per cent.[11]

Differential diagnosis

In the assessment of the patient with angina, other causes of chest pain should be considered. These include costochondritis, panic attack, pulmonary embolism, aortic dissection, reflux, pericarditis and pneumothorax. In a study of 399 episodes of chest pain presenting in primary care,[24] musculoskeletal chest pain was the cause in 20 per cent of all diagnoses, reflux oesophagitis in 13 per cent, costochondritis in 13 per cent, stable angina in 10 per cent and unstable angina or myocardial infarction in 2 per cent. A detailed history, physical examination and selected investigations would differentiate the cause of the presenting symptom.

Management

Medical treatment of CHD has two main objectives,[25] namely secondary prevention of further CVD or death and the reduction of symptoms, principally chest pain. Treatments for the prevention of major coronary events, i.e. myocardial infarction and death, include:

▷ antiplatelet agents – aspirin with clopidogrel. Clopidogrel is used if aspirin is absolutely contraindicated or following STEMI or stenting
▷ beta-blockers
▷ cholesterol-lowering therapy
▷ ACE inhibitor (or angiotensin II receptor blockers if intolerant to ACE inhibitor).

Treatment of other cardiovascular risk factors should be initiated in order to halt or delay progression of atherosclerosis and reduce the risk of major CHD events, as shown on Table 3.6 (see p. 88). Hyperlipidaemia, hypertension and diabetes all require optimal control. Weight reduction and cessation of smoking also should be instituted. This is discussed further in Chapter 2.

Reduction of symptoms of angina

▷ Use sublingual nitroglycerin or nitroglycerin spray for the immediate relief of angina. The tablets (0.3–0.6 mg) or spray (0.4 mg nitroglycerin per puff) can be used every 5 minutes, and up to a maximum of three tablets or puffs may be required for the relief of angina. Spray is more practical as it has a longer shelf life. If pain persists after this or if it recurs after a short interval, the patient should go to the nearest emergency facility as this may indicate an acute coronary event.[26]

Table 3.6 ○ *Risk factors and relative risk reduction in major CHD events*

Risk factor and goal	Recommended agent(s)	Change in risk factor	Relative risk reduction
LDL cholesterol <2.6 mmol/L	High-dose statin and diet	≥ ↓50%	48%
BP <140/90 (130/80 in diabetes)	Diuretic Beta-blocker ACE inhibitor	Systolic ↓20 mmHg or diastolic ↓10 mmHg	46–49%
Platelet function	Aspirin 75–81 mg/day		42%
Beta-blocker post-myocardial infarction	Non-cardioselective; no sympathomimetic activity		23% CHD death
ACE inhibitor post-MI			20%
Sudden death post-MI	Omega-3 fish oil 1000 mg/day		30% CHD death
Cardiac rehabilitation	Individual prescription	↑ Moderate aerobic physical activity	26% CHD death
Diet	Mediterranean	↑ Fruits, vegetables, legumes, nuts, whole grains, fish, monounsaturated oils	52–72% 33% CHD deaths

Source: Robinson JG, Maheshwari N. A 'poly-portfolio' for secondary prevention: a strategy to reduce subsequent events by up to 97% over five years.[27]

Copyright Elsevier. Used with permission.

▷ Add a beta-blocker unless there are contraindications such as asthma or bradycardia.
▷ Use long-acting calcium antagonist or long-acting nitrates when the use of beta-blockers is clearly contraindicated.
▷ Use long-acting calcium antagonist or long-acting nitrates in combination with beta-blockers when beta-blockers alone are unsuccessful [*note*: verapamil should not be co-prescribed with beta-blockers].

Referral

The need for angiography and revascularisation should be evaluated in all patients. Evidence suggests invasive treatment offers symptomatic relief but does not appear to decrease the risk of myocardial infarction.[28] The decision to refer should be undertaken with the patient's views and concerns in mind, and the patient should be aware of the possible consequences. Discussion with a cardiologist may be helpful to guide the subsequent treatment, especially in cases where the diagnosis is unclear.

Box 3.2 ○ **Indications for referral**

▶ When diagnosis is uncertain or new-onset angina.

▶ Evidence of continuing extensive ischaemia (e.g. a strongly positive exercise test).

▶ Angina that is increasing in frequency or severity.

▶ Angina that persists despite optimal medical therapy and lifestyle advice.

Source: Department of Health. *National Service Framework for Coronary Heart Disease.*[29]

Acute coronary syndrome

Definition

Acute coronary syndrome (ACS) encompasses unstable angina, NSTEMI and STEMI. Previously, angina was classified as stable and unstable, whereas myocardial infarction was classified as Q-wave and non-Q-wave infarction. With the development of newer and more sensitive diagnostic tests, it has become increasingly difficult to differentiate between NSTEMI and unstable angina. The differentiation depends on whether the ischaemia was severe enough to cause release of detectable quantities of biomarkers of myocardial necrosis.[30]

Figure 3.2 ○ **Defining acute coronary syndrome**

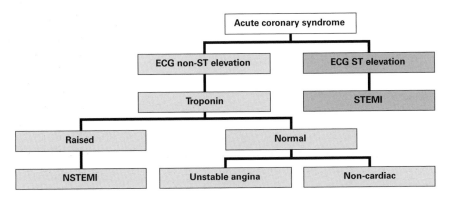

Unstable angina and NSTEMI

Longitudinal studies indicate that prognosis for the two conditions is different, with NSTEMI being more similar to STEMI.[31,32] The European Society of Cardiology (ESC) and the American College of Cardiology (ACC) changed the classification of acute coronary syndrome in 2002.[33–35] Table 3.7 shows the difference in the new definition from the previous World Health Organization (WHO) definition.[36,37]

Table 3.7 ○ *Definition of myocardial infarction*

WHO	ESC and ACC
Two of three:	Acute/recent myocardial infarction
■ clinical history	Biomarker of necrosis and one of:
■ typical ECG changes	■ ischaemic symptoms
■ raised cardiac enzymes	■ new Q-waves
	■ ischaemic ECG changes
	■ coronary intervention
	Established myocardial infarction
	■ new Q-waves or two of four of above

Symptoms

Box 3.3 ○ *The presentation of acute coronary syndrome*

▶ Prolonged (>20 min) angina pain at rest.
▶ New-onset severe angina.
▶ Recent change of previously stable angina (accelerated angina).
▶ Post-myocardial infarction angina.

The typical presentation of ACS is chest pain occurring at rest. Note though that chest pain may be absent. A study considering 20,881 patients with ACS found that 1763 (9 per cent) presented without chest pain. Of these, 49 per

90

cent had dyspnoea, 26 per cent had diaphoresis, 24 per cent had nausea or vomiting and 19 per cent had syncope/presyncope (total exceeds 100 per cent as there were patients with more than one dominant symptom). Moreover, the diagnosis can be missed as nearly a quarter of these patients were not initially recognised as having ACS. The morbidity and mortality in patients without chest pain were significantly higher than that of patients with typical symptoms.[38]

Investigations

Unlike chronic stable angina, the resting ECG is of key importance. In NSTEMI, ECG changes include ST depression, T-wave inversion and other non-specific changes. However, 1–6 per cent of patients with a normal ECG still have NSTEMI. Serial ECG increases diagnostic sensitivity for ACS (sensitivity 34.2 per cent; specificity 99.4 per cent; (LR+):57; (LR–):0.66).[39]

GP management

Urgent assessment

The main role of the GP is to recognise the condition and initiate urgent management and referral. Early and rapid transfer to secondary care is advisable, as opposed to waiting for the results of investigations.[40]

The steps are summarised briefly below and elaborated on further in the management of STEMI:

▷ stabilisation with oxygen and monitoring of vital signs
▷ analgesia (preferably intravenous (IV) opiates)
▷ aspirin 300 mg stat
▷ urgent referral with ambulance transfer.

Rehabilitation

After discharge, management should consist of:[41]

▷ use of medication, including aspirin, clopidogrel (for 12 months post-event), beta-blockers, ACE inhibitors and statins
▷ treatment of behavioural risk factors such as therapeutic lifestyle changes including smoking cessation and exercise.

Adherence

Poor adherence to treatment for secondary prevention may be due to both patient and physician factors.[42]

PHYSICIAN NON-ADHERENCE

In the REACH registry,[43] only 79 per cent of patients at high risk of an atherothrombotic event were given antiplatelets therapy. Physician adherence to antiplatelets prescribing was best in the group of patients with coronary artery disease (86 per cent) and worst in the group with ≥ 3 risk factors (54 per cent).

PATIENT NON-ADHERENCE

In the PREMIER study,[44] more than 1 in 5 patients discontinued use of aspirin, beta-blockers or statins, and 1 in 8 discontinued use of all three medications 1 month after an AMI. Treatment discontinuation was associated with higher mortality (hazards ratio 3.81; 95% CI, 1.88–7.72). On discharge, the GP should ensure that the patient understands the reasons for continuing medication and how adherence affects outcomes.

ST-segment elevation myocardial infarction

Symptoms

The symptoms of STEMI are more severe, are not relieved by rest and last longer, typically presenting with central crushing chest pain. Atypical presentations include epigastric pain, which can go unrecognised and lead to fatal outcomes. Myocardial infarctions can also be silent and only recognised from the characteristic Q-waves on routine ECGs, or after complications such as heart failure arise. In the National Registry of Myocardial Infarction, in the US, 33 per cent of patients with confirmed myocardial infarction were found to have presented without chest pain.[45] Other symptoms such as diaphoresis, nausea, vomiting, weakness and syncope may be present.[46]

92

Table 3.8 ○ *Clinical features increasing the probability of STEMI in patients presenting with acute chest pain*

Clinical feature	LR+ (95% CI)
Chest pain radiation	
■ both arms with pain	9.7 (4.6–20)
■ left arm pain	2.2 (1.6–3.1)
■ right shoulder pain	2.9 (1.4–6.0)
Third heart sound on auscultation	3.2 (1.6–6.5)
Hypotension (systolic blood pressure ≤80 mmHg)	3.1 (1.8–5.2)
Pulmonary crackles on auscultation	2.1 (1.4–3.1)
Diaphoresis	2.0 (1.9–2.2)
Nausea or vomiting	1.9 (1.7–2.3)
History of myocardial infarction	1.5–3.0*

Source: Simel DL, Rennie D, Keitz SA (eds). *The Rational Clinical Examination: evidence-based clinical diagnosis* New York: McGraw-Hill, 2009[46] Reproduced with permission of The McGraw-Hill Companies.

* Heterogeneous studies so LR is reported as a range.

Features such as pleuritic chest pain, sharp or stabbing chest pain, positional chest pain and chest pain reported by palpation decrease the probability of a myocardial infarction but do not exclude it.

Early recognition is vital for acute management as, during this time, serious complications such as arrhythmias may occur and thrombolytic therapy should not be delayed from the initial 'window' period. Thrombolytic therapy initiated within 70 minutes of symptom onset was associated with a mortality of 1.2 per cent compared with treatment initiated between 70–180 minutes, which had a mortality of 8.7 per cent.[47]

What can a GP do?

As with ACS, the role of the primary care physician in the acute management of a STEMI is primarily in the recognition and stabilisation of the patient. Investigations are of secondary concern.

There is good evidence that the following interventions can influence outcome.

Ambulance

Every hour delay decreases the benefits of fibrinolytic therapy by 2 lives/1000 infarcts ('minutes mean muscle').[48–49] Early ambulance transfer is therefore essential. Pre-hospital thrombolysis is also an option, particularly in rural settings. In a meta-analysis of pre-hospital thrombolysis versus in-hospital thrombolysis, the time difference to thrombolysis was approximately 60 minutes.[50] This study showed that pre-hospital thrombolysis for AMI significantly decreased all-cause hospital mortality.

Aspirin

Aspirin that is started immediately and continued for 1 month reduces vascular events by 29 per cent (95% CI, 65–77).[51] The evidence is substantial, with 135,000 randomised patients from 287 analysed studies.

Analgesia

The use of IV opiates reduces pain, anxiety and helps treat acute left ventricular failure.[52]

Over and above these interventions, stabilisation of the patient's condition is imperative. Oxygen should be delivered to reduce cardiac ischaemia. Monitoring of blood pressure, pulse rate, oxygen saturation and continuous ECG is initiated and subsequently maintained. IV access should be established as soon as possible to allow immediate delivery of drugs.

Shock and arrhythmias are typical complications of an AMI and should be treated accordingly. GPs should ensure that they are up-to-date with resuscitative measures and check that they are competent with the use of resuscitative equipment and that the equipment is checked regularly. Basic cardiopulmonary resuscitation is discussed further in Chapter 11.

Suffering an AMI is a very stressful situation during which the patient and family members often feel overwhelmed. The GP should explain to them what is causing the pain, how this can best be dealt with and what will happen next.

Hospital management

It is helpful for the GP to be aware of the hospital management of STEMI if only to be able to communicate to the patient and the family of the continuum of care.

Fibrinolytic therapy

Fibrinolysis given to patients with STEMI or bundle branch block saves 38 lives per 1000 patients treated and the mortality benefits are sustained at 10 years.[48,53]

Clopidogrel

Clopidogrel in addition to aspirin was associated with an additional 20 per cent relative reduction in the composite of cardiovascular death, non-fatal myocardial infarction or stroke at 1 year.[54] The COMMIT trial,[55] which included 45,852 patients with suspected AMI, showed that allocation to clopidogrel in addition to aspirin for 4 weeks produced a 9 per cent reduction in death, reinfarction or stroke. This corresponded to nine fewer events per 1000 patients treated for about 2 weeks.

Angiography and percutaneous coronary intervention

In patients with STEMI, it is the availability of interventional cardiology facilities that determines the care pathway.[56] For facilities that can offer percutaneous coronary intervention (PCI), the literature suggests that this approach is superior to pharmacological reperfusion. However, if the expected door-to-balloon time exceeds the door-to-needle time by more than 60 minutes, fibrinolytic treatment should be considered. Once thrombolysis has commenced then any subsequent PCI may be delayed so careful local protocols for both are vital.

IV beta-blockade

Early IV beta-blockers reduce the size of the infarct and the combined end-point of reinfarction, cardiac arrest and mortality by approximately 16 per cent (95% CI, 9–23).[57–59]

ACE inhibitors and angiotensin II receptor blockers

ACE inhibitors[60] given within 36 hours of onset of symptoms reduce the 30 days' mortality by 7 per cent (95% CI, 2–11).

Statin therapy

Patients should be treated with a statin following a myocardial infarction. The lipid targets set by NICE are lower for patients with a history of ischaemic heart disease with a target cholesterol level of less than 4 mmol/L and LDL less than 2.0 mmol/L, or a 25 per cent reduction in total cholesterol and 30 per cent reduction in LDL, whichever achieves the lowest figure.[61]

Investigations

Investigations are secondary to the patient's stabilisation and management. ECGs should be done and repeated serially. Ischaemic changes include ST elevation, T-wave inversion and, later, the appearance of Q-waves. Table 3.9[46] indicates ECG features that increase the probability of a myocardial infarction in a patient with chest pain. ST segment depression and new T-wave peaking or inversions were three times as likely to occur in patients with AMI.

Table 3.9 ○ **ECG features that increase the probability of a myocardial infarction in a patient with chest pain**

ECG feature	LR+ (95% CI)
Any ST segment elevation	11 (7.1–18)
New ST segment elevation ≥1 mm	5.7–54[a]
New conduction defect	6.3 (2.5–16)
New Q-wave	5.3–25[a]
Any Q-wave	3.9 (2.7–5.7)
Any ST segment depression	3.2 (2.5–4.1)
T-wave peaking or inversion ≥1 mm	3.1[b]
New ST segment depression	3.0–5.2[a]
Any conduction defect	2.7 (1.4–5.4)
New T-wave inversion	2.4–2.8[a]

Notes: **a** Heterogeneous studies so LR is reported as a range; **b** Data not available for calculation of CI.

Source: Simel DL, Rennie D, Keitz SA (eds). *The Rational Clinical Examination: evidence-based clinical diagnosis* New York: McGraw-Hill, 2009[46] Reproduced with permission of The McGraw-Hill Companies.

Management post-discharge

Management is similar to that of NSTEMI and the GP plays a central role to ensure evidence-based therapies for patients discharged from hospital have been initiated and, if not, to initiate the treatment and ensure maintenance for the appropriate duration.

Summary of management of AMI (NSTEMI and STEMI)

Smoking cessation

At 9 years of smoking cessation, the cardiovascular risk of ex-smokers is equal to that of lifelong non-smokers.[62]

Aspirin and clopidogrel

After an AMI, aspirin prevents approximately 40 vascular events, i.e. death, myocardial infarction and stroke per 100 patients treated.[51] Adding clopidogrel for the first 4 weeks gives an additional 9 per cent reduction in death, reinfarction and stroke.[55]

Beta-blocker

Long-term beta-blockade after an AMI reduces all-cause mortality by 23 per cent (95% CI, 15–30).[57–59]

ACE inhibitor

In patients with heart failure, long-term ACE inhibition reduces mortality by 23 per cent (95% CI, 12–33).[63,64] In patients with normal left ventricular function, ACE inhibition reduces the composite of cardiovascular death, stroke, or myocardial infarction by 22 per cent (95% CI, 14–30).

Cholesterol-lowering therapy

Statin therapy reduces the 5-year incidence of major coronary events, coronary revascularisation and stroke by about one-fifth per mmol/L reduction in LDL cholesterol.[65]

Exercise

Randomised clinical trials of cardiac rehabilitation following myocardial infarction have shown a relative risk reduction for cardiovascular death of 21 per cent (95% CI, 6–34) in the rehabilitation group compared with the control group. However, there was no significant difference for non-fatal recurrent myocardial infarction.[66]

Case-based discussion

Box 3.4 ○ *Case scenario 1*

Mrs Brown is a 49-year-old Caucasian woman who is registered with your practice. She presents to the clinic complaining of shortness of breath and palpitations while making her breakfast this morning. On looking at her records, you note that there is a 3-year history of hypertension and diabetes for which she is receiving medication. Mrs Brown used to be a heavy smoker but stopped 15 years ago. There is a family history of diabetes and myocardial infarction (mother at age 65). She lives alone.

On examination, she appears to be sweating profusely. Her blood pressure is 140/90 mmHg and her pulse rate is 90 b.p.m. regular.

1 ▶ What is the likely diagnosis?

2 ▶ How will you proceed?

This patient has diabetes and risk factors for ischaemic heart disease, so hypoglycaemia secondary to diabetic medication or a myocardial infarction are both likely diagnoses. Diabetic patients may not experience chest pain during a myocardial infarction. The patient is likely to feel very frightened by these distressing symptoms. The doctor should acknowledge this and explore what the patient may feel is happening and what she is worried about. An appropriate explanation of further action is required, which might include checking her blood sugar. If it is low, the GP should correct the hypoglycaemia, start oxygen if available, monitor vitals signs, initiate an ECG, consider aspirin if there is no contraindication and arrange urgent transfer to nearest emergency unit via ambulance as appropriate. It would be helpful to ask if the patient has anyone she would like the practice team to contact, to make them aware she is being transferred to hospital.

Box 3.5 ○ *Case scenario 2*

Mr White is a 55-year-old man who presents to your clinic with a history of central chest pain radiating to the left arm. This occurs on exertion and is relieved by rest. It started about 1 year ago and has not got any worse.

He has no history of hypertension, diabetes or hyperlipidaemia that you are aware of, but he rarely visits the practice. He does not smoke. There is no family history of ischaemic heart disease but his mother was hypertensive from the age of 60.

On examination, he is comfortable. His blood pressure is 140/90 with a pulse rate of 85 b.p.m. regular. His BMI is 32 kg/m².

1 ▶ **What is the likely diagnosis?**

2 ▶ **What investigations would you perform?**

3 ▶ **Would a stress ECG be helpful?**

4 ▶ **What else would you discuss with the patient in this consultation?**

From this history this patient is likely to have stable angina. Although he has no known modifiable cardiovascular risk factors, he is a 55-year-old male and his cardiovascular risk has not been formally assessed. This is not uncommon. Vascular health checks are important to identify patients with hypertension, diabetes or hyperlipidaemia, or who are overweight, or smokers who may be at risk of ischaemic heart disease. This allows risk factor modification prior to development of symptomatic disease.

It would be helpful to explore the patient's ideas about what he feels may be causing his symptoms. Patients are becoming increasingly aware of the symptoms of heart disease and the patient may suspect a diagnosis of angina. The complaint of chest pain also needs to be considered within the psychosocial context, so it would be important to find out the patient's occupation and home situation. The doctor should give a careful explanation of what angina is and what appropriate next steps are needed. It would also be important to explore lifestyle factors such as diet and exercise, which may influence cardiovascular risk. Investigations should include fasting lipid profile and glucose.

This patient should be referred for further investigation. A positive stress ECG would be helpful as his pre-test probability is likely to be high with a typical history of stable angina in a 55-year-old male. Depending on the results of the exercise test, further investigation such as an angiogram may be appropriate, and it may be helpful to discuss this possibility with the patient depending on how much detail he wishes to have at this stage. It may be helpful to start aspirin and glyceryl trinitrate (GTN) spray as needed, pending further investigations. It would also be important to ensure the patient has a clear understanding of what to do should the symptoms get worse or persist at rest. The GP should emphasise the need to call an ambulance rather than using other medical services if pain is severe or not relieved by GTN, to ensure timely intervention as required.

Summary

CHD is a leading cause of death in the UK. Modifiable risk factors include smoking, diabetes, hypertension and hyperlipidaemia. Characteristic clinical features include crushing central chest pain, although atypical presentations are not uncommon. The role of the GP is to address risk factors in those at risk of CHD, identify those with probable CHD and arrange timely referral. GPs should also follow up patients after coronary events to ensure appropriate evidence-based treatment is optimised.

100

References

1 • World Health Organization. *The Global Burden of Disease: 2004 update* Geneva: WHO, 2008.

2 • Stuckler D. Population causes and consequences of leading chronic diseases: a comparative analysis of prevailing explanations *Milbank Quarterly* 2008; **86(2)**: 273.

3 • Allender S, Peto V, Scarborough P, *et al. Coronary Heart Disease Statistics* London: British Heart Foundation, 2008.

4 • Padwal R, Straus SE, McAlister FA. Evidence based management of hypertension. Cardiovascular risk factors and their effects on the decision to treat hypertension: evidence based review *British Medical Journal* 2001; **322(7292)**: 977–80.

5 • D'Agostino RB Snr, Vasan RS, Pencina MJ, *et al.* General cardiovascular risk profile for use in primary care: the Framingham Heart Study *Circulation* 2008; **117(6)**: 743–53.

6 • Fuster V, Lewis A. Conner Memorial Lecture. Mechanisms leading to myocardial infarction: insights from studies of vascular biology *Circulation* 1994; **90(4)**: 2126–46.

7 • Gibbons RJ, Abrams J, Chatterjee K, *et al. ACC/AHA 2002 Guideline Update for the Management of Patients with Chronic Stable Angina: a report of the American College of Cardiology/ American Heart Association Task Force on Practice Guidelines (Committee to Update the 1999 Guidelines for the Management of Patients with Chronic Stable Angina)*, 2002, www.americanheart.org/downloadable/heart/1044991838085StableAnginaNewFigs.pdf [accessed September 2010].

8 • Nawar EW, Niska RW, Xu J. National Hospital Ambulatory Medical Care Survey: 2005 emergency department summary *Advance Data* 2007; **386**: 1–32.

9 • Nilsson S, Scheike M, Engblom D, *et al.* Chest pain and ischaemic heart disease in primary care *British Journal of General Practice* 2003; **53(490)**: 378–82.

10 • Hemingway H, Langenberg C, Damant J, *et al.* Prevalence of angina in women versus men: a systematic review and meta-analysis of international variations across 31 countries *Circulation* 2008; **117(12)**: 1526–36.

11 • Fox K, Garcia MA, Ardissino D, *et al.*; Task Force on the Management of Stable Angina Pectoris of the European Society of Cardiology; ESC Committee for Practice Guidelines (CPG). Guidelines on the management of stable angina pectoris: executive summary: the Task Force on the Management of Stable Angina Pectoris of the European Society of Cardiology *European Heart Journal* 2006; **27(11)**: 1341–81.

12 • Epstein O, Perkin GD, Cookson J, *et al. Clinical Examination* (fourth edn) Oxford: Mosby Elsevier, 2008.

13 • Diamond GA, Staniloff HM, Forrester JS, *et al.* Computer-assisted diagnosis in the noninvasive evaluation of patients with suspected coronary disease *Journal of the American College Cardiology* 1983; **1(2 pt 1)**: 444–55.

14 • Katz DA, Williams GC, Brown RL, *et al.* Emergency physicians' fear of malpractice in evaluating patients with possible acute cardiac ischemia *Annals of Emergency Medicine* 2005; **46(6)**: 525–33.

15 • Schattner A. The unbearable lightness of diagnostic testing: time to contain inappropriate test ordering *Postgraduate Medical Journal* 2008; **84(998)**: 618–21.

16 • Verstappen WHJM, van der Weijden T, Sijbrandij J, *et al.* Effect of a practice-based strategy on test ordering performance of primary care physicians: a randomized trial *Journal of the American Medical Association* 2003; **289(18)**: 2407–12.

17 • Ridker PM, Paynter NP, Rifai N, *et al.* C-reactive protein and parental history improve global cardiovascular risk prediction: the Reynolds Risk Score for men *Circulation* 2008; **118(22)**: 2243–51.

18 • Ridker PM, Buring JE, Rifai N, *et al.* Development and validation of improved algorithms for the assessment of global cardiovascular risk in women: the Reynolds Risk Score *Journal of the American Medical Association* 2007; **297(6)**: 611–19.

19 • World Health Organization *Definition and Diagnosis of Diabetes Mellitus and Intermediate Hyperglycaemia: report of a WHO/IDF consultation* Geneva: WHO, 2006, www.who.int/diabetes/publications/Definition%20and%20diagnosis%20of%20diabetes_new.pdf [accessed September 2010].

20 • American Diabetes Association. Standards of medical care in diabetes – 2009 *Diabetes Care* 2009; **32(Suppl 1)**: S13–61.

21 • Stone NJ, Bilek S, Rosenbaum S. Recent National Cholesterol Education Program Adult Treatment Panel III Update: adjustments and options. *American Journal of Cardiology* 2005; **96(4 suppl 1)**: 53–9.

22 • Dendukuri N, Chiu K, Brophy JM. Validity of electron beam computed tomography for coronary artery disease: a systematic review and meta-analysis *BMC Medicine* 2007; **25(5)**: 35.

23 • Hoffmann U, Ferencik M, Cury RC, *et al.* Coronary CT angiography *Journal of Nuclear Medicine* 2006; **47(5)**: 797–806.

24 • Klinkman MS, Stevens D, Gorenflo DW. Episodes of care for chest pain: a preliminary report from MIRNET. Michigan Research Network *Journal of Family Practice* 1994; **38(4)**: 345–52.

25 • Snow V, Barry P, Fihn SD, *et al.*; American College of Physicians; American College of Cardiology Chronic Stable Angina Panel. Primary care management of chronic stable angina and asymptomatic suspected or known coronary artery disease: a clinical practice guideline from the American College of Physicians *Annals of Internal Medicine* 2004; **141(7)**: 562–7.

26 • Thadani U. Role of nitrates in angina pectoris *American Journal of Cardiology* 1992; **70(8)**: B43–53.

27 • Robinson JG, Maheshwari N. A 'poly-portfolio' for secondary prevention: a strategy to reduce subsequent events by up to 97% over five years *American Journal of Cardiology* 2005; **95(3)**: 373–8.

28 • Kuukasjarvi P, Malmivaara A, Halinen M, *et al.* Overview of systematic reviews on invasive treatment of stable coronary artery disease *International Journal of Technology Assessment in Health Care* 2006; **22(2)**: 219–34.

29 • Department of Health. *National Service Framework for Coronary Heart Disease: modern standards and service models* London: DoH, 2000.

30 • Anderson JL, Adams CD, Antman EM, *et al.* ACC/AHA 2007 guidelines for the management of patients with unstable angina/non-ST-elevation myocardial infarction: a report of the American College of Cardiology/American Heart Association Task Force on Practice Guidelines (Writing Committee to Revise the 2002 Guidelines for the Management of Patients With Unstable Angina/Non-ST-Elevation Myocardial Infarction) developed in collaboration with the American College of Emergency Physicians, the Society for Cardiovascular Angiography and Interventions, and the Society of Thoracic Surgeons endorsed by the American Association of Cardiovascular and Pulmonary Rehabilitation and the Society for Academic Emergency Medicine *Journal of the American College of Cardiology* 2007; **50(7)**: e1–157.

31 • Aguirre FV, Younis LT, Chaitman BR, *et al.* Early and 1-year clinical outcome of patients' evolving non Q-wave versus Q-wave myocardial infarction after thrombolysis: results form the TIMI II Study *Circulation* 1995; **91(10)**: 2541–8.

32 • Zareba W, Moss AJ, Raubertas RF. Risk of subsequent cardiac events in stable convalescing patients after first non Q-wave and Q-wave myocardial infarction: the limited role of non-invasive testing. The Multicenter Myocardial Ischemia Research Group *Coronary Artery Disease* 1994; **5(12)**: 1009–18.

33 • Myocardial infarction redefined: a consensus document of the Joint European Society of Cardiology/American College of Cardiology Committee for the redefinition of myocardial infarction *European Heart Journal* 2000; **21(18)**: 1502–13.

34 • Leupker RV, Apple FS, Christenson RH, *et al.* Case definitions for acute coronary heart disease in epidemiology and clinical research studies: a statement from the AHA Council on Epidemiology and Prevention; AHA Statistics Committee; World Heart Federation Council on Epidemiology and Prevention; Centers for Disease Control and Prevention; and the National Heart, Lung, and Blood Institute *Circulation* 2003; **108(20)**: 2543–9.

35 • Thygesen K, Alpert JS, White HD, *et al.* Universal definition of myocardial infarction *Circulation* 2007; **116(22)**: 2634–53.

36 • Nomenclature and criteria for diagnosis of ischemic heart disease: report of the Joint International Society and Federation of Cardiology/World Health Organization task force on standardization of clinical nomenclature *Circulation* 1979; **59(3)**: 607–9.

37 • Tunstall-Pedoe H, Kuulasmaa K, Amouyel P, *et al.* Myocardial infarction and coronary deaths in the World Health Organization MONICA Project: registration procedures, event rates, and case-fatality rates in 38 populations from 21 countries in four continents *Circulation* 1994; **90(1)**: 583–612.

38 • Brieger D, Eagle KA, Goodman SG, *et al.*; GRACE Investigators. Acute coronary syndromes without chest pain, an underdiagnosed and undertreated high-risk group *Chest* 2004; **126(2)**: 461–9.

39 • Fesmire FM, Percy RF, Bardoner JB, *et al.* Usefulness of automated serial 12-lead ECG monitoring during the initial emergency department evaluation of patients with chest pain *Annals of Emergency Medicine* 1998; **31(1)**: 3–11.

40 • Sodi R, Hine T, Shenkin A. General practitioner (GP) cardiac troponin test requesting: findings from a clinical laboratory audit *Annals of Clinical Biochemistry* 2007; **44(pt 3)**: 290–3.

41 • Peters RJ, Mehta S, Yusuf S. Acute coronary syndromes without ST segment elevation *British Medical Journal* 2007; **334(7606)**: 1265–9.

42 • Husted S. Evidence-based prescribing and adherence to antiplatelet therapy: how much difference do they make to patients with atherothrombosis? *International Journal of Cardiology* 2009; **134(2)**: 150–9.

43 • Bhatt DL, Steg PG, Ohman EM, *et al.* International prevalence, recognition, and treatment of cardiovascular risk factors in outpatients with atherothrombosis *Journal of the American Medical Association* 2006; **295(2)**: 180–9.

44 • Ho PM, Spertus JA, Masoudi FA, *et al.* Impact of medication therapy discontinuation on mortality after myocardial infarction *Archives of Internal Medicine* 2006; **166(17)**: 1842–7.

45 • Canto JG, Shlipak MG, Rogers WJ, *et al.* Prevalence, clinical characteristics, and mortality among patients with myocardial infarction presenting without chest pain *Journal of the American Medical Association* 2000; **283(24)**: 3223–9.

46 • Simel DL, Rennie D, Keitz SA (eds). *The Rational Clinical Examination: evidence-based clinical diagnosis* New York: McGraw-Hill, 2009.

47 • Weaver WD, Cerqueira M, Hallstrom AP, *et al.* Prehospital-initiated *vs* hospital-initiated thrombolytic therapy *Journal of the American Medical Association* 1993; **270(10)**: 1211–16.

48 • Indications for fibrinolytic therapy in suspected acute myocardial infarction: collaborative overview of early mortality and major morbidity results from all randomized trials of more than 1000 patients. Fibrinolytic Therapy Trialists' (FTT) Collaborative Group *Lancet* 1994; **343(8893)**: 311–22.

49 • Ahmad RA, Bond S, Burke J, *et al.* Patients with suspected myocardial infarction: effect of mode of referral on admission time to a coronary care unit *British Journal of General Practice* 1992; **42(357)**: 145–7.

50 • Morrison LJ, Verbeek PR, McDonald AC, *et al.* Mortality and prehospital thrombolysis for acute myocardial infarction: a meta-analysis *Journal of the American Medical Association* 2000; **283(20)**: 2686–92.

51 • Collaborative overview of randomized trials of antiplatelet therapy – I: prevention of death, myocardial infarction and stroke by prolonged antiplatelet therapy in various categories of patients. Antiplatelet Trialists' Collaboration *British Medical Journal* 1994; **308(6921)**: 81–106.

52 • Theroux P, Cairns JA. Unstable angina and NSTEMI. In: S Yusuf, JA Cairns, AJ Camm, *et al.* (eds). *Evidence Based Cardiology* (second edn) London: BMJ Books, 2003, pp. 397–425.

53 • Baigent C, Collins R, Appleby P, *et al*. ISIS-2: 10 year survival among patients with suspected acute myocardial infarction in randomized comparison of intravenous streptokinase, oral aspirin, both, or neither. The ISIS-2 (Second International Study of Infarct Survival) Collaborative Group *British Medical Journal* 1998; **316(7141)**: 1337–43.

54 • Yusuf S, Zhao F, Metha SR, *et al*. Effects of clopidogrel in addition to aspirin in patients with acute coronary syndromes without ST-segment elevation *New England Journal of Medicine* 2001; **345(7)**: 494–502.

55 • Chen ZM, Jiang LX, Chen YP, *et al*. Addition of clopidogrel to aspirin in 45,852 patients with acute myocardial infarction: randomised placebo-controlled trial *Lancet* 2005; **366(9497)**: 1607–21.

56 • Antman EM, Anbe DT, Armstrong PW, *et al*. ACC/AHA guidelines for the management of patients with ST-elevation myocardial infarction – executive summary: a report of the American College of Cardiology/American Heart Association Task Force on Practice Guidelines (Writing Committee to Revise the 1999 Guidelines for the Management of Patients with Acute Myocardial Infarction) *Circulation* 2004; **110(5)**: 588–636.

57 • The Beta-Blocker Pooling Project (BBPP): subgroup findings from randomized trials in post infarction patients. The Beta-Blocker Pooling Project Research Group *European Heart Journal* 1988; **9(1)**: 8–16.

58 • Hjalmarson A. Effects of beta blockade on sudden cardiac death during acute myocardial infarction and the postinfarction period *American Journal of Cardiology* 1997; **80(9B)**: 35J–39J.

59 • Yusuf S, Peto R, Lewis J, *et al*. Beta blockade during and after myocardial infarction: an overview of the randomized trials *Progress in Cardiovascular Diseases* 1985; **27(5)**: 335–71.

60 • Indications for ACE inhibitors in the early treatment of acute myocardial infarction: systematic overview of individual data from 100,000 patients in randomized trials. ACE Inhibitor Myocardial Infarction Collaborative Group *Circulation* 1998; **97(22)**: 2202–12.

61 • National Institute for Health and Clinical Excellence. *Secondary Prevention in Primary and Secondary Care for Patients Following a Myocardial Infarction* London: NICE, 2007.

62 • Doll R, Peto R, Boreham J, *et al*. Mortality from cancer in relation to smoking: 50 years observations on British doctors *British Journal of Cancer* 2005; **92(3)**: 426–9.

63 • Garg R, Yusuf S. Overview of randomized trials of angiotensin-converting enzyme inhibitors on mortality and morbidity in patients with heart failure. Collaborative Group on ACE Inhibitor Trials *Journal of the American Medical Association* 1995; **273(18)**: 1450–6.

64 • Yusuf S, Sleight P, Pogue J, *et al*. Effects of an angiotensin-converting-enzyme inhibitor, ramipril, on cardiovascular events in high-risk patients. The Heart Outcomes Prevention Evaluation Study Investigators *New England Journal of Medicine* 2000; **342(3)**: 145–53.

65 • Baigent C, Keech A, Kearney PM, *et al*. Efficacy and safety of cholesterol-lowering treatment: prospective meta-analysis of data from 90,056 participants in 14 randomised trials of statins *Lancet* 2005; **366(9493)**: 1267–78.

66 • Oldridge NB, Guyatt GH, Fischer ME, *et al*. Cardiac rehabilitation after myocardial infarction. Combined experience of randomized clinical trials *Journal of the American Medical Association* 1988; **260(7)**: 945–50.

Stroke and transient ischaemic attack

4

Jonathan Mant

Aims

The aim of this chapter is to review the role of the GP in the management of people with stroke and transient ischaemic attack (TIA).

Key learning points

▶ The risk of a stroke within a few days of a TIA is high, but circumstantial evidence suggests prompt action can substantially reduce this risk.
▶ Carotid endarterectomy is effective at reducing risk of stroke in people who have had a TIA and have significant carotid artery stenosis, but the benefit declines the longer the operation is delayed after the TIA.
▶ People with acute stroke should be managed in hospital.
▶ People who have had a previous stroke or TIA remain at increased long-term risk of further vascular events. Control of vascular risk factors, in particular blood pressure and cholesterol, can reduce this risk.
▶ Many people with stroke have long-term problems, both physical and psychological. The primary care team could play a key role in making sure these long-term issues are addressed.

Introduction

Stroke may be defined as:

a clinical syndrome characterised by an acute loss of local cerebral function with symptoms lasting more than 24 hours or leading to death, and which is thought to be due to either spontaneous haemorrhage into the brain substance (haemorrhagic stroke) or inadequate cerebral blood supply to a part of the brain (ischaemic stroke) as a result of low blood flow, thrombosis or embolism associated with diseases of the blood vessels (arteries or veins), heart or blood.[1]

The advantage of this recently proposed definition over the traditional World Health Organization definition[2] is that it excludes subarachnoid haemorrhage, which may present with the clinical features of stroke, but is pathologically distinct and is managed quite differently. Most stroke is ischaemic – for example in the South London Stroke Register between 1995 and 2004, excluding subarachnoid haemorrhage, 77 per cent of strokes were ischaemic, 15 per cent were haemorrhagic and 8 per cent were unclassified.[3] Haemorrhagic strokes tend to be more severe, and are associated with higher mortality in the first 3 months after the event (but not thereafter).[4]

Mortality from stroke is declining in the UK, but it remains the third most common cause of death, accounting for over 50,000 (about 10 per cent of total) deaths in England and Wales in 2005.[5] The fall in mortality reflects a reduction in incidence[6] and improvement in survival following stroke.[7,8] This downward trend goes back to the early part of the twentieth century,[9] and may be due to improvements in population health as a result of improved living conditions, shifts in diet (e.g. less use of salt as a preservative; greater use of polyunsaturated fats) and in more recent years medical interventions such as blood pressure lowering and statins.[9,10]

Notwithstanding the decline in incidence and mortality from stroke, the condition will remain a major issue for health services and society in the future for three reasons. The incidence of stroke rises with age,[6] so, while age-specific incidence is falling, overall incidence may increase in the future as the proportion of older people in our population rises.[7] Second, stroke is the most common cause of adult disability – it has been estimated that there are about 300,000 people in England living with moderate or severe problems.[11] Third, the costs of stroke are high. A recent study calculated that the total cost to the UK of stroke was of the order of £9 billion per annum, including £4.4 billion of direct NHS costs, £2.4 billion of costs of informal care, £1.3 billion of lost productivity, and £0.8 billion in benefits payments.[12]

Stroke has been the subject of a major national strategy document published in 2007,[11] and of national clinical guidelines published in 2008.[13,14] This chapter will seek to put this national strategy and the clinical guidelines within the context of primary care. From a primary care perspective, acute stroke and TIA is relatively uncommon – each GP might expect to see only one patient with a TIA per annum and three or four people with a new stroke.[7] On the other hand, prevalence is high, with 8 per cent of people over the age of 65 having suffered a past stroke or TIA,[15] and about 1.5 per cent of a typical practice population has had a stroke or TIA.[16] Therefore, much of the workload in primary care is directed at the ongoing management of someone with a stroke or TIA and indeed at the primary prevention of stroke, which is the subject of other chapters in this book. Nevertheless, the general practitioner may have an important part to play in acute management, particularly of TIA.

Early management of TIA

A TIA is conventionally defined as 'a clinical syndrome characterised by an acute loss of focal cerebral or monocular function with symptoms lasting less than 24 hours and which is thought to be due to inadequate cerebral or ocular blood supply'.[1] The distinction between TIA and a minor stroke is somewhat arbitrary, with duration of symptoms being the key difference rather than (as perhaps was originally intended) whether there is underlying cerebral infarction.[17] However, from a pragmatic point of view, the primary care management of someone who has had focal neurological symptoms that have resolved is the same whether or not there has been underlying cerebral damage, and whether or not the final diagnosis is TIA or minor stroke.

Risk of stroke after TIA

It has been recognised in recent years that the risk of a stroke following a TIA is high: of the order of 8 per cent in the first 7 days after the event, 12 per cent after 1 month, and 17 per cent after 3 months, with the risks of recurrence following minor stroke even higher.[18] It is likely that the risks in the past were under-estimated because of selection bias (patients who went on to have an early stroke after a TIA will not have entered studies that recruit people from non-urgent out-patient clinics) and because temporary neurological symptoms preceding a stroke were not differentiated from the subsequent event.[19–21]

Amongst people with TIA, it is possible to use a simple clinical score to identify people who are at particularly high risk of stroke following a TIA. The score that has been adopted by NICE is the ABCD^2 score (see Table 4.1 on p. 108).[13,22] This gives a score between 0 and 7 on the basis of the patient's age, blood pressure, clinical features, duration of symptoms and presence of diabetes. The risk of stroke rises with the ABCD^2 score. This is illustrated in Figure 4.1, which shows the risk of stroke within 7 days of the TIA by ABCD^2 score. People with ABCD^2 scores of 3 or less are at lower risk of stroke – about 1 per cent risk by 7 days; people with scores of 4 or 5 are at moderate risk of stroke (about 5 per cent risk by 7 days); and people with scores of 6 or 7 are at high risk of stroke (over 10 per cent risk by 7 days). In the data-sets from which this score was derived and validated, 93 per cent of strokes within 7 days of a TIA occurred in people with ABCD^2 scores of

4 or more, which represented two thirds of the study population.[22] This has been operationalised in the NICE clinical guideline, which recommends that 'people who have had a suspected TIA who are at high risk of stroke (that is, with an ABCD^2 score of 4 or above) should have specialist assessment and investigation within 24 hours of onset of symptoms'.[13]

Table 4.1 ○ **The ABCD^2 score**

Age	60 years or over	1 point
Blood pressure	Raised on first assessment after TIA: ≥140 mmHg systolic OR ≥90 mmHg diastolic	1 point
Clinical features of TIA	Unilateral weakness of one or more of face, arm, hand or leg OR	2 points
	speech impairment (dysarthria or dysphasia) without weakness	1 point (max. 2 pts)
Duration of TIA	≥60 minutes 10–59 minutes	2 points 1 point
Diabetes		1 point

Source: adapted from Johnston SC, Rothwell PM, Nguyen-Huynh MN, *et al*. Validation and refinement of scores to predict very early stroke risk after transient ischaemic attack.[22]

Figure 4.1 ○ **ABCD^2 score and risk of stroke at 7 days**

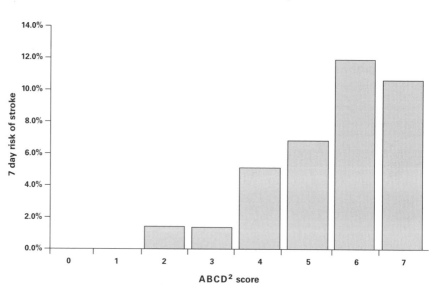

Source: adapted from Johnston SC, Rothwell PM, Nguyen-Huynh MN, *et al*. Validation and refinement of scores to predict very early stroke risk after transient ischaemic attack.[22]

Diagnosis of TIA

The diagnosis of TIA remains essentially a clinical one, though a substantial proportion of TIAs (between 35 per cent and 50 per cent)[23] have abnormalities on diffusion weighted imaging (DWI) MRI scans, which may persist for a couple of weeks after the event.[24] The key clinical features are: sudden onset; symptoms of loss of focal neurological function; symptoms maximal at onset; and short duration.[1] The focal symptoms reflect a carotid-lesion vascular event in about 80 per cent of TIAs, and a vertebrobasilar vascular event in up to 20 per cent.[25] Classic carotid focal symptoms are unilateral weakness or clumsiness in face, arm or leg, speech disturbance and loss of vision in one eye. Vertebrobasilar symptoms and signs include hemianopia, vertigo, ataxia and diplopia, but also often include hemiparesis.[26] Although the definition allows for symptoms to persist for up to 24 hours, over half of TIAs will resolve in less than 1 hour.[27] Factors that make a diagnosis of TIA less likely include non-focal neurological symptoms such as fainting or loss of consciousness, and headache.[28] Migraine and syncope are the most common non-TIA diagnosis in people referred with suspected TIA.[25]

Treatment of TIA

There are two interventions (aspirin and carotid endarterectomy) of proven benefit in the early management of acute cerebrovascular disease, but there is also circumstantial evidence suggesting that early medical intervention in the first few days after the event might have an important role in reducing risk of early stroke.

Evidence for the use of aspirin comes predominantly from two mega-trials: the International Stroke Trial (IST) and the Chinese Acute Stroke Trial (CAST).[29,30] Commencing aspirin within 48 hours of the onset of symptoms of acute stroke is associated with a 5 per cent reduction in the risk of death or dependency – the equivalent of needing to treat 79 people to prevent one case of death or dependency.[31] While this evidence was gathered in the context of acute stroke, it seems reasonable to apply the evidence to TIA. NICE took this approach with its recommendation that people with suspected TIA should immediately be started on aspirin (dose of 300 mg).[13] The dose reflects the value of obtaining rapid and complete inhibition of platelet cyclo-oxygenase – the subsequent maintenance dose can be lower, e.g. 75 mg daily.

Carotid endarterectomy for patients with a recent TIA or minor stroke who have a 70 per cent or greater stenosis in the ipsilateral carotid artery is associated with a 60 per cent reduction in the relative risk of stroke at 5 years (including risks of operative strokes or death) – the equivalent of preventing one stroke for every six operations performed.[32] However, the benefit of surgery is closely related to how soon after the TIA/stroke that the procedure is performed, with one stroke prevented for every three operations performed (for 70 per cent or greater stenosis) if carried out within 2 weeks, rising to 11 if done after 12 weeks.[33] Indeed, if it is performed within 2 weeks, the procedure is also effective for people with 50–69 per cent stenosis, with one stroke prevented for every seven operations, though the benefit in this group attenuates rapidly over time, and does not appear to be effective if performed outside the 2-week window.[33] A review of studies looking at safety of carotid surgery in relation to timing of the event found no evidence, contrary to perceived wisdom, that operating in the subacute phase after stroke/TIA is associated with any increased risk of stroke attributable to surgery.[34] This evidence is very much reflected in the NICE guideline, which recommends:

people with stable neurological symptoms from acute non-disabling stroke or TIA who have symptomatic carotid stenosis of 50–99 per cent according to the NASCET (North American Symptomatic Carotid Endarterectomy Trial) criteria should be assessed and referred for carotid endarterectomy within 1 week of onset of stroke or TIA symptoms and undergo surgery within a maximum of 2 weeks of onset of stroke or TIA symptoms.[13]

While this operation is highly effective, in practice few patients are eligible. Thus, in one series of 580 consecutive patients with TIA/minor stroke referred to a specialist clinic, only 32 (5.5 per cent) went on to have a carotid endarterectomy.[35]

The circumstantial evidence for early medical intervention comes from two observational studies: the EXPRESS study, and the SOS-TIA study.[35, 36] EXPRESS was a 'before and after' study set up to assess the impact of changes in the organisation of a daily TIA clinic in Oxford. In phase 1, GPs made urgent referrals to the clinic, where a diagnosis would be made and treatment recommendations sent back to the GP to initiate treatment. In phase 2, no appointments were necessary and treatments were initiated at the specialist clinic. Between phase 1 and phase 2, the median delay from symptom onset to initiation of medical treatment was reduced from 20 days to less than 1 day. The treatment that was initiated comprised simvastatin (40 mg daily), blood pressure lowering unless the systolic blood pressure was less than 130 mmHg, aspirin 300 mg, clopidogrel 300 mg (if at high risk of stroke), and anticoagulation if indicated (e.g. because of atrial fibrillation). This approach was associated with an 80 per cent reduction in the risk of stroke at 90 days, from 10 per cent to 2 per cent. There is some randomised evidence to support the use of clopidogrel early in the management of TIA and minor stroke from the FASTER study.[37] In this trial, patients were randomised within 24 hours of symptom onset to clopidogrel or placebo and simvastatin or placebo (all received aspirin). Dual therapy was associated with a 30 per cent reduction in risk of stroke at 90 days. Conversely, FASTER found no evidence of benefit from early initiation of statin therapy.

In the SOS-TIA study, the effect of a 'round-the-clock' service for patients with symptoms of TIA in Paris was evaluated by comparing the observed stroke rate after 3 months with the expected rate from the ABCD^2 score.[36] Over half of the patients were seen within 24 hours of onset of symptoms, and a treatment regime similar to that in the EXPRESS study was used (but without dual anti-platelet therapy). The expected stroke rate at 90 days was 6 per cent, the observed rate 1 per cent – a similar effect to that seen in EXPRESS. Given this evidence, NICE recommends that measures for secondary prevention should be introduced as soon as the diagnosis (of TIA/minor stroke) is confirmed, including discussion of individual risk factors.[13] It is also on the basis of this evidence that the National Stroke Strategy has prioritised the urgent referral of people with suspected TIA to specialist rapid-access clinics (see Box 4.1).[11]

111

Box 4.1 ○ *Markers of a quality service for TIA and minor stroke – the English National Stroke Strategy*

▶ Immediate referral for appropriately urgent specialist assessment and investigation is considered in all patients presenting with a recent TIA or minor stroke.

▶ A system that identifies as urgent those with early risk of potentially preventable full stroke – to be assessed within 24 hours in high-risk cases; all other cases are assessed within 7 days.

▶ Provision to enable brain imaging within 24 hours and carotid intervention, echocardiography and ECG within 48 hours where clinically indicated.

Role of primary care in management of TIA

The first contact that most people with TIA or minor stroke have with the health service is with their GP.[38,39] What should the GP do? If symptoms are evolving or are not resolving, then the patient should be referred urgently to hospital with suspected stroke. If the symptoms have resolved then the patient should be referred to a TIA clinic, using the ABCD^2 score to decide the degree of urgency with which this should be done (if ABCD$^2 \geq 4$, refer for specialist review within 24 hours). In terms of treatment, a 300 mg aspirin tablet should be given if the patient is not already on aspirin, followed by 75 mg daily. If the symptoms have not resolved, then aspirin may be withheld, in case the symptoms are caused by intracerebral haemorrhage (which will require brain imaging to exclude). Current guidance is that further secondary prevention treatments such as additional antiplatelet therapy, and cholesterol- and blood pressure-lowering agents are not given until the diagnosis has been confirmed.[13] The patient should be told not to drive for 4 weeks, unless an alternative diagnosis is established.[40]

Early management of stroke

The emphasis of both the NICE guideline and the National Stroke Strategy is that stroke should be seen as a medical emergency to be managed in hospital.[11,13] There are two key drivers behind this strategic approach. First, proven acute treatments are available for ischaemic stroke that require hospital admission, not least because brain scanning is required to exclude haemorrhagic stroke. These treatments are aspirin[31] (see above) and thrombolysis with alteplase.[41] There is a narrow therapeutic time window within which alteplase can be given – NICE recommends within 3 hours of onset of symptoms, though recent evidence suggests it may be of some benefit if administered within 4 and a half hours.[42] Second, there is good evidence that stroke unit care is associated with better long-term outcomes following stroke.[43] In this context, the only people with stroke that will not require admission to hospital are those where the event has largely resolved at the time of first contact with health services, who should be managed as per TIA above, and those where the family would feel a hospital admission was inappropriate in the context of end-of-life care.

Role of primary care in management of acute stroke

Since the aim in suspected acute stroke is to initiate transfer to hospital as soon as possible, people with symptoms suggestive of this diagnosis should be encouraged to dial 999 for an ambulance rather than to see a GP. In those cases where a GP does see a patient, a simple screening tool that can facilitate diagnosis is the FAST (Face, Arm, Speech Test), which comprises three items – facial weakness, arm weakness and speech disturbance (see Table 4.2).[44] Paramedics using this tool achieve similar levels of accuracy to GPs and A&E doctors in diagnosing stroke. In a study in Newcastle, paramedics using the tool were correct in 78 per cent (positive predictive value) of cases that they labelled as having stroke, as compared with 71 per cent correct referrals by GPs or A&E doctors.[44] The most common non-stroke diagnoses in people with suspected stroke are seizures, syncope and infections with associated confusion.[44,45]

Table 4.2 ○ *Aids in the diagnosis of stroke: FAST*

Facial movements	Ask patient to smile or show teeth. Look for new lack of symmetry
Arm movements	Lift the patient's arms together to 90° if sitting, 45° if supine and ask him or her to hold the position for 5 seconds and then let go. Does one arm drift down or fall rapidly?
Speech	If the patient attempts a conversation: ■ look for new disturbance of speech ■ check with companion ■ look for slurred speech ■ look for word-finding difficulties (which can be confirmed by asking names of commonplace items nearby) ■ if severe visual disturbance, place object in patient's hand and ask what it is

Source: Harbison J, Hossain O, Jenkinson D, *et al*. Diagnostic accuracy of stroke referrals from primary care, emergency room physicians, and ambulance staff using the Face, Arm, Speech Test.[44]

A more accurate tool, albeit designed primarily for use in A&E rather than in the community, is the ROSIER scale (Recognition of Stroke in the Emergency Room) (see Table 4.3). This is a tool to exclude hypoglycaemia, an important treatable cause of a stroke mimic. It includes the elements of the FAST test, and adds assessment of leg weakness and visual field defects, and looks for features that would reduce the likelihood of stroke (seizures or syncope). Validation of ROSIER showed that it had high diagnostic accuracy, with a sensitivity of 93 per cent, a specificity of 83 per cent and a positive predictive value of 90 per cent.[45]

Table 4.3 ○ *Aids in the diagnosis of stroke: ROSIER scale*

	If yes, score:
Has there been loss of consciousness of syncope?	−1
Has there been seizure activity?	−1
Is there new acute onset (or on awakening from sleep) of:	
■ asymmetric facial weakness	+1
■ asymmetric arm weakness	+1
■ asymmetric leg weakness	+1
■ speech disturbance	+1
■ visual field defect	+1

Total score greater than zero indicates stroke

Source: Nor AM, Davis J, Sen B, *et al*. The Recognition of Stroke in the Emergency Room (ROSIER) scale: development and validation of a stroke recognition instrument.[45]

Secondary prevention

People with a history of minor stroke or TIA have increased risk of further vascular events over the long term, of the order of 44 per cent over 10 years for someone aged 65–9.[46,47] Follow-up of people with a first stroke (mean age 72) in the Oxford Community Stroke Project showed that such people remain at increased risk (approximately twofold) of death as compared with an age- and sex-matched general population over the long term.[48] After the first year of follow-up, non-stroke cardiovascular disease was the commonest cause of death. These data indicate the potential importance of secondary prevention in people who have had a stroke or TIA and that, in the long term, the emphasis should be on prevention of all types of vascular events rather than simply stroke.

The principles of secondary prevention of vascular events in people who have had a stroke or TIA are the same as those in primary prevention. The main difference between secondary and primary prevention is that the absolute risk of a vascular event is generally higher in people with existing disease, so the potential benefit of treatment is greater. The long-term issues to consider are: lifestyle modification; blood pressure lowering; cholesterol lowering; and anti-thrombotic treatment. The evidence underpinning lifestyle modifications are considered in Chapter 2. The National Clinical Guideline for Stroke recommendations are summarised in Table 4.4.[14]

Table 4.4 ○ *Lifestyle modification for people who have had a stroke or TIA*

Smoking cessation	Individualised strategies may include pharmacological agents and/or psychological support
Exercise	The aim should be to achieve moderate physical activity (sufficient to become slightly breathless) for 20–30 minutes each day
Diet	■ Five or more portions of fruit and vegetables per day ■ Two portions of fish per week, one of which should be oily (salmon, trout, herring, pilchards, sardines, fresh tuna) ■ Reduce and replace saturated fats with polyunsaturated or monounsaturated fats – use of low-fat dairy products; use of vegetable and plant oils rather than butter/lard; less meat ■ Weight loss if overweight or obese ■ Reduce salt intake
Alcohol	Keep within recognised safe drinking limits: ≤3 units per day for men; ≤two units per day for women

Source: Intercollegiate Stroke Working Party. *National Clinical Guideline for Stroke*.[14]

114

Blood pressure lowering

The main evidence for lowering blood pressure in people who have had a stroke or TIA comes from the PROGRESS trial.[49] In this study, over 6000 people with a history of stroke or TIA were randomised to a blood pressure-lowering regime involving an angiotensin-converting enzyme (ACE) inhibitor +/- a diuretic and followed up for an average of 4 years. There was no blood pressure entry criterion, i.e. people with 'normal' blood pressure could be entered. A feature of the trial that has made subsequent interpretation problematic was that prior to randomisation the participating clinician would decide whether to randomise to single therapy versus placebo or to double therapy versus double placebo. Thus, the intensity of blood pressure lowering in the trial was determined not by chance but by physician choice, which in turn will have been influenced by patient factors. Overall, patients allocated active treatment had a 9/4 mmHg reduction in blood pressure as compared with the placebo group, and this reduction was associated with a 26 per cent reduction in the risk of major vascular events. The size of the effect was what would be anticipated given the degree of blood pressure lowering that was achieved, suggesting that this was a general effect of blood pressure lowering, rather than of the specific agents used.[50] This is consistent with systematic reviews that have found that impact of blood pressure-lowering agents on cardiovascular events is largely determined by the reduction in blood pressure that is achieved.[51,52] Subgroup analysis demonstrated that this effect was of similar magnitude regardless of baseline blood pressure.[53] However, this effect was seen entirely in patients who received combination therapy (who had a 40 per cent reduction). Patients who only received the ACE inhibitor experienced a non-significant 4 per cent reduction in risk, even though they had a 5/3 mmHg lower blood pressure. This suggests either that the ACE inhibitor was ineffective, or that there is a subgroup of people with stroke/TIA (40 per cent of the PROGRESS study population) who do not benefit from blood pressure lowering.

The more recent PRoFESS trial in 20,000 people with recent stroke did not find any benefit from use of an angiotensin receptor blocker (telmisartan) as compared with placebo. Though follow-up was shorter in this study (mean 2.5 years), there was only a 3.8/2.0 mmHg lower blood pressure achieved by active treatment, 30 per cent non-adherence by the end of the study, and greater use of other antihypertensives in people in the placebo arm.[54]

There is some concern about the applicability of the PROGRESS evidence to all people with cerebrovascular disease in primary care. People on a typical general practice TIA/stroke register are on average 12 years older than the participants of PROGRESS (76 versus 64 years old),[16] and the relative

115

size of the observed benefit in PROGRESS decreased with age.[55] Notwithstanding this reservation, the overall message to take from the PROGRESS trial is that important reductions in risk of vascular events can be achieved by blood pressure lowering in people who have had a stroke or TIA. The National Clinical Guideline recommends that a target of 130/80 mmHg is aimed for in people with established cardiovascular disease.[14]

Cholesterol lowering

Randomised controlled trials have demonstrated that statins lower total cholesterol, in particular low-density lipoprotein (LDL) cholesterol, and reduce cardiovascular events and all-cause mortality.[56] This effect is seen in people with a history of stroke or TIA. For example, in the Heart Protection Study, which included over 3000 patients with a history of cerebrovascular disease, there was a 20 per cent reduction in the risk of major vascular events in people treated with 40 mg of simvastatin as compared with placebo.[57] Interestingly, there was no reduction in recurrent stroke, though there was a reduction in first strokes. This perhaps is partly a reflection of the complex relationship between cholesterol and stroke, with epidemiological studies showing no clear association between total cholesterol (or LDL cholesterol) and stroke risk.[58] While the SPARCL trial has demonstrated that use of high-dose statins (80 mg of atorvastatin) can lead to a small reduction (16 per cent risk reduction) in stroke recurrence if used in people with a history of stroke or TIA,[59] it is interesting to note that the overall reduction in major cardiovascular events (20 per cent) achieved in SPARCL was similar to that achieved with just 40 mg simvastatin in people with stroke or TIA in the Heart Protection Study. NICE recommends that, for secondary prevention, patients should be prescribed 40 mg simvastatin, and consideration should be given to increasing this dose if the total cholesterol remains above 4 mmol/L or the LDL cholesterol above 2 mmol/L.[60] The National Clinical Guideline for Stroke notes, however, that statins should be avoided in people who have had a haemorrhagic stroke.[14] This reflects the observational evidence that lower cholesterol is associated with increased risk of haemorrhagic stroke in people over the age of 60,[58] and the evidence from SPARCL that high-dose atorvastatin increased the risk of haemorrhagic stroke.[59]

Anti-thrombotic treatment

Aspirin is effective in the secondary prevention of serious vascular events. Unlike in primary prevention, there is clear net benefit, with an overall reduction of 1.5 per cent serious vascular events per annum.[61] There have been a number of trials in recent years exploring whether dual antiplatelet therapy confers greater benefit than the single agent. The MATCH trial randomised people with recent ischaemic stroke or TIA to clopidogrel plus placebo or clopidogrel plus aspirin.[62] While there was a small non-significant reduction in the incidence of serious vascular events (15.7 per cent versus 16.7 pre cent) after 18 months of follow-up, this was offset by a significant increase in the risk of major haemorrhage (2.6 per cent versus 1.3 per cent). The CHARISMA trial randomised people with a history of cardiovascular disease or multiple vascular risk factors, including over 4000 people with a history of stroke or TIA, to aspirin plus placebo or aspirin plus clopidogrel.[63] As in MATCH, dual therapy was associated with a non-significant reduction in the primary endpoint after an average of 28 months' follow-up, but a non-significant increase in major bleeding. In ESPRIT, patients with TIA or minor stroke were randomised to aspirin or aspirin plus extended-release dipyridamole.[64] After a mean of 3.5 years' follow-up, there was a 20 per cent reduction of the primary endpoint (which was a composite of major vascular events or major bleeding complication) in people on dual antiplatelet therapy. Finally, the PRoFESS trial compared aspirin and extended-release dipyridamole with clopidogrel in patients with previous ischaemic stroke.[65] Rates of stroke and of major haemorrhage were essentially similar in the two arms of the trial. However, the study used a relatively low dose of aspirin (25 mg b.d.), so it is difficult to place this result in the context of the existing evidence base. NICE guidance is that the combination of modified-release (MR) dipyridamole and aspirin is recommended for people who have had an ischaemic stroke or a TIA for a period of 2 years from the most recent event.[66]

Another aspect of anti-thrombotic therapy is whether patients should be anticoagulated. Atrial fibrillation is a clear indication for anticoagulation in people who have had a stroke/TIA. History of stroke/TIA is a strong indicator of risk of stroke in atrial fibrillation,[67] anticoagulation is significantly more effective than aspirin at reducing this risk,[68] and this evidence has been shown to be applicable in elderly patients in primary care settings.[69] Trials of aspirin versus warfarin post-myocardial infarction have shown that warfarin is at least as effective as aspirin in preventing ischaemic heart disease events, so there is no need to prescribe aspirin as well for thromboprophylaxis in such patients, since risk of haemorrhage is higher on dual therapy.[70]

117

Longer-term care

Qualitative and quantitative research has identified significant long-term problems facing people with stroke and their families.[71-73] Psychosocial problems predominate (for carers as well as patients), and there may be a feeling of abandonment after the early rehabilitation phase has been completed. Unfortunately, the evidence base for how to deal with these problems remains limited. There is some evidence for a variety of community-based rehabilitation interventions,[74,75] but access to such interventions remains patchy. There is little evidence for how to address the psychosocial problems, including post-stroke depression.[76] Provision of information can improve patient knowledge, and when delivered actively can have positive effects on mood.[77] In particular, active training of caregivers can lead to better patient and carer psychosocial outcomes.[78] Similarly, access to Family Support Services by organisations such as the Stroke Association can prove beneficial to carers, but access to these services is usually limited to the first year after stroke.[79]

Longer-term support services remain poorly developed. The primary care team is the main contact that many stroke patients have with formal healthcare services. While secondary prevention remains important, the other aspects of holistic care need to be considered. The aspiration of the National Stroke Strategy is that a range of services are in place and easily accessible to support the individual long-term needs of individuals and their carers.[11] It recognises that a co-ordinated approach is needed between health and social care, involving housing, transport, employment, education and leisure services, and the voluntary sector.

Summary

While the care of the patient with acute stroke will increasingly be managed in the hospital sector, the GP will continue to play a major role in the management of stroke, in particular with regard to secondary prevention, which has a strong evidence base, and with regard to longer-term care, where the evidence base is less well established.

Self-assessment questions

1 ▷ A first-year medical student has joined the practice and is observing your surgery. The first patient you see is Mr AB who had a history of TIA last year. The medical student asks what a TIA is and what might cause it. Which of the following statements is **not** true?

   a. TIA is a clinical diagnosis.
   b. Atrial fibrillation is associated with an increased risk of TIA.
   c. TIA is most often due to an inherited hypercoagulable state.
   d. 80 per cent of TIAs are caused by abnormalities in carotid artery circulation.
   e. 20 per cent of TIAs are due to abnormalities in the vertebro-basilar circulation.

2 ▷ The patient from question 1, Mr AB, is a 65-year-old man who had a TIA last year. He describes the symptoms of TIA to your medical student. Which of the following features would **not** be typical for a history of TIA?

   a. Headache.
   b. Slurred speech.
   c. Monocular visual loss.
   d. Symptoms resolved within 24 hours.
   e. One-sided facial paralysis.

3 ▷ Mr AB describes the symptoms of his TIA to the medical student. 'I couldn't speak, just couldn't get my words out, for about an hour and a half. But then I was back to normal. I went to see the GP that afternoon and he said my blood pressure was up too.' His BP was recorded as 150/95. What would have been the best course of action for the GP to take?

   a. Refer to hospital.
   b. Refer to TIA clinic to be seen within 24 hours.
   c. Refer to TIA clinic to be seen in 2 weeks.
   d. Start clopidogrel, aspirin and simvastatin.
   e. Review the next day to see if symptoms recurred.

4 ▷ Regarding treatment for Mr AB during the consultation that day, what would have been most appropriate for the GP to prescribe?

a. Aspirin 300 mg.
b. Aspirin 300 mg and clopidogrel 300 mg.
c. Aspirin, statin and clopidogrel.
d. Clopidogrel 300 mg.
e. None of the above.

5 ▷ Mr AB drives to the shops and back but doesn't drive long distances. At the time of his TIA, what advice should Mr AB have received about driving?

a. He should not drive again.
b. He should not drive for a week following TIA.
c. There are no restrictions on driving as long as he doesn't drive long distances.
d. He should not drive for 4 weeks following TIA.
e. He should not drive for 6 months following TIA.

6 ▷ You are on call and have a telephone call from the daughter of Mrs BE, a 70-year-old woman who lives alone in a house about 5 minutes from the surgery. Mrs BE's daughter went to visit her mother this morning and while they were having a cup of tea, about 10 minutes ago, Mrs BE became unable to articulate her words and the left side of her face appeared to droop. She is alert and breathing. Mrs BE's daughter asks if you could do a home visit. What would you do?

a. Agree you will visit in the next half an hour.
b. Agree to visit immediately.
c. Ask the daughter if it's possible to bring Mrs BE to the surgery.
d. Call an ambulance.
e. Ask Mrs BE's daughter to call back in half an hour to see if the patient's symptoms have resolved.

7 ▷ Mrs BE has a CT scan that shows an ischaemic stroke. If there are no contraindications, within what time window from onset of symptoms would it not be appropriate to consider thrombolysis?

a. 30 minutes.
b. 1 hour.
c. 2 hours.
d. 3 hours.
e. 6 hours.

8 ▷ Mrs BE makes a good recovery and is discharged home. Secondary prevention is important to reduce the risk of further stroke. According to the National Clinical Guideline for stroke in the UK, what is the blood pressure target for patients with a history of stroke?

a. Less than 100/70.
b. Less than 120/80.
c. Less than 130/80.
d. Less than 140/90.
e. Less than 150/90.

9 ▷ Regarding antiplatelet therapy, what treatment should Mrs BE receive according to latest evidence and guidelines?

a. Aspirin for 1 year.
b. Aspirin and clopidogrel for 6 months.
c. Aspirin and clopidogrel for 12 months.
d. Dipyridamole for 12 months.
e. Aspirin and dipyridamole for 2 years.

10 ▷ Mrs BE also enquires about cholesterol tablets after reading an article in the newspaper. Which of the following statements is true?

a. Patients should receive 40 mg simvastatin if they have a high cholesterol after a stroke.
b. All patients should receive 80 mg atorvastatin following stroke.
c. Statins are ineffective in the prevention of stroke.
d. Patients with haemorrhagic stroke should not receive statins.
e. All stroke patients should receive 10 mg simvastatin.

Answers

1 = c ▷ Inherited hypercoaguable states are associated with TIA but this is not the most common cause.

2 = a ▷ Headache is not usually associated with TIA. Migraine is a differential diagnosis that is more commonly associated with headache.

3 = b ▷ Mr AB had an $ABCD^2$ score of 5 so should have been seen within 24 hours in the TIA clinic.

4 = a ▷ If symptoms have resolved, the evidence suggests aspirin 300 mg should be given, but further additional antiplatelet therapy, statin and blood pressure-lowering medication should be reserved until a formal assessment and diagnosis of TIA has been made.

5 = d ▷ Patients should not drive for 4 weeks following TIA.

6 = d ▷ This patient has probably acute stroke, which is a medical emergency requiring admission to hospital as soon as possible.

7 = e ▷ Thrombolysis can be effective if given within 3 hours of onset of symptoms although recent evidence suggests that thrombolysis within 4.5 hours may also be effective.

8 = c ▷ The National Clinical Guideline for stroke published in 2008 suggests a blood pressure target of less than 130/80 for patients with a history of stroke.

9 = e ▷ Evidence from the ESPRIT trial suggests treatment with aspirin and dipyridamole for 2 years after stroke will effectively reduce the risk of further events.

10 = d ▷ Evidence from the SPARCL study suggests statins may increase risk of haemorrhagic stroke.

References

1 • Warlow C, van Gijn J, Dennis M, *et al*. Is it a vascular event and where is the lesion? *Stroke: Practical Management* (third edn) Oxford: Blackwell Publishing, 2008, pp. 35–130.

2 • Hatano S. Experience from a multicentre stroke register: a preliminary report *Bulletin of the World Health Organization* 1976; **54(5)**: 541–53.

3 • Heuschmann PU, Grieve AP, Toschke AM, *et al*. Ethnic group disparities in 10-year trends in stroke incidence and vascular risk factors: the South London Stroke Register (SLSR) *Stroke* 2008; **39(8)**: 2204–10.

4 • Andersen KK, Olsen TS, Dehlendorff C, *et al.* Haemorrhagic and ischemic strokes compared: stroke severity, mortality, and risk factors *Stroke* 2009; **40(6)**: 2068–72.

5 • Office for National Statistics. *Mortality Statistics Cause: review of the Registrar General on deaths by cause, sex and age, in England and Wales, 2005* London: ONS, 2006.

6 • Rothwell PM, Coull AJ, Giles MF, *et al.* Change in stroke incidence, mortality, case-fatality, severity, and risk factors in Oxfordshire, UK from 1981 to 2004 (Oxford Vascular Study) *Lancet* 2004; **363(9425)**: 1925–33.

7 • Mant J, Wade DT, Winner S. Health care needs assessment: stroke. In: A Stevens, J Raftery, J Mant, *et al.* (eds). *Health Care Needs Assessment: the epidemiologically based needs assessment reviews, First Series* (second edn) Oxford: Radcliffe Medical Press, 2004, pp. 141–244.

8 • Lewsey JD, Gillies M, Jhund PS, *et al.* Sex differences in incidence, mortality, and survival in individuals with stroke in Scotland, 1986 to 2005 *Stroke* 2009; **40(4)**: 1038–43.

9 • Charlton J, Murphy M, Khaw K, *et al.* Cardiovascular diseases. In: J Charlton, M Murphy (eds). *The Health of Adult Britain 1841–1994*, vol. 2, London: The Stationery Office, pp. 60–81.

10 • Capewell S, O'Flaherty M. Trends in cardiovascular disease: are we winning the war? *Canadian Medical Association Journal* 2009; **180(13)**: 1285–6.

11 • Department of Health. *National Stroke Strategy* London: DoH, 2007.

12 • Saka O, McGuire A, Wolfe C. Cost of stroke in the United Kingdom *Age and Ageing* 2009; **38(1)**: 27–32.

13 • National Institute for Health and Clinical Excellence. *Clinical Guideline 68, Stroke: diagnosis and initial management of acute stroke and transient ischaemic attack (TIA)* London: Royal College of Physicians, 2008, www.nice.org.uk/CG68 [accessed September 2010].

14 • Intercollegiate Stroke Working Party. *National Clinical Guideline for Stroke* (third edn) London: Royal College of Physicians, 2008.

15 • Mant J, McManus RJ, Hare R, *et al.* Identification of stroke in the community: a comparison of three methods *British Journal of General Practice* 2003; **53(492)**: 520–4.

16 • Mant J, McManus RJ, Hare R. Applicability to primary care of national clinical guidelines on blood pressure lowering for people with stroke: cross sectional study *British Medical Journal* 2006; **332(7542)**: 635–7.

17 • Easton JD, Saver JL, Albers GW, *et al.* Definition and evaluation of transient ischaemic attack. A scientific statement for healthcare professionals from the American Heart Association/American Stroke Association Stroke Council; Council on Cardiovascular Surgery and Anaesthesia; Council on Cardiovascular Radiology and Intervention; Council on Cardiovascular Nursing; and the Interdisciplinary Council on Peripheral Vascular Disease *Stroke* 2009; **40(6)**: 2276–93.

18 • Coull AJ, Lovett JK, Rothwell PM on behalf of the Oxford Vascular Study. Population based study of early risk of stroke after transient ischaemic attack or minor stroke: implications for public education and organisation of services *British Medical Journal* 2004; **328(7435)**: 326–8.

19 • Lovett JK, Dennis MS, Sandercock PAG, *et al.* Very early risk of stroke after a first transient ischemic attack *Stroke* 2003; **34(8)**: e138–42.

20 • Giles MF, Rothwell PM. Risk of stroke early after transient ischaemic attack: a systematic review and meta-analysis *Lancet Neurology* 2007; **6(12)**: 1063–72.

123

21 • Selvarajah JR, Smith CJ, Hulme S, *et al.* Prognosis in patients with transient ischaemic attack (TIA) and minor stroke attending TIA services in the North West of England: the NORTHSTAR study *Journal of Neurology, Neurosurgery and Psychiatry* 2008; **79(1)**: 38–43.

22 • Johnston SC, Rothwell PM, Nguyen-Huynh MN, *et al.* Validation and refinement of scores to predict very early stroke risk after transient ischaemic attack *Lancet* 2007; **369(9588)**: 283–92.

23 • Saver JL, Kidwell C. Neuroimaging in TIAs *Neurology* 2004; **62(8 suppl 6)**: s22–5.

24 • Schulz UG, Briley D, Meagher T, *et al.* Diffusion-weighted MRI in 300 patients presenting late with subacute transient ischemic attack or minor stroke *Stroke* 2004; **35(11)**: 2459–65.

25 • Dennis MS, Bamford JM, Sandercock PAG, *et al.* Incidence of transient ischemic attacks in Oxfordshire, England *Stroke* 1989; **20(3)**: 333–9.

26 • Marx JJ, Mika-Gruettner A, Thoemke F, *et al.* Diffusion weighted magnetic resonance imaging in the diagnosis of reversible ischaemic deficits of the brainstem *Journal of Neurology, Neurosurgery and Psychiatry* 2002; **72(5)**: 572–5.

27 • Rothwell PM, Giles MF, Flossman E, *et al.* A simple score (ABCD) to identify individuals at high early risk of stroke after transient ischaemic attack *Lancet* 2005; **366(9479)**: 29–36.

28 • Dawson J, Lamb KE, Quinn TJ, *et al.* A recognition tool for transient ischaemic attack *QJM* 2009; **102(1)**: 43–9.

29 • International Stroke Trial Collaborative Group. The International Stroke Trial (IST): a randomised trial of aspirin, subcutaneous heparin, both, or neither among 19435 patients with acute ischaemic stroke *Lancet* 1997; **349(9065)**: 1569–81.

30 • CAST (Chinese Acute Stroke Trial) Collaborative Group. A randomised placebo-controlled trial of early aspirin use in 20,000 patients with acute ischaemic stroke *Lancet* 1997; **349(9066)**: 1641–9.

31 • Sandercock PAG, Counsell C, Gubitz GJ, *et al.* Antiplatelet therapy for acute ischaemic stroke *Cochrane Database of Systematic Reviews* 2008; **3**: CD000029.

32 • Rothwell PM, Eliasziw M, Gutnikov AS, *et al.* Analysis of pooled data from the randomised controlled trials of endarterectomy for symptomatic carotid stenosis *Lancet* 2003; **361(9352)**: 107–16.

33 • Rothwell PM, Eliasziw M, Gutnikov AS, *et al.* Endarterectomy for symptomatic carotid stenosis in relation to clinical subgroups and timing of surgery *Lancet* 2004; **363(9413)**: 915–24.

34 • Rerkasem K, Rothwell PM. Systematic review of the operative risks of carotid endarterectomy for recently symptomatic stenosis in relation to the timing of surgery *Stroke* 2009; **40(10)**: e564–72.

35 • Rothwell PM, Giles MF, Chandratheva A, *et al.* Effect of urgent treatment of transient ischaemic attack and minor stroke on early recurrent stroke (EXPRESS study): a prospective population-based sequential comparison *Lancet* 2007; **370(9596)**: 1432–42.

36 • Lavallée PC, Meseguer E, Abboud H, *et al.* A transient ischaemic attack clinic with round-the-clock access (SOS-TIA): feasibility and effects *Lancet Neurology* 2007; **6(11)**: 953–60.

37 • Kennedy J, Hill MD, Ryckborst KJ, *et al.* for the FASTER Investigators. Fast assessment of stroke and transient ischaemic attack to prevent early recurrence (FASTER): a randomised controlled pilot trial *Lancet Neurology* 2007; **6(11)**: 961–9.

38 • Giles MF, Flossman E, Rothwell PM. Patient behaviour immediately after transient ischaemic attack according to clinical characteristics, perception of the event, and predicted risk of stroke *Stroke* 2006; **37(5)**: 1254–60.

39 • Lasserson DS, Chandratheva A, Giles MF, *et al*. Influence of general practice opening hours on delay in seeking medical attention after transient ischaemic attack (TIA) and minor stroke: prospective population based study *British Medical Journal* 2008; **337**; a1569.

40 • Lasserson DS. Initial management of suspected transient cerebral ischaemia and stroke in primary care: implications of recent research *Postgraduate Medical Journal* 2009; **85(1006)**: 422–7.

41 • National Institute for Health and Clinical Excellence. *Alteplase for the Treatment of Acute Ischaemic Stroke: NICE technology appraisal guidance 122* London: NICE, 2007.

42 • Hacke W, Kaste M, Bluhmki E, *et al.*; ECASS Investigators. Thrombolysis with alteplase 3 to 4.5 hours after acute ischaemic stroke *New England Journal of Medicine* 2008; **359(13)**: 1317–29.

43 • Stroke Unit Trialists' Collaboration. Organised inpatient (stroke unit) care for stroke *Cochrane Database of Systematic Reviews* 2007; **4**: CD000197.

44 • Harbison J, Hossain O, Jenkinson D, *et al*. Diagnostic accuracy of stroke referrals from primary care, emergency room physicians, and ambulance staff using the Face Arm Speech Test *Stroke* 2003; **34(1)**: 71–6.

45 • Nor AM, Davis J, Sen B, *et al*. The recognition of stroke in the Emergency Room (ROSIER) scale: development and validation of a stroke recognition instrument *Lancet Neurology* 2005; **4(11)**: 727–34.

46 • van Wijk I, Kappelle LJ, van Gijn J, *et al*. for the LILAC study group. Long-term survival and vascular event risk after transient ischaemic attack of minor ischaemic stroke: a cohort study *Lancet* 2005; **365(9477)**: 2098–104.

47 • Clark TG, Murphy MFG, Rothwell PM. Long term risks of stroke, myocardial infarction, and vascular death in 'low risk' patients with a non-recent transient ischaemic attack *Journal of Neurology, Neurosurgery and Psychiatry* 2003; **74(5)**: 577–80.

48 • Dennis MS, Burn JPS, Sandercock PAG, *et al*. Long-term survival after first ever stroke: the Oxfordshire Community Stroke Project *Stroke* 1993; **24(6)**: 796–800.

49 • PROGRESS Collaborative Group. Randomised trial of a perindopril-based blood-pressure lowering regimen among 6,105 individuals with previous stroke or transient ischaemic attack *Lancet* 2001; **358(9287)**: 1033–41.

50 • Staessen JA, Wang J-G, Thijs L. Cardiovascular prevention and blood pressure reduction: a quantitative overview updated until 1 March 2003 *Journal of Hypertension* 2003; **21(6)**: 1055–76.

51 • Blood Pressure Lowering Treatment Trialists' Collaboration. Effects of different blood pressure lowering regimens on major cardiovascular events: results of prospectively designed overviews of randomised trials *Lancet* 2003; **362(9395)**: 1527–35.

52 • Law MR, Morris JK, Wald NJ. Use of blood pressure lowering drugs in the prevention of cardiovascular disease: meta-analysis of 147 randomised trials in the context of expectations from prospective epidemiological studies *British Medical Journal* 2009; **338**: b1665.

53 • Arima H, Chalmers J, Woodward M, *et al*. Lower target blood pressures are safe and effective for the prevention of recurrent stroke: the PROGRESS trial *Journal of Hypertension* 2006; **24(6)**: 1201–8.

54 • Yusuf S, Diener H-C, Sacco R, *et al*. Telmisartan to prevent recurrent stroke and cardiovascular events *New England Journal of Medicine* 2008; **359(12)**: 1225–37.

55 • Rodgers A, Chapman N, Woodward M, *et al*. Perindopril-based blood pressure lowering in individuals with cerebrovascular disease: consistency of benefits by age, sex and region *Journal of Hypertension* 2004; **22(3)**: 653–9.

56 • Cholesterol Treatment Trialists' (CTT) Collaborators. Efficacy and safety of cholesterol-lowering treatment: prospective meta-analysis of data from 90,056 participants in 14 randomised trials of statins *Lancet* 2005; **366(9493)**: 1267–78.

57 • Heart Protection Study Collaborative Group. Effects of cholesterol-lowering with simvastatin on stroke and other major vascular events in 20,536 people with cerebrovascular disease or other high-risk conditions *Lancet* 2004; **363(9411)**: 757–67.

58 • Prospective Studies Collaboration. Blood cholesterol and vascular mortality by age, sex, and blood pressure: a meta-analysis of individual data from 61 prospective studies with 55,000 vascular deaths *Lancet* 2007; **370(9602)**: 1829–39.

59 • The Stroke Prevention by Aggressive Reduction in Cholesterol Levels (SPARCL) Investigators. High-dose atorvastatin after stroke or transient ischaemic attack *New England Journal of Medicine* 2006; **355(6)**: 549–59.

60 • National Institute for Health and Clinical Excellence. *Clinical Guideline 67, Lipid Modification* London: NICE, 2008, www.nice.org.uk/CG067 [accessed September 2010].

61 • Antithrombotic Trialists' (ATT) Collaboration. Aspirin in the primary and secondary prevention of vascular disease: collaborative meta-analysis of individual participant data from randomised trials *Lancet* 2009; **373(9678)**: 1849–60.

62 • Diener H-C, Bougousslavsky J, Brass LM, *et al*. Aspirin and clopidogrel compared with clopidogrel alone after recent ischaemic stroke or transient ischaemic attack in high-risk patients (MATCH): randomised, double-blind, placebo-controlled trial *Lancet* 2004; **364(9431)**: 331–7.

63 • Bhatt DL, Fox KAA, Hacke W, *et al*. for the CHARISMA investigators. Clopidogrel and aspirin versus aspirin alone for the prevention of atherothrombotic events *New England Journal of Medicine* 2006; **354(16)**: 1706–17.

64 • The ESPRIT Study Group. Aspirin plus dipyridamole versus aspirin alone after cerebral ischaemia of arterial origin (ESPRIT): randomised controlled trial *Lancet* 2006; **367(9523)**: 1665–73.

65 • Sacco RL, Diener H-C, Yusuf S, *et al*. for the PRoFESS Study Group. Aspirin and extended-release dipyridamole versus clopidogrel for recurrent stroke *New England Journal of Medicine* 2008; **359(12)**: 1238–51.

66 • National Institute for Health and Clinical Excellence. *Clopidogrel and Modified-Release Dipyridamole in the Prevention of Occlusive Vascular Events* [Technology Appraisal 90] London: NICE, 2005, www.nice.org.uk/TA090 [accessed September 2010].

67 • Hart R, Pearce LA. Current status of stroke risk stratification in patients with atrial fibrillation *Stroke* 2009; **40(7)**: 2607–10.

68 • EAFT (European Atrial Fibrillation Trial) Study Group. Secondary prevention in non-rheumatic atrial fibrillation after transient ischaemic attack or minor stroke *Lancet* 1993; **342(8882)**: 1255–62.

69 • Mant J, Hobbs FD, Fletcher K, *et al.* on behalf of the BAFTA investigators. Warfarin versus aspirin for stroke prevention in an elderly community population with atrial fibrillation (the Birmingham Atrial Fibrillation Treatment of the Aged Study, BAFTA): a randomized controlled trial *Lancet* 2007; **370(9586)**: 493–503.

70 • Hurlen M, Abdelnoor M, Smith P, *et al.* Warfarin, aspirin, or both after myocardial infarction *New England Journal of Medicine* 2002; **347(13)**: 969–74.

71 • Hare R, Rogers H, Lester H, *et al.* What do stroke patients and their carers want from community services? *Family Practice* 2006; **23(1)**: 131–6.

72 • Murray J, Ashworth R, Forster A, *et al.* Developing a primary care based stroke service: a review of the qualitative literature *British Journal of General Practice* 2003; **53(487)**: 137–42.

73 • Murray J, Young J, Forster A, *et al.* Developing a primary care-based stroke model: the prevalence of longer-term problems experienced by patients and carers *British Journal of Medical Practice* 2003; **53**: 803–7.

74 • Logan PA, Gladman JRF, Avery A, *et al.* Randomised controlled trial of an occupational therapy intervention to increase outdoor mobility after stroke *British Journal of General Practice* 2004; **329(7479)**: 1372–5.

75 • Green J, Forster A, Bogle S, *et al.* Physiotherapy for patients with mobility problems more than one year after stroke: a randomised controlled trial *Lancet* 2002; **359(9302)**: 199–203.

76 • Hackett ML, Anderson CS, House A, *et al.* Interventions for treating depression after stroke *Cochrane Database of Systematic Reviews* 2008; **4**: CD003437.

77 • Smith J, Forster A, House A, *et al.* Information provision for stroke patients and their caregivers *Cochrane Database of Systematic Reviews* 2008; **2**: CD001919.

78 • Kalra L, Evans A, Perez I, *et al.* Training carers of stroke patients: randomised controlled trial *British Medical Journal* 2004; **328(7488)**: 1099.

79 • Mant J, Carter J, Wade DT, *et al.* Family support for stroke: a randomised controlled trial *Lancet* 2000; **356(9232)**: 808–13.

127

Peripheral vascular disease and erectile dysfunction

5

Michael Kirby

Aims

The aim of this chapter is to highlight the importance of peripheral vascular disease (PVD) and erectile dysfunction (ED) as common cardiovascular problems seen in general practice. In the first part of the chapter, we give an overview of the epidemiology and main risk factors for PVD, clinical presentation, investigation and appropriate management in primary care. In the second part of the chapter, we discuss the assessment and management of ED in more detail.

Peripheral vascular disease

Key learning points

▶ Understand the underlying cause of PVD.
▶ Realise the cost implications of PVD.
▶ Understand how to identify and assess patients in primary care.
▶ Treat and refer patients with PVD appropriately.
▶ Guideline 89 from the Scottish Intercollegiate Guidelines Network (SIGN) provides an excellent resource for the management of PVD.[1]

Introduction

PVD, sometimes known as peripheral arterial disease (PAD) in the UK, presents a major health problem in the UK and is often overlooked because many patients are asymptomatic. PVD prevalence rises markedly in diabetes.

In a primary care setting, the methods of diagnosis and the criteria for referral to a specialist vary between GPs. National guidelines are available from

SIGN.[1] The SIGN guidelines have been used as a resource for this chapter.

In patients with PVD, limitations due to restricted mobility may result in a significantly reduced quality of life.[2] Optimal management, including lifestyle advice, drug therapy and support, can help patients maintain their quality of life and prevent deterioration.

Overview of peripheral vascular disease

PVD is atherosclerosis and atherothrombosis of the distal aorta and/or leg arteries causing arterial stenosis or blockage, restricting blood flow to the legs. PVD is a term that encompasses asymptomatic and symptomatic disease. Atherosclerosis is rarely limited to a single territory and therefore may also affect the arteries of the arms, the neck, the kidneys, the heart and the brain. The disease may not cause symptoms until the atherosclerosis has progressed to a stage where the arteries are sufficiently narrowed and the disease declares itself. Symptoms will depend on which arteries are affected and the severity of the disease.

The most common presentation of symptomatic PVD is intermittent claudication, characterised by calf pain or occasionally thigh or even buttock pain on walking, which resolves with rest. These symptoms result from a failure of the lower-extremity arterial supply to meet the metabolic demands of the muscles during walking.[3] Patients will report a diminishing quality of life as walking distance and speed are reduced, compromising their mobility and independence. About 15–20 per cent of patients with lower-extremity arterial disease, equating to an estimated 150–200 per million of the UK population, will progress from intermittent claudication to chronic limb ischaemia (CLI). This may be characterised by pain at rest, ulceration and gangrene. CLI endangers the viability of the leg and may necessitate surgical revascularisation or amputation.[4,5]

Patients diagnosed with PVD, including those who are asymptomatic, are at increased risk of mortality, myocardial infarction (MI) and stroke, with relative risks two to three times that of age-matched groups.[1,6,7]

PVD is an indicator of diffuse and significant atherosclerotic disease in people aged over 55 years,[4] and sufferers are six times more likely to die within 10 years than the general population.[8] Hence, PVD whether symptomatic or not is an important prognostic marker.

In Europe and North America, the prevalence of PVD is estimated at 27 million, based on current epidemiological projections (16 per cent of the population aged 55 years and over). An estimated 10.5 million people are symptomatic, and the majority (16.5 million) are asymptomatic.[4] Unfortunately, accurate estimation is compromised because asymptomatic patients are usually undiagnosed.

In the UK, at least 720,000 people suffer from symptomatic PVD[9] and over 102,000 are newly diagnosed with PVD each year.[10] It has been estimated that approximately 5 per cent of people over the age of 60 years, which equates to 600,000 people in the UK, suffer from intermittent claudication as a result of PVD.[11] Less than half the patients with PVD are aware they have it, and GPs are only aware of it in around 30 per cent of their patients who have the condition.[12]

Some patients with symptomatic PVD do not seek treatment, because the early symptoms of intermittent claudication often manifest as fatigue, discomfort or pain in the muscles of the legs on exercise, particularly when walking up hills or stairs, and are assumed to be a normal part of the ageing process. Prevalence estimates vary due to differences in definition and method of diagnosis. A critical review of the subject found evidence of asymptomatic lower-extremity arterial disease in the 55–74 age group of 10 per cent using ABI (ankle brachial index) <0.9 as a cut-off, and 4.6 per cent in the same age group when a questionnaire was used. They concluded that the prevalence of intermittent claudication is highly dependent on age, sex and geographic location. The prevalence increases with age and the male predominance diminishes after 70 years of age.[4]

Prevalence increases with age. A study of patients aged ≥70 years (or 50–69 with a history of smoking or diabetes) detected PVD in 29 per cent, concluding that it is commonplace within primary care practices, but physician awareness is low.[13] In the Edinburgh Artery Study, 4.5 per cent of the population aged 55–74 had intermittent claudication, but non-invasive investigations revealed a further 8 per cent had significant symptomatic disease and 16 per cent had moderately abnormal asymptomatic results.[14] This study also found that 21 per cent of patients with diabetes or impaired glucose tolerance had evidence of PVD compared with 12.5 per cent in the general population.[14] Investigators in a European study found that asymptomatic PVD was present in one-third of patients with diabetes.[15] Mean levels of smoking, systolic blood pressure and triglycerides are often higher in patients with diabetes, which may explain the higher incidence.[16]

The population with diabetes has worse angiographic findings, more amputations and higher mortality than the non-diabetic population.[17] Two independent sources of data (the Danish Amputation Register and the Diabetes Control Activity in the US) demonstrated that major amputation rates in people with diabetes is 3000–3900 per million per year, compared with 200–280 per million per year among people without diabetes.[4] These complications are preventable and avoidable, with evidence to suggest that more than 50 per cent of amputations could be avoided by appropriate screening and education.[18] The identification of patients who are developing arterial disease provides the opportunity for other risk factors to be treated and diabetic care to be intensified. Primary care therefore has a very important role in preventing both primary and secondary vascular disease through the early detection of PVD.

Risk factors for PVD are the same as those for other cardiovascular disease (CVD), and include advancing age, smoking and diabetes. Diabetes and smoking carry a three- to four-fold relative increased risk of PVD.[19] After 18 years of follow-up in the Framingham study, 78 per cent of intermittent claudication cases were attributable to smoking.[7] Other risk factors include hypertension, hyperlipidaemia, hyperhomocysteinaemia,[20] elevated plasma fibrinogen levels, impaired glucose tolerance and a history of CVD, previous MI or stroke.[21]

Cost

Community orientation regarding resources

The consequences of PVD represent a cost not only in health care but also a cost due to reduced productivity. Symptomatic PVD carries a 30 per cent risk of death within 5 years, rising to almost 50 per cent within 10 years, mainly due to MI (60 per cent) and stroke (12 per cent). These risks are doubled in patients with severe disease requiring surgery. Patients with asymptomatic PVD have a two- to five-fold increased risk of non-fatal cardiovascular events.[22] Approximately half of patients presenting with symptomatic PVD also have symptoms of ischaemic heart disease,[23] which is responsible for a quarter of premature deaths and is estimated to cost the UK economy a total of £7055 million per year in direct and indirect costs.[24]

PVD that is not diagnosed or is under-treated may lead to a fatal ischaemic event that could have been prevented by an opportunistic case-finding strategy. This would provide the opportunity to address a preventive intervention including lifestyle advice, management of risk factors and antiplatelet therapy.

One-year data from the REACH registry showed that PVD was associated with a higher incidence of cardiovascular events than both coronary artery disease (CAD) and cerebrovascular disease. This study involved 68,266 patients with established atherosclerotic disease (cerebrovascular disease, CAD, PAD), or multiple (≥ 3) risk factors for atherosclerosis. Results showed that the incidences of the endpoint of cerebrovascular disease death, MI or stroke, or hospitalisation for atherosclerotic events, were 14.5 per cent for cerebrovascular disease, 15.2 per cent for CAD, and 21.1 per cent for

PAD patients with established disease.[25] UK data extracted from the registry show a similar pattern of both morbidity and mortality.

Classification

SIGN guidance [1] refers to the Fontaine classification,[25] which described PVD as follows:

▷ **stage 1** ▶ asymptomatic
▷ **stage 2** ▶ intermittent claudication
▷ **stage 3** ▶ rest pain/nocturnal pain
▷ **stage 4** ▶ necrosis/gangrene.

Diagnostic features of peripheral vascular disease

Primary care management, working in a multidisciplinary team, and specific problem-solving skills

Careful medical examination is essential in the diagnosis of PVD and it is important to identify which vessel territory is affected. The classical history typical of intermittent claudication is muscle pain brought on by exercise and relieved by rest. The location of the pain is determined by the degree of atheroma and the site at which the vessel is affected. The pain most commonly occurs in the calf; however, it can occur in the foot indicating disease in the femoro-popliteal segment or lower. Disease at the aorto-iliac level may produce pain in the buttock, hip or thigh, and is often associated with ED in males. The symptoms tend to be similar on a daily basis at a similar level of exercise. Therefore, careful palpation of the femoral, popliteal, posterior tibial and dorsalis pedis pulses is essential; however, the presence of foot pulses does not exclude PVD.[1,26]

In the ischaemic foot there may be nail changes or lack of hair on the toes. There may be evidence of muscle wasting, wounds and ulcers may be slow to heal, the foot may feel cold and look pale (or red in critical impairment of the circulation), and elevation of the limb may increase the pallor. There may also be loss of vibration sense and light touch sensation, and/or reduced capillary filling after blanching with light finger pressure.[27]

Peripheral vascular insufficiency may produce a positive Buerger's sign. This can be demonstrated when the patient is supine, the limb blanches and appears pale on elevation, then appears red when lowered over the edge of the bed. Auscultation of the arteries for bruits may indicate a stenotic area.

A systolic bruit may be audible over the kidneys in renal artery stenosis, and it is essential to listen to the neck for carotid or vertebral artery bruits. A general examination may provide evidence of other risk factors for athero-sclerosis. A corneal arcus or xanthelasma may be present, and lipid deposits may be observed within the Achilles, triceps or finger extensor tendons indicating hyperlipidaemia. The arterioles and capillary bed can be examined for abnormalities in the retina with an ophthalmoscope. The abdomen should be palpated for aortic aneurysm.

Specific questionnaires that have been validated for use in patients with intermittent claudication may be useful for determining health status. An example of this is the King's College questionnaire.[28]

The ABPI (ankle brachial pressure index) is the most useful indicator of PVD. This simple non-invasive test can be performed in a non-clinical environment and is usually a good predictor of subsequent cardiovascular events.[21,29,30] However, it cannot give an accurate reading on calcified arteries where occlusion of the blood flow by the cuff is not possible (e.g. in diabetes) and as a result of this may miss small-vessel disease. ABPI cannot be used to measure the effectiveness of preventive treatment, because the index does not reduce despite the risk reductions afforded by antiplatelet therapy.[21] Annex 1 in the SIGN guideline[1] presents a recommended method for measurement of ABPI.

Arterial calcification can often be asymptomatic but may be visible on radiography of the feet. It is important to document this, because, when calcification is present, results of Doppler studies may be misleading. Exercise testing is sometimes useful to detect mild forms of PVD in patients with normal resting ABPI values and typical symptoms.[31] A resting ABPI cut point of 0.9 has been shown in several clinical studies to be up to 95 per cent sensitive in detecting angiogram-positive disease and around 99 per cent specific in identifying supposedly healthy subjects.[1,32] Although highly sensitive and specific for PVD, a normal ABPI at rest, in combination with classic symptoms, requires referral for an ABPI measurement after exercise and/or imaging to confirm or refute a possible diagnosis.[1]

The ABPI of patients with intermittent claudication typically lies between 0.5 and 0.9. Critical-limb ischaemia Fontaine stage III or IV is generally associated with an ABPI of less than 0.5.[1] District nurses are trained to perform ABPI for venous ulceration; as a result of this ABPI is commonly performed in the community, and it is a skill that could be used by practice nurses.

The impact on quality of life will depend on many factors, including the co-morbidities. Many patients with claudication, for example, will have chronic knee, hip and back pain due to degenerative conditions.

Referral to secondary care

The SIGN guideline [1] recommends that patients with suspected PVD should be referred to secondary care if:

▷ the primary care team is not confident of making the diagnosis, lacks the resources necessary to institute and monitor best medical treatment or is concerned that symptoms may have an unusual cause
▷ risk factors are unable to be managed to recommended targets
▷ a patient has symptoms that limit lifestyle and objective signs of arterial disease such as clinical signs and low ABPI
▷ young and otherwise healthy adults are presenting prematurely with claudication; they should be referred to exclude entrapment syndromes and other rare disorders such as venous claudication, neurogenic claudication and osteoarthritis leading to referred pain.

Treatment strategies

Cardiovascular risk reduction

PRIMARY CARE MANAGEMENT AND PRACTISING HOLISTICALLY

There is a wealth of information which suggests that risk factor management is treated less aggressively for patients with PVD as opposed to those with CHD.[13,33,34] The SIGN guideline[1] recommends that patients with PVD should be referred within primary care to the practice cardiovascular clinic so that risk factor modification and long-term follow-up can be properly monitored. Second, when a diagnosis of peripheral vascular disease is made, the patient should have a full cardiovascular risk assessment carried out. Optimal management of cardiovascular risk factors is clearly very important and current advice for patients with PVD is to stop smoking, keep walking, achieve blood pressure and lipid targets, and to take antiplatelet therapy. Lifestyle management may include an exercise programme and/or a weight loss programme.

Exercise training programmes can increase pain-free and maximal walking distances; a meta-analysis found exercise training increased maximal walking distance by 179 metres.[21] Smoking cessation slows progression to CLI and reduces the risk of MI and cardiovascular risk, but it is uncertain whether it relieves intermittent claudication and it does not improve treadmill walking distances.[20]

SIGN guidance[1]

Person-centred care, a comprehensive approach and practising holistically

▷ All patients with PVD should be actively discouraged from smoking.

▷ Lipid-lowering therapy with a statin is recommended for patients with PVD and a total cholesterol level greater than 3.5 mmol/L.

▷ Optimal glycaemic control is recommended for patients with PVD and diabetes, in order to reduce the incidence of cardiovascular events.

▷ Obese patients with PVD should be treated to reduce their weight.

▷ Hypertensive patients with PVD should be treated to reduce their blood pressure.

▷ Antiplatelet therapy is recommended for symptomatic PVD.

Despite all the evidence that antiplatelet therapy reduces the incidence of vascular events in patients with atherothrombotic disease,[21] under-treatment is common. In the PARTNERS programme only 54 per cent of patients with prior PVD and 33 per cent with newly diagnosed PVD received antiplatelet therapy compared with 71 per cent of patients with CVD.[13] The benefits and risks of using antiplatelet agents in patients undergoing surgical intervention need to be taken into consideration. For patients undergoing stents, peripheral angioplasty or peripheral bypass surgery, guidelines recommend that aspirin can be continued peri-procedure unless there are particular concerns over operative bleeding. Consideration should be given to stopping clopidogrel in patients 5 days before surgery. There is no published evidence to show that antiplatelet therapy improves limb salvage in patients with CLI; however, their high risk of MI and stroke justifies prophylactic antiplatelet therapy.[35] The management of patients with CLI usually involves revascularisation, which is a cost-effective method of preserving the limb, associated with lower morbidity and mortality than amputation.[5]

SIGN guidance[1] on drug therapy for PVD is summarised below. The five drugs licensed in the UK for the treatment of intermittent claudication are cilostazol, naftidrofuryl, oxpentifylline, inositol nicotinate and cinnarizine.

Cilostazol appears to have both antiplatelet and vasodilatory effects.[36] It inhibits phosphodiesterase II and increases cyclic adenosine monophosphate levels causing vasodilation.[37] It also reduces the proliferative response to a number of pro-atherogenic growth factors.[38] Two large randomised controlled trials, which assessed the efficacy of cilostazol in improving mean walking distance and quality of life, found that the drug increased walking distance by 50–76 per cent compared with 20 per cent with placebo, and significantly improved quality of life. However, adverse effects led to its withdrawal in 16 per cent of the study population versus 8 per cent with placebo.[39,40] SIGN recommends the consideration of treatment with this drug in patients with intermittent claudication, particularly when it occurs over a short distance. It should be stopped if it is ineffective after 3 months or if side effects prevent compliance with therapy.[1]

Naftidrofuryl is considered to have vasodilatory effects. It works at tissue level to improve oxygenation, increase adenosine triphosphate levels and reduce lactic acid.[41] Studies have shown that naftidrofuryl improved walking distance by 92 per cent (versus 17 per cent with placebo) in patients who had already undertaken exercise training[42] and positively affected quality of life.[43,44] SIGN recommends consideration of this drug for treatment in people with intermittent claudication and poor quality of life.[1]

Oxpentifylline, inositol nicotinate and cinnarizine all have vasodilatory effects. Oxpentifylline and inositol nicotinate may also affect the composition of the blood. Due to a lack of efficacy evidence, SIGN does not currently recommend these drugs for the treatment of intermittent claudication.[1]

SIGN recommends that in the absence of a good body of trial evidence for both endovascular and surgical intervention, the guidelines drafted by the TransAtlantic Intersociety Consensus on the management of peripheral arterial disease (TASC) should be considered.[1] The TASC guidelines have recently been updated with a new consensus document, TASC III.[45]

SIGN guidance[1] recommends that:

▷ for the majority of patients with intermittent claudication, endovascular and surgical intervention are not recommended
▷ for those patients with severe disability or deteriorating symptoms, referral to a vascular specialist is recommended
▷ advice for patients about possible interventions should be based on the TASC guidelines.

Follow-up

Primary care management and working in a multidisciplinary team to provide person-centred, holistic care

Structured care and follow-up should be offered to patients with chronic disease. The SIGN[1] guideline suggests that all patients with PVD should be included in the systematic disease management arrangement and the optimal management of risk factors. This should be done in primary care and can be enhanced by brief motivational interventions.

Brief motivational interventions include the following:

▷ feedback on personal risk
▷ highlighting the responsibilities of the patient
▷ looking for and examining the patient's pros and cons for changing behaviours
▷ advice on changing behaviour from a professional perspective
▷ compiling a menu 'of ways to reduce risks'
▷ positive empathic counselling style
▷ highlighting the profession's confidence in the patient's ability to change.

Qualities of a practitioner using brief motivational interventions include the following:

▷ positive, optimistic outlook
▷ compassionate style
▷ empathic
▷ able to create good rapport.

The aim of the approach is to avoid provoking defensiveness in the patient and to generate enthusiasm for making the change.[46]

Summary

PVD is a common disorder that often co-exists with other CVD due to the underlying pathological process of atherosclerosis, which can affect multiple organs. Effective management of underlying risk factors such as diabetes, hypertension and hyperlipidaemia is fundamental to management of these patients in primary care. However, patients presenting with symptoms and signs of significant PVD require further investigation and appropriate timely referral to secondary care for investigation and, potentially, surgical management to improve blood supply or remove non-viable tissue.

Case-based discussion

Box 5.1 ○ *Case scenario*

Patient CD is a 70-year-old man who lives in a first-floor flat. He has been a smoker for 40 years and his two brothers both died in their sixties from 'heart problems'. He has a history of hypertension. His current medication is bendrofluazide 2.5 mg once daily. Recent bloods show a fasting glucose of 5.3 mmol/L, cholesterol level of 7.8 mmol/L and high-density lipoprotein cholesterol (HDLC) 0.9 mmol/L with normal renal and liver function tests. He has been able to live an independent lifestyle up until recently when he has noticed increasing amounts of pain in his calves on walking. He can no longer get to the local shop, which is less than 100 yards from his flat. He also gets pain in his legs at night but this goes away if he hangs his legs over the side of the bed. He has also noticed the second toe on his left foot has gone black and is oozing. He can't reach his toes to cover this up. He is struggling to get up the stairs in his flat but 'doesn't want to go into a home'. He wonders what you can do to help.

On examination he has black discolouration of his second left toe. The left foot is pink but his toes have a capillary refill time of about 5 seconds. Posterior tibial and dorsalis pedis pulses on the left are absent. Buerger's sign is negative. Pulse is 80 regular and BP is 130/80 mmHg.

1 ▶ What are the main issues in this case?

2 ▶ What is the likely diagnosis?

3 ▶ What investigations might you arrange?

4 ▶ Who else might you involve?

Practising holistically

The main issue here for the patient is maintaining his independence. He has risk factors for arterial disease that need appropriate management. He gives a clear history of intermittent claudication and rest pain with gangrene of his second left toe. He has social issues around how he is managing at home that need to be addressed.

Data gathering and making a diagnosis

This patient has a classic history and examination-finding of PVD. He has the complication of gangrene in the left toe.

Clinical management

This patient requires management of cardiovascular risk factors. A statin for his high cholesterol would be appropriate. His blood pressure is currently well controlled and he is not diabetic. Aspirin would also be beneficial.

Assessment of ABPI and referral to a vascular surgeon would also be appropriate for definitive treatment of his underlying arterial disease. The patient does not have significant past medical history so may be a candidate for surgery if this was deemed necessary. The district nurse should be involved to dress the toe and the tissue viability nurse could also be consulted. Social services should also be involved to provide any support required to keep this patient in his own home.

Managing medical complexity

This case is reasonably straightforward. However, many patients with PVD have a more complex medical history and may not be fit for surgery. Conservative management to address risk factors, control pain and manage skin breakdown involving the multidisciplinary team, which may include pain specialists, is vital for optimal management of these patients.

Primary care administration

Appropriate documentation and effective communication between teams is vital to ensure a co-ordinated and effective care plan.

Working with colleagues and in teams

This patient requires multidisciplinary team involvement as described above, including GP, district nurse, tissue viability nurse, vascular surgeon and social worker. Patients with other coexisting CVD may require input from other experts such as cardiologists or stroke specialists.

Maintaining an ethical approach

This patient is keen to stay in his own home and his autonomy should be respected and every effort made to make this possible through a multidisciplinary team approach. This would also reduce costs to society if the patient remained independent in his own home rather than requiring expensive care in a residential home. He would benefit from treatment with a statin and aspirin, and referral to secondary care; this would also reduce harm such as spreading gangrene or worsening pain, which could result from inaction.

Fitness to practise

Ensuring the safety of the patient in his own home whilst respecting his wishes to stay there is crucial. Putting the patient as your first concern and working with the multidisciplinary team to provide effective care is required as part of the duties of a doctor.

Self-assessment questions

1 ▷ Regarding the causes of PVD, which of the statements is **not** correct?

   a. PVD is more common in patients with hypertension.
   b. PVD is 20 times more common in diabetics.
   c. PVD is most commonly due to atherosclerosis.
   d. Patients with a history of MI are more likely to have PVD.
   e. Smoking is an important risk factor in PVD.

2 ▷ Which of the following is **not** a symptom of PVD?

   a. Calf pain on walking.
   b. Rest pain.
   c. Skin discolouration.
   d. Erectile dysfunction.
   e. Rash all over the body.

3 ▷ Which dorsalis pedis systolic/brachial systolic pressure ratio would be considered normal?

   a. Less than 0.9.
   b. Less than 0.7.
   c. Greater than 0.9.
   d. Greater than 0.7.
   e. None of the above.

4 ▷ Which of the following is **not** a clinical feature of hyperlipidaemia?

   a. Corneal arcus.
   b. Xanthomata.
   c. Family history.
   d. Yellow skin.
   e. Xanthelasma.

5 ▷ Regarding Buerger's sign, which of the following is correct?

    a. Is always found in patients with significant ischaemia.

    b. Involves pallor of the limb on elevation.

    c. Is only found in the presence of gangrene.

    d. Can be used instead of pressure indices.

    e. An angiogram is not required if Buerger's sign is negative.

Answers

1 = b ▷ Patients with diabetes have a three- to four-fold increased risk of PVD.

2 = e ▷ Rash is not commonly associated with PVD.

3 = c ▷ The systolic pressure in the feet should be at least 90 per cent of that of the arm.

4 = d ▷ Yellow skin is commonly associated with jaundice, which is usually due to liver disease.

5 = b ▷ Buerger's sign may be positive in patients with significant PVD. However, a negative Buerger's test does not exclude the presence of PVD.

Further information

☐ **British Heart Foundation**
Greater London House, 180 Hampstead Road, London NW1 7AW
Tel: 020 7554 0000 • Fax: 020 7554 0100
Heart Information Line: 0300 330 3311 (local rate number, available Mon–Fri, 9 a.m.–6 p.m., a free service for those seeking information on heart health issues) • **www.bhf.org.uk**

☐ **Circulation Foundation** (formerly the British Vascular Foundation)
c/o Royal College of Surgeons of England, 35–43 Lincoln's Inn Fields, London WC2A 3PE
Tel: 020 7304 4779 • **www.circulationfoundation.org.uk**

☐ **Patient UK** • **www.patient.co.uk**
A useful website with links to leaflets, support groups, information about medicines and drugs, etc.

Erectile dysfunction

Key learning points

▶ Understanding the physiological mechanisms leading to ED.

▶ Assessing the patient with ED and asking appropriate questions.

▶ Identifying the probable cause of ED using the results of diagnostic tests.

▶ Advising the patient on the various treatment options.

▶ National guidelines from the British Society of Sexual Medicine[47] are available on its website.

Introduction

Importance of a comprehensive, holistic approach

ED in older men is recognised as a marker of underlying vascular disease. Primary care has an important role in the identification and management of vascular disease and the prevention of secondary events.

The process of normal erectile function is complex. It requires the co-ordination of a number of psychological, hormonal, neurological and vascular factors. ED is the inability to achieve or maintain an erection sufficient for sexual activity. The increasing wealth of research surrounding the causes and effects of ED leaves little doubt that ED can be hugely detrimental to a man's self esteem and overall quality of life. The availability of new and effective therapies has made it possible for this extremely common medical condition to be increasingly understood and managed in primary care.

The most common physical causes of ED are conditions that impair arterial flow to the erectile tissues or disrupt the nervous system, such as atherosclerosis, hypertension or diabetes. ED may often be the first presenting symptom in men with previously undiagnosed chronic conditions, such as CVD and diabetes. The proactive identification of ED can not only help restore a sexual relationship, but also allow underlying diseases to be diagnosed at an earlier stage. This will improve treatment outcomes and prevent long-term complications.

ED and CVD share the same vascular risk factors (see Box. 5.2, overleaf).

Box 5.2 ○ *Shared risk factors for ED and CVD*

▶ Male gender.

▶ Age.

▶ Dyslipidaemia.

▶ Hypertension.

▶ Diabetes.

▶ Obesity.

▶ Sedentary lifestyle.

▶ Smoking.

▶ Depression.

The underlying common denominator is endothelial dysfunction and there is increasing evidence that ED can precede a cardiac event or predict subclinical CAD,[48] and this has led to a consensus that a man with ED is a vascular patient until proved otherwise.[49]

Diabetes

Diabetes significantly increases the risk of CVD and ED. Middle-aged men with diabetes are around five times more likely to die of CVD than men without diabetes.[50] Cardiovascular and neurological complications associated with diabetes increase the risk of developing ED by a complex mechanism that interferes with the interaction between the endothelium and the smooth muscle cells.

Over 50 per cent of men with diabetes will have suffered from ED at some time and as many as 39 per cent suffer from ED all the time.[51] The onset of ED in men with diabetes usually occurs gradually, and often 10–15 years earlier than those without diabetes.

The metabolic syndrome consists of a cluster of risk factors that increase the risk of cardiovascular disease and Type 2 diabetes.[52] It is also associated with an increased incidence of moderate to severe ED in men over the age of 50.[53] The metabolic syndrome was reviewed in the West of Scotland Coronary Prevention Study (WOSCOPS), which evaluated 6000 men over 5 years. Interestingly, the metabolic syndrome was associated with a 3.7-fold increased risk of coronary heart disease and a 24.5-fold increased risk for the development of diabetes.[54]

To establish whether diabetes is the underlying cause in men with ED, dipstick testing alone is not adequate. It has been found that if the dipstick test alone is used to identify the presence of diabetes in men with ED, four out of five new cases of diabetes will be missed (80 per cent).[55] Fasting blood glucose should be undertaken to diagnose diabetes reliably in men with ED.

Hypertension

ED is not only more prevalent in patients with hypertension than in age-matched controls, it is also more severe in those with hypertension than in the general population. In men with hypertension, mild ED was found in 7.7 per cent, moderate ED in 15.4 per cent and severe ED in 45.2 per cent.[56]

Treatment of hypertension can exacerbate the situation. A series of studies[57-59] found that the incidence of ED in hypertensive patients ranged from 17 per cent in patients with untreated hypertension, to 25 per cent (rising to 68 per cent) in patients with treated hypertension. Antihypertensive drugs affect not only the blood pressure but also the compliance of the erectile tissue, resulting in a functional venous leak. They impair erectile function as much as the atherosclerotic changes of the vascular system secondary to the hypertension itself.[60,61]

The angiotensin II receptor blocker drugs (ARBs) are the treatment of choice in these patients, and a study using valsartan[58] showed that the drug did not induce ED compared with the combined beta- and alpha-blocker carvedilol. An alternative to the ARB drugs is doxazosin, which also minimises the risk of ED developing as an adverse effect.[59]

Previous myocardial infarction

A history of MI is associated with the development of ED. Studies have found that the incidence of ED ranges from 44–64 per cent in patients who have previously had an MI.[57,62]

Smoking

The Massachusetts Male Aging Study (MMAS)[63] showed that men who smoked at baseline increased their risk of developing moderate to total ED to 24 per cent compared with non-smokers (14 per cent). And in the Health Professionals study[64] smoking increased the risk of developing ED by 50 per cent.

Smoking interferes with the cavernous veno-occlusive mechanism and adversely affects the erectile response to intracavernosal injections.[65,66]

Smoking cessation should therefore be a prime objective in any man pre-senting with ED. Other lifestyle measures are also very important.

Physical activity

The Health Professionals follow-up study[64] confirmed the important impact of obesity, physical activity, alcohol use and smoking on ED. Over 14 years 22,086 men aged 40–75 were followed up; 17.7 per cent developed ED dur-ing follow-up. Obesity nearly doubled the risk of ED, while physical activity reduced the risk of ED. The least active men, with higher levels of sedentary behaviour, were more likely to develop ED. Running for at least 2.5 hours per week was associated with a 30 per cent relative risk reduction for ED when compared with no regular activity; 1.5 hours of running or 3 hours of rigorous outdoor work reduced the relative risk by 20 per cent.

Lifestyle measures are therefore extremely important in men troubled by ED and this was underscored in the Princeton Consensus,[49] which empha-sised the importance of lifestyle intervention in those men with both vas-cular disease and ED.

Impact on relationships

Ensuring a person-centred approach and practising holistically

The impact of ED on the couple can be enormous. In one study of men with ED and partners, nearly three-quarters of women said that the man usually initiated sexual activity.[67] However, a man with ED may withdraw from sexual activity completely, fearing that he may be 'unable to perform'. The following disturbing statistics were found in a study of men with ED and their partners:[68]

▷ only 10 per cent of couples had experienced any sexual kissing or caressing in the 4 weeks before presentation
▷ almost half the couples had not experienced any sexual activity for 2.5 years
▷ almost 84 per cent of men rated sexual intercourse as important, compared with only 20 per cent of women. However, both men and women overestimated the importance their respective partners placed on intercourse
▷ there was clinical evidence of urogenital atrophy in one-third of women (over 46 years).

Broaching the subject of ED

A disturbingly high number of men suffer needlessly with their ED without seeking treatment. Many men who are embarrassed to raise the subject would like to be asked about their erectile function by a healthcare professional. A few alarming statistics are shown in Box 5.3.

Box 5.3 ○ *Issues around broaching the subject of erectile dysfunction*

▶ Only one in ten men with ED aged between 18–59 years seeks medical attention for ED.[69]

▶ Nearly 60 per cent of men with ED have not previously received treatment for their ED.[70]

▶ Of these, 69 per cent wish to be treated and 58 per cent want the physician to discuss the subject of their erections.

▶ Despite regular clinic visits, only 33 per cent of diabetic patients with ED had discussed the problem with their GP.[51]

▶ Although patients with hypertension visit physicians regularly for antihypertensive treatment, many do not receive treatment for ED (33 per cent).[56]

▶ Only 14 per cent of men with diabetes and 8 per cent of men without diabetes had been asked by their physician about sexual problems.[71]

▶ However, nearly 50 per cent of men with diabetes and 47 per cent of men without diabetes felt that they should routinely be asked about their sexual health.[71]

Why aren't health professionals initiating discussions about sex?

Ensuring a person-centred approach and practising holistically

Research suggests that health professionals also have difficulties discussing sexuality. Research has shown that 47 per cent of adult patients have never been asked by their primary care physicians whether they have had sexual relationships.[72] Although nearly three-quarters of doctors said that they routinely asked 80–100 per cent of their male patients about ED, doctors actually initiated discussions about ED in just 17 per cent of men with hypertension, 18 per cent with diabetes and 30 per cent of those aged over 65 years.[73] If the subject of erectile function is discussed in a consultation, it is most often raised by the patient (85 per cent of the time).[74] The prescribing policy related to Schedule 2 may cause confusion for both doctors and patients.

Open questions are vital if the real route of a sexual problem is to be uncovered. The first few questions are critical for putting the patient at ease, reassuring him that any problems can be discussed and encouraging him to be comfortable about his sexual function. Introducing the subject as a problem that commonly coexists with heart disease or diabetes and explaining that asking about ED is a routine part of that assessment is perhaps the most appropriate approach.

If it is felt that the patient does have ED, supplementary questions can then determine the extent and the exact nature of the problem. For example, the next question could be 'Do you have erections when you wake up in the morning or during the night?' The partner's attitude to the problem should also be established. A key question is obviously whether the impairment of erections is consistent rather than situational. Libido is usually preserved in men presenting with ED but a decline of sexual drive may suggest an endocrinological cause of the problem.

Ejaculation is much less commonly affected than the erection itself but enquiries should be made as to whether ejaculation is premature, delayed, dry (as commonly occurs following transurethral resection of the prostate) or absent altogether. Previous medical history should include a brief survey of sexual history, previous surgery and enquiry about multisystem disorders. Alcoholism, thyroid dysfunction and other system disorders should be borne in mind. A detailed history of all concomitant medications is important in the evaluation of patients with ED.

A comprehensive approach

The Sexual Health Inventory for Men (SHIM) is a structured questionnaire that can be used to identify possible ED, as shown in Box 5.4 (see p. 149).

Physical examination

Specific problem-solving skills and a comprehensive approach

A thorough physical examination is important as part of the basic assessment of the man with ED. Care should be taken to look for clinical signs of thyroid under-activity, liver disease or anaemia. Hypertension and other serious cardiovascular pathology must also be excluded. A focused neurological examination is valuable. Examination of the external genitalia should be performed with a view to excluding a genital or acquired abnormality of the penis itself and an assessment of the size of the testicles.

Box 5.4 ○ *The Sexual Health Inventory for Men (SHIM)*

Each question has several different responses. Circle the number of the response that best describes your own situation. Please be sure that you select one and only one response for each question.

Over the past 6 months:

How do you rate your *confidence* that you could get and keep an erection?

1 ▶ Very low

2 ▶ Low

3 ▶ Moderate

4 ▶ High

5 ▶ Very high

When you had erections with sexual stimulation, *how often* were your erections hard enough for penetration (entering your partner)?

0 ▶ No sexual activity

1 ▶ Almost never or never

2 ▶ A few times (much less than half the time)

3 ▶ Sometimes (about half the time)

4 ▶ Most times (more than half the time)

5 ▶ Almost always or always

During sexual intercourse, *how often* were you able to maintain your erections after you had penetrated (entered) your partner?

0 ▶ Did not attempt intercourse

1 ▶ Almost never or never

2 ▶ A few times (much less than half the time)

3 ▶ Sometimes (about half the time)

4 ▶ Most times (much more than half the time)

5 ▶ Almost always or always

During sexual intercourse, *how difficult* was it to maintain your erection to completion of intercourse?

0 ▶ Did not attempt intercourse

1 ▶ Extremely difficult

2 ▶ Very difficult

3 ▶ Difficult

4 ▶ Slightly difficult

5 ▶ Not difficult

When you attempted sexual intercourse, *how often* was it satisfactory for you?

0 ▶ Did not attempt intercourse

1 ▶ Almost never or never

2 ▶ A few times (much less than half the time)

3 ▶ Sometimes (about half the time)

4 ▶ Most times (much more than half the time)

5 ▶ Almost always or always

Add the numbers corresponding to questions 1–5. If your score is 21 or less, you may be showing signs of erectile dysfunction and may want to speak with your doctor.

Source: Sexual Health Inventory for Men (SHIM).[75]

149

In men with associated lower urinary tract symptoms, a digital rectal examination should be performed to assess prostate size and consistency, and a prostate-specific antigen (PSA) test may also be helpful.

Special investigations

Specific problem-solving skills and a comprehensive approach

Baseline, haematological and biochemical screening are necessary, which should exclude diabetes, liver abnormalities and a 9.00 a.m. testosterone. Many clinicians dealing with ED routinely measure prolactin and sex hormone-binding globulin in addition.

In conclusion, the initial basic assessment of ED is important and is the main opportunity for the physician to establish a rapport with the patient. The advent of new, effective, non-invasive therapies for ED have put the ball firmly in the court of the primary care physician, and the importance of excluding other important pathologies such as diabetes, hypertension or pituitary tumour should not be underestimated.

Management of ED

Practising holistically and a community-oriented approach regarding resources

According to the *British Society for Sexual Medicines Guidelines on the Management of Erectile Dysfunction*[47] the primary goal in the management of ED is to enable the patient and his partner to enjoy a satisfactory sexual experience. This involves:

▷ the identification and treatment of any curable causes of ED
▷ initiating lifestyle change and risk factor modification
▷ the provision of education and counselling for both patients
  and their partners.

While ED may be associated with other causes of CVD including endothelial dysfunction, dyslipidaemia and hypertension, it may be the first presentation of serious medical conditions such as hypertension or diabetes.

ED can be managed, or even cured in some cases, with current treatments. Investigations for ED should involve the identification of any modifiable risk factors. Lifestyle factors include psychosocial issues, adverse effects of non-prescription drugs and any influential co-morbidities. Risk factors are shown in Box 5.2. Lifestyle and risk factor modifications should accompany any pharmacotherapy or psychological therapy. Pharmacotherapy should not be withheld, however, if lifestyle changes are not made.[47]

To qualify for prescriptions at NHS expense, ED should be associated with (but not necessarily caused by) the medical conditions shown in Box 5.5.[1]

```
┌──────────────────────────────────────────────────────────────────┐
│  Box 5.5 ○ NHS qualifiers for prescribing drugs that treat ED      │
├──────────────────────────────────────────────────────────────────┤
│  ▶ Diabetes.                                                       │
│  ▶ Multiple sclerosis.                                             │
│  ▶ Parkinson's disease.                                            │
│  ▶ Poliomyelitis.                                                  │
│  ▶ Prostate cancer.                                                │
│  ▶ Prostatectomy (including TURP).                                 │
│  ▶ Radical pelvic surgery.                                         │
│  ▶ Renal failure treated by dialysis or transplant.                │
│  ▶ Severe pelvic injury.                                           │
│  ▶ Single-gene neuronal disease.                                   │
│  ▶ Spinal cord injury.                                             │
│  ▶ Spina bifida.                                                   │
└──────────────────────────────────────────────────────────────────┘
```

In addition, a patient qualifies if he:[47]

▷ was receiving a course of NHS drug treatment on 14 September 1998
▷ is suffering 'severe distress' on account of his ED.

The decision on whether to refer the patient to specialist services is down to the clinical judgement of the GP. The Department of Health recommends referral if the GP is satisfied that the man is suffering from impotence and that the impotence is causing him severe distress. Severe distress can be defined as:[47]

▷ significant disruption of normal social and occupational activities
▷ marked effect on mood, behaviour, social and environmental awareness
▷ marked effect on interpersonal relationships.

The following algorithm shows the treatment strategy of erectile dysfunction.[74, 76]

The objective of treatment is not just to restore a rigid erection, but also to restore a satisfactory sexual relationship.

Step 1

a. Educate the patient about risk factors and co-morbidities, together with
b. Counselling of the patient, and partner if possible
c. Consideration of the treatment options
d. Initiate medical treatment

Select treatment according to the medical and psychological contraindications, patient preference and availability:

▷ PDE5 inhibitors [the preferred treatment option in the majority of patients]
▷ other oral treatment
▷ local therapies
▷ pharmacological
▷ mechanical.

If not satisfactory, go to **Step 2**.

Step 2

Re-evaluate and adjust therapy:
▷ dose titration
▷ advise patient on optimal use of treatment.

If not satisfactory, go to **Step 3**.

Step 3

Consider alternative oral or local therapy as above. If still not satisfactory, go to **Step 4**.

Step 4

Refer to a specialist. Depending on the predominant aetiology and circumstances the specialist could be a:

▷ urologist – penile prosthesis, penile revascularisation, correction of penile deformity
▷ psychosocial therapist or psychiatrist – treatment of complicated psychosexual problems
▷ other medical specialist.

152

Summary

Traditionally, ED has been one of those hidden conditions that patients and health professionals have often ignored. With the progressive increase in life expectancy, and increasing quality of health and life in older people, the number of men who suffer from ED is also increasing. The advent of effective oral therapy and the surrounding publicity has brought ED into the public domain. Therapy for ED was the domain of hospital specialists, but it is increasingly clear that many men are best managed in the community. The proactive identification of ED can not only help restore a sexual relationship, but also enable underlying disease to be detected. The recognition of ED as a warning sign of vascular disease has led to the concept that a man with ED and no cardiac symptoms is a cardiac or vascular patient until proven otherwise.[48]

Self-assessment questions

Answer the questions below as either true or false:

1 ▷ ED may be a marker for a number of conditions including CVD and diabetes.

2 ▷ Men with ED do not require any special tests.

3 ▷ A random glucose test can reliably diagnose diabetes in men with ED.

4 ▷ A man's quality of life can be substantially diminished by ED.

5 ▷ ED has a very negative impact on marital relationships.

6 ▷ Patients with CVD and diabetes should be routinely asked about ED.

7 ▷ GPs and nurses are in an ideal position to proactively discuss ED and its ramifications.

8 ▷ A physical examination need not form part of the basic assessment of a man presenting with ED.

9 ▷ PDE5 inhibitors are the preferred treatment option in the majority of ED patients.

10 ▷ Lifestyle and risk factor modification should accompany any pharmacological or psychological therapy for ED.

Answers

1 = True
2 = False
3 = False
4 = True
5 = True
6 = True
7 = True
8 = False
9 = True
10 = True

☐ Some content of this chapter has been previously published in Kirby M. Erectile dysfunction *GM2 Gender (Men's Health)* 2008; **38**: 11–15 ☐ and in Kirby M. *Erectile Dysfunction and Vascular Disease* Oxford: Blackwell, 2003. Used with permission.

Further reading

☐ *British Society for Sexual Medicine Guidelines on the Management of Erectile Dysfunction* Fisherwick: BSSM, 2007. **www.bssm.org.uk/downloads/ BSSM_ED_Management_Guidelines_ 2007.pdf** [accessed October 2010].

☐ The Sexual Health Inventory for Men (SHIM). Available at **www.njurology.com/_forms/shim.pdf** [accessed September 2010].

Further information

☐ **British Association for Sexual and Relationship Therapy** (BASRT)
Tel: 020 8543 2707 • Email: info@basrt.org.uk • **www.basrt.org.uk**

☐ **Men's Health Forum**
32–6 Loman Street, London SE1 0EH
Tel: 020 7922 7908 • **www.menshealthforum.org.uk**

☐ **Relate**
Regional office locator:
www.relate.org.uk/find-your-nearest-service/index.html
Relateline: 0845 130 4010 ☐ Email: enquiries@relate.org.uk
www.relate.org.uk/home/index.html

□ **Sexual Advice Association**

Suite 301, Emblem House, London Bridge Hospital, 27 Tooley Street, London SE1 2PR

Helpline: 020 7486 7262 • info@sexualadviceassociation.co.uk

www.impotence.org.uk

References

1 • Scottish Intercollegiate Guidelines Network. *SIGN Guideline 89, Diagnosis and Management of Peripheral Arterial Disease* Edinburgh: SIGN, 2006. www.sign.ac.uk/pdf/sign89.pdf [accessed September 2010].

2 • Dumville JC, Lee AJ, Smith FB, *et al*. The health related quality of life in people with peripheral arterial disease in the community: Edinburgh Artery Study *British Journal of General Practice* 2004; **54(508)**: 826–31.

3 • Hiatt WR, Hirsch AT, Regensteiner JG, *et al*. The Vascular Clinical Trialists. Clinical trials for claudication. Assessment of exercise performance, functional status, and clinical endpoints *Circulation* 1995; **92(3)**: 614–21.

4 • Weitz LI, Byrne J, Claggett GP, *et al*. Diagnosis and treatment of chronic arterial insufficiency of the lower extremities: a critical review *Circulation* 1996; **94(11)**: 3026–49.

5 • Santilli JD, Santilli SM. Chronic critical limb ischaemia: diagnosis, treatment and prognosis *American Family Physician* 1999; **59(7)**: 1899–908.

6 • Dormandy JD, Heeck L, Vig S. The natural history of claudication: risk to life and limb *Seminars in Vascular Surgery* 1999; **12(2)**: 123–37.

7 • Fowkes FGR. Epidemiology of atherosclerotic arterial disease in the lower limbs *European Journal of Vascular Surgery* 1988; **2(5)**: 283–91.

8 • Criqui M, Langer RD, Fronek A, *et al*. Mortality over a period of 10 years in patients with peripheral arterial disease *New England Journal of Medicine* 1992; **326(6)**: 381–6.

9 • Norgren L, Hiatt WR, Dormandy JA, *et al*. Inter-Society Consensus for the Management of Peripheral Arterial Disease (TASC II) *European Journal of Vascular and Endovascular Surgery* 2007; **33(Suppl 1)**: S1–75.

10 • National Institute for Health and Clinical Excellence. *Clopidogrel and Dipyridamole for the Prevention of Atherosclerotic events* [Technical Appraisal 90] London: NICE, 2005, www.nice.org.uk/TA090 [accessed September 2010].

11 • Meijer W, Hoes AW, Rutgers D, *et al*. Peripheral arterial disease in the elderly: the Rotterdam Study *Arteriosclerosis, Thrombosis, and Vascular Biology* 1998; **18(2)**: 185–92.

12 • Novo S. Classification, epidemiology, risk factors and natural history of peripheral arterial disease *Diabetes, Obesity and Metabolism* 2002; **4(Suppl 2)**: S1–6.

13 • Hirsch AT, Criqui MH, Treat-Jacobson D, *et al*. Peripheral arterial disease detection, awareness, and treatment in primary care *Journal of the American Medical Association* 2003; **286(11)**: 1317–24.

14 • Fowkes FG, Housley E, Cawood EH, *et al*. Edinburgh Artery study: prevalence of asymptomatic and symptomatic peripheral arterial disease in the general population *International Journal of Epidemiology* 1991; **20(2)**: 384–92.

155

15 • Elhadd TA, Robb R, Jung RT, *et al*. Pilot study of prevalence of asymptomatic peripheral arterial occlusive disease in patients with diabetes attending a hospital clinic *Practical Diabetes International* 2003; **16(6)**: 163–6.

16 • MacGregor AS, Price JF, Hau CM, *et al*. Role of systolic blood pressure and plasma triglycerides in diabetic peripheral arterial disease *Diabetes Care* 1999; **22(3)**: 453–8.

17 • Jude EB, Oyibo SO, Chalmers N, *et al*. Peripheral arterial disease in diabetic and nondiabetic patients: a comparison of severity and outcome *Diabetes Care* 2001; **24(8)**: 1433–7.

18 • Boulton AJ. Why bother educating the multi-disciplinary team and the patient: the example of prevention of lower extremity amputation in diabetes *Patient Education and Counseling* 1995; **26(1–3)**: 183–8.

19 • Krentz AJ, Mani R, Shearman CP. Peripheral arterial disease in diabetes: time for a co-ordinated approach to management *British Journal of Diabetes and Vascular Disease* 2003; **3**: 92–6.

20 • Hiatt WR. Medical treatment of peripheral arterial disease and claudication *New England Journal of Medicine* 2001; **344(21)**: 1608–21.

21 • Belch J, Topol E, Agnelli G, *et al*. Critical issues in peripheral arterial disease detection and management *Archives of Internal Medicine* 2003; **163(8)**: 884–92.

22 • Tierny S, Fennessy F, Hayes DB. ABC of arterial and vascular disease. Secondary prevention of peripheral vascular disease *British Medical Journal* 2000; **320(7244)**: 1262–5.

23 • Aronow WS, Ahn C. Prevalence of coexistence of coronary artery disease, peripheral arterial disease, and atherothrombotic brain infarction in men and women ≥62 years of age *American Journal of Cardiology* 1994; **74(1)**: 64–5.

24 • Peterson S, Peto V, Rayner M. *Coronary Heart Disease Statistics*, 2004, www.heartstats.org/datapage.asp?id=1652 [accessed September 2010].

25 • Steg PG, Bhatt DL, Wilson PW, *et al*. One-year cardiovascular event rates in outpatients with atherothrombosis *Journal of the American Medical Association* 2007; **297(11)**: 1197–206.

26 • Fontaine R, Kim M, Kieny R. Die chirurgissche Behandlung de periphen Durch-blutungsstorungen *Helvetica chirurgica acta* 1995; **21(5–6)**: 499–533.

27 • Shaw JE, Zimmet PZ. The epidemiology of diabetic neuropathy *Diabetes Reviews* 1999; **7**: 245–52.

28 • Morgan MB, Crayford T, Murrin B, *et al*. Developing the Vascular Quality of Life Questionnaire: a new disease-specific quality of life measure for use in lower limb ischaemia *Journal of Vascular Surgery* 2001; **33(4)**: 679–87.

29 • Papamichael CM, Lekakis JP, Stamatelopoulos KS, *et al*. Ankle-brachial index as a predictor of the extent of coronary atherosclerosis and cardiovascular events in patients with coronary artery disease *American Journal of Cardiology* 2000; **86(6)**: 615–18.

30 • Vowden P, Vowden K. Doppler Assessment and ABPI: interpretation in the management of leg ulceration. www.worldwidewounds.com/2001/march/Vowden/Doppler-assessment-and-ABPI.html [accessed September 2010].

31 • Hiatt WR, Hoag S, Hamman RF. Effect of diagnostic criteria on the prevalence of peripheral arterial disease *Circulation* 1995; **91(5)**: 1472–9.

32 • Fowkes FGR. The measurement of atherosclerotic peripheral arterial disease in epidemiological surveys *International Journal of Epidemiology* 1988; **17(2)**: 248–54.

33 • Meijer WT, Cost B, Bernsen RMD, *et al.* Incidence and management of intermittent claudication in primary care in the Netherlands *Scandinavian Journal of Primary Health Care* 2002; **20(1)**: 33–4.

34 • Cassar K, Coull R, Bachoo P, *et al.* Management of secondary risk factors in patients with intermittent claudication *European Journal of Vascular and Endovascular Surgery* 2003; **26(3)**: 262–6.

35 • Peripheral Arterial Diseases Antiplatelet Consensus Group. Antiplatelet therapy in peripheral arterial disease. Consensus statement *European Journal of Vascular and Endovascular Surgery* 2003; **26(1)**: 1–16.

36 • Takahashi S, Oida K, Fujiwara R, *et al.* Effect of Cilostazol, a cyclic amp phosphodiesterase inhibitor, on the proliferation of rat aortic smooth muscle cells in culture *Journal of Cardiovascular Pharmacology* 1992; **20(6)**: 900–6.

37 • Matousovic K, Grande JP, Chini CC, *et al.* Inhibitors of cyclic nucleotide phosphodiesterase isozymes type-III and type-IV suppress mitogenesis of rat mesangial cells *Journal of Clinical Investigation* 1995; **96(1)**: 401–10.

38 • Reilly MP, Mohler IE. Cilostazil: Treatment of intermittent claudication *Annals of Pharmacotherapy* 2001; **35(1)**: 48–56.

39 • Thompson PD, Zimmet R, Forbes WP, *et al.* Meta analysis of results from eight randomised placebo-controlled trials on the effect of cilostazol on patients with intermittent claudication *American Journal of Cardiology* 2002; **90(12)**: 1314–19.

40 • Regensteiner JG, Ware JE Jr, McCarthy WJ, *et al.* Effect of cilostazol on treadmill walking, community-based walking ability, and health-related quality of life in patients with intermittent claudication due to peripheral arterial disease: meta-analysis of six randomised controlled trials *Journal of the American Geriatrics Society* 2002; **50(12)**: 1939–46.

41 • Lehert P, Comte S, Gamand S, *et al.* Naftidrofuryl in intermittent claudication: a retrospective analysis *Journal of Cardiovascular Pharmacology* 1994; **23(Suppl 3)**: S48–52.

42 • Boccalon H, Lehert P, Mosnier M. Effect of naftidrofuryl on physiological walking distance in patients with intermittent claudication. Findings of the Naftidrofuryl Clinical Ischaemia Study (NCIS) *International Angiology* 2001; **20(1)**: 58–65.

43 • D'Hooge D, Lehert P, Clement DL. Naftidrofuryl in quality of life (NIQOL). A Belgian study *International Angiology* 2001; **20(4)**: 288–94.

44 • Spengel F, Clement D, Boccolon H, *et al.* Findings of the Naftidrofuryl in Quality of Life (NIQOL) European Study Program *International Angiology* 2002; **21(1)**: 20–7.

45 • Norgren L, Hiatt WR, Dormandy JA, *et al.* Inter-Society Consensus for the Management of Peripheral Arterial Disease (TASC II) *European Journal of Vascular and Endovascular Surgery* 2007; **33(Suppl 1)**: S1–75.

46 • Maclean C. Using brief motivational interventions in practice *British Journal of Primary Care Nursing* 2009; **6(1)**.

47 • *British Society for Sexual Medicine Guidelines on the Management of Erectile Dysfunction* Fisherwick: BSSM, 2007, www.bssm.org.uk/downloads/BSSM_ED_Management_Guidelines_2007.pdf [accessed September 2010)

48 • Vlachopoulos C, Aznaouridis K, Ioakeimidis N *et al.* Unfavourable endothelial and inflammatory state in erectile dysfunction patients with or without coronary artery disease *European Heart Journal* 2006; **27(22)**: 2640–8.

49 • Jackson G, Rosen RC, Kloner RA, *et al.* The second Princeton consensus on sexual dysfunction and cardiac risk: new guidelines for Sexual Medicine *Journal of Sexual Medicine* 2006; **3(1)**: 28–36.

50 • British Heart Foundation Statistics Database. www.heartstats.org/homepage.asp [accessed September 2010]. 2002.

51 • Hacket GI. Impotence: the most neglected complication of diabetes *Diabetes Research* 1995; **28**: 75–83.

52 • Balon R, Yerangani VK, Pohl R, *et al.* Sexual dysfunction during antidepressant treatment *Journal of Clinical Psychiatry* 1993; **54(6)**: 209–12.

53 • Roose SP. Sexual activity and cardiac risk: is depression a contributing factor? *American Journal of Cardiology* 2000; **86(2A)**: 38F–40F.

54 • Sattar N, Gaw A, Scherbakova O, *et al.* Metabolic syndrome with and without C-reactive protein as a predictor of coronary heart disease and diabetes in the West of Scotland Coronary Prevention Study *Circulation* 2003; **108(4)**: 414–19.

55 • Sairam K, Kulinskaya E, Boustead GB, *et al.* Prevalence of undiagnosed diabetes mellitus in male erectile dysfunction *BJU International* 2001; **88(1)**: 68–71.

56 • Burchardt M, Burchardt T, Baer L, *et al.* Hypertension is associated with severe erectile dysfunction *Journal of Urology* 2000; **164(4)**: 1188–91.

57 • Wabrek AJ, Burchell RC. Male sexual dysfunction associated with coronary heart disease *Archives of Sexual Behavior* 1980; **9(1)**: 69–75.

58 • Alexander WD. Sexual function in diabetic men. In: JC Pickup, G Williams (eds). *Textbook of Diabetes* (second edn) Oxford: Blackwell Science, 1997, pp. 1–59.

59 • Bulpitt CJ, Dollery CT, Carne S. Change in symptoms of hypertensive patients after referral to hospital clinic *British Heart Journal* 1976; **38(2)**: 121–8.

60 • Fogari R, Zoppi A, Polett L, *et al.* Sexual activity in hypertensive men treated with valsartan and carvedilol: a crossover study *American Journal of Hypertension* 2001; **14(1)**: 27–31.

61 • Jackson G. Erectile dysfunction and hypertension *International Journal of Clinical Practice* 2002; **56(7)**: 491–2.

62 • Bortolotti A, Parazzini E, Colli E, *et al.* The epidemiology of erectile dysfunction and its risk factors *International Journal of Andrology* 1997; **20(6)**: 323–34.

63 • Johannes CB, Araujo AB, Fieldman HA, *et al.* Incidence of erectile dysfunction in men aged 40 to 69 years old: longitudinal results from the Massachusetts Male Aging Study *Journal of Urology* 2000; **163(2)**: 460–3.

64 • Bacon CG, Mittleman MA, Kawachi I, *et al.* A prospective study of risk factors for erectile dysfunction *Journal of Urology* 2006; **176(1)**: 217–21.

65 • Glina S, Reichelt AC, Leão PP, *et al.* Impact of cigarette smoking on papaverine-induced injection *Journal of Urology* 1988; **140(3)**: 523–4.

66 • Juenemann KP, Lue TF, Luo JA, *et al.* The effect of cigarette smoking on penile erection *Journal of Urology* 1987; **138(2)**: 438–41.

67 • Carroll JL, Bagley DH. Evaluation of sexual satisfaction in partners of men experiencing erectile failure *Journal of Sex and Marital Therapy* 1990; **16(2)**: 70–8.

68 • Riley A, Riley E. Behavioural and clinical findings in couples where the man presents with erectile disorder: a retrospective study *International Journal of Clinical Practice* 2000; **54(4)**: 220–4.

69 • Laumann EO, Paik A, Rosen RC. Sexual dysfunction in the United States: prevalence and predictors *Journal of the American Medical Association* 1999; **281(6)**: 537–44.

70 • Impotence Association Survey. London: 2000 and 2001.

71 • Nicolosi A, Glasser D, Brock G, *et al.* Diabetes and sexual function in older adults: results of an international survey *British Journal of Diabetes and Vascular Disease* 2002; **2(4)**: 336–9.

72 • Matthews WC, Linn LS. AIDS prevention in primary care clinics: testing the market *Journal of General Internal Medicine* 1989; **4(1)**: 34–8.

73 • Perttula E. Physician attitudes and behaviour regarding erectile dysfunction in at-risk patients from a rural community *Postgraduate Medical Journal* 1999; **75(880)**: 83–5.

74 • Broekman CPM, van der Werff ten JJ, Slob AK. The patient with erection problems and his general practitioner *International Journal of Impotence Research* 1994; **6(2)**: 59–65.

75 • The Sexual Health Inventory for Men (SHIM). Available at www.njurology.com/_forms/shim.pdf [accessed September 2010].

76 • Lue T, Giuliano F, Khoury S, *et al.* (eds). *Clinical Manual of Sexual Medicine. Sexual Dysfunction in Men. Based on the Reports of the 2nd International Consultation on Sexual Dysfunction. Paris, June 28–July 1st, 2003*. Health Publications Ltd, 2004.

Cardiac arrhythmias

6

Patrick Heck and Simon Fynn

Introduction

Patients presenting with cardiac arrhythmias vary from those with highly symptomatic, but benign, premature ventricular complexes (PVCs), through to those who experience no symptoms in the setting of sustained episodes of ventricular tachycardia (VT). The most common cardiac arrhythmia is atrial fibrillation and is dealt with in Chapter 7.

161

This chapter will detail the remaining more common cardiac arrhythmias seen in general practice. For the purposes of this chapter, arrhythmias can be conveniently subdivided into the following categories:

▷ extrasystoles
  ◻ premature atrial complexes
  ◻ premature ventricular complexes
▷ bradyarrhythmias
  ◻ sinus bradycardia
  ◻ sick sinus syndrome
  ◻ atrioventricular block
▷ tachyarrhythmias
  ◻ supraventricular tachycardias
  ◻ ventricular tachycardias.

Key learning points

▶ Typical symptoms and presentation of different arrhythmias.
▶ Possible causes and types of patient in which different arrhythmias may occur.
▶ Initial investigations that may be useful.
▶ Outline of management for different arrhythmias.

Extrasystoles

Premature complexes, or extrasystoles, are the most common cause of an irregular pulse, particularly in younger patients. Extrasystoles can originate from any area of the heart, but arise more commonly from the ventricles (PVC) than from the atria (premature atrial complex, PAC).

Presentation

The majority of people with PACs or PVCs are asymptomatic and the ectopics are incidental findings on routine electrocardiograms (ECGs). When symptomatic, the most common sensation is of an 'extra beat'. The early nature of the extrasystoles reduces ventricular filling time and hence systolic output, such that the radial pulsation of an extrasystole is often greatly reduced or even absent, causing the sensation of 'missed beats'. In contrast, the post-PVC beat has a longer filling time, hence more vigorous ventricular contraction, which is felt by some patients.

Causes

Extrasystoles can arise in normal hearts, but are more often associated with structural heart disease, and increase in frequency with age. They can occur in the setting of ischaemia, infection or inflammation, or can be provoked by alcohol, caffeine, tobacco or stress, as well as electrolyte or metabolic disturbances.

ECG and other investigations

PACs appear on an ECG as a premature P-wave that usually has a different morphology from the sinus P-wave, due to its different origin within the atria. The QRS accompanying the PAC is normally narrow (see Figure 6.1).

Figure 6.1 ○ *Premature atrial complex*

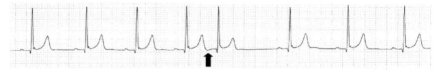

Note: Premature P-wave with abnormal morphology (indicated by arrow). Following QRS is premature and narrow.

162

A PVC is readily identifiable on an ECG as an early QRS complex that has an abnormal morphology and is broad (QRS >120 msec). The subsequent sinus beat is usually delayed and this is called a compensatory pause (see Figure 6.2). The term *bigeminy* refers to the occurrence of a PVC following every normal complex (see Figure 6.3); likewise, *trigeminy* describes a PVC following every two normal complexes.

Figure 6.2 ○ **Premature ventricular complex**

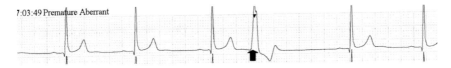

Note: Premature complex with broad QRS (indicated by arrow). Followed by compensatory pause.

Figure 6.3 ○ **Ventricular bigeminy**

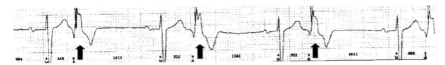

Note: The ECG strip shows a PVC (indicated by arrow) following every sinus beat.

The need for additional investigations in the context of extrasystoles depends on the clinical setting. If the history or examination suggest underlying heart disease, such as hypertension, valvular disease or ischaemia, then these should be investigated appropriately. If the patient is taking medication such as a diuretic then electrolyte imbalance should be excluded.

Management and prognosis

In normal hearts extrasystoles have no impact on mortality.[1,2] Such patients should be reassured, although a beta-blocker (BB) or a calcium channel blocker (CCB) can be used with some success to suppress the extrasystoles if symptomatic. In patients who have underlying heart disease or are found to have a predisposing cause, such as infection or electrolyte disturbance, treatment should focus on this, rather than on the extrasystoles. Should this fail to suppress the extrasystoles and the patient is symptomatic, BBs again remain the anti-arrhythmic of choice.

Referral to a specialist is rarely required unless highly symptomatic and refractory to simple drug therapy, or unless there are concerns about underlying cardiac disease.

Bradyarrhythmias

Bradycardia is often arbitrarily defined as a heart rate of ≤40 b.p.m. Bradyarrhythmias can result from disease anywhere along the conduction pathways of the heart, although typically due to disease either within the sinoatrial (SA) node or at the atrioventricular (AV) node.

Sinus bradycardia

PRESENTATION

Sinus bradycardia alone rarely causes symptoms unless the heart rate is unusually low or it slows suddenly. Advanced SA disease can result in severe bradycardias or prolonged sinus pauses that may cause symptoms such as presyncope, dizziness or syncope, although only pauses of longer than 3 to 4 seconds are generally symptomatic. A failure of the diseased SA node to adequately increase heart rate with activity, termed chronotropic incompetence, can result in fatigue and dyspnoea with exercise.

CAUSES

Asymptomatic sinus bradycardia frequently occurs in healthy young adults, particularly in athletes, is physiological and is not associated with conduction tissue disease.

Sinus bradycardia may be iatrogenic, caused by drugs that slow the SA node, namely BBs, amiodarone, some CCBs and ivabradine. The most common cause of SA disease is age-related idiopathic fibrosis, which can affect any part of the conduction system. Other causes are listed in Table 6.1.

Table 6.1 ○ *Causes of sinus bradycardia*

Physiological	SA disease
Drugs	Idiopathic fibrosis
Hypothermia	Ischaemic heart disease
Vasovagal	Amyloidosis
Hypoxia	Pericardial disease
Hypothyroidism	Post-cardiac surgery

ECG AND OTHER INVESTIGATIONS

Sinus bradycardia may be intermittent and often requires ambulatory ECG monitoring for accurate diagnosis (see Figure 6.4). Invasive electrophysiological studies contribute little as measurements of SA function add minimally to the management of this arrhythmia.

Figure 6.4 ○ *Sinus bradycardia*

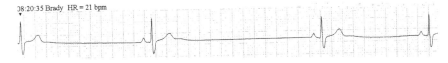

08:20:35 Brady HR = 21 bpm

Note: Every P-wave is conducted and the PR interval is normal.

Few additional investigations are required and are concerned with excluding the reversible causes of sinus bradycardia, such as drug-induced ones or hypothyroidism.

MANAGEMENT AND PROGNOSIS

Asymptomatic sinus bradycardia seldom requires treatment and is a benign arrhythmia. In the presence of symptoms and in the absence of any reversible causes, sinus bradycardia can be treated with permanent pacing.[3] Such patients should be referred to a specialist for assessment. If warranted, pacing is ideally achieved by insertion of a rate-responsive single-chamber atrial pacemaker, but in many patients there is also evidence of AV conduction disease, requiring placement of a ventricular lead as well (dual-chamber pacemaker).

Sick sinus syndrome

The sick sinus syndrome (SSS), also referred to as the tachy-brady syndrome, describes a combination of sinus bradycardia with paroxysms of atrial tachyarrhythmias, most notably atrial fibrillation.

PRESENTATION

The SSS typically presents with symptoms from the tachyarrhythmias. The bradycardias are revealed incidentally on ambulatory monitoring or with symptoms following initiation of rate-slowing medication to treat the tachyarrhythmia.

CAUSES

The cause is usually idiopathic fibrosis of the SA node, making it more common in the elderly. It can also occur in association with other structural heart disease and so can occasionally be seen in children with congenital heart disease.

ECG AND OTHER INVESTIGATIONS

As the arrhythmias are paroxysmal, ambulatory monitoring is invariably required.

Additional investigations are concerned with the stratification of thromboembolic risk, if atrial fibrillation is present, and the assessment of any underlying heart disease.

MANAGEMENT AND PROGNOSIS

Treatment of SSS varies depending on the predominant rhythm problem. Bradyarrhythmias will often require permanent pacing[3] and tachyarrhythmias require drug therapy. As almost all anti-arrhythmics used for the tachyarrhythmias will worsen SA function and exacerbate bradycardias, drug therapy and pacing are frequently used in combination. Accordingly, SSS is usually best managed jointly with a specialist.

Appropriate thromboembolic protection must also be used in patients with SSS and atrial fibrillation or flutter.

Atrioventricular block

AV block is classified as first, second or third degree depending on the extent of the block:

▷ **first-degree block** ▶ conduction time is prolonged (>0.2 sec) but all impulses are conducted
▷ **second-degree block** ▶ impulses are intermittently blocked. Second-degree AV block is further subclassified as either Mobitz type I (Wenckebach), with progressive lengthening of the conduction time until an impulse is not conducted, or Mobitz type II, where there is occasional or repetitive block of an impulse without prior lengthening of conduction time
▷ **third-degree block** ▶ all impulses are blocked (complete AV block) and an escape rhythm is present.

167

PRESENTATION

First-degree AV block is asymptomatic except in rare cases when the PR interval is prolonged to such an extent that there is effective mechanical AV dissociation.

With second-degree AV block symptoms depend on the number of conducted impulses, with the majority of patients being asymptomatic. Some patients will report subjective feelings of 'missed beats' and those with persistent 2:1 AV block can report symptoms similar to sinus bradycardia.

In third-degree (complete) AV block the rate and stability of the escape rhythm dictates the extent of symptoms, which includes those of bradycardia mentioned above, but also presyncope and syncope. Exertional fatigue and dyspnoea are more common due to a failure of the heart rate to increase with effort. The slow escape rates present in complete AV block can also sometimes cause VTs. Rarely, third-degree AV block can result in sudden death from ventricular asystole.

CAUSES

The commonest cause of AV block in the Western world is idiopathic fibrosis followed by ischaemic heart disease. Other causes are listed in Table 6.2 (p. 168).

First-degree and Mobitz type I AV block can occur in normal, healthy children, as well as in well-trained athletes, particularly when monitored overnight, and is likely due to increased resting vagal tone.

Table 6.2 ○ *Causes of AV block*

Idiopathic fibrosis	Cardiomyopathy
Ischaemic heart disease	Infection (Chagas, TB, endocarditis)
Drugs	Hypothermia
Congenital AV block	Cardiac surgery
Increased vagal tone	Radiotherapy
Connective tissue disease	Hypothyroidism

ECG AND OTHER INVESTIGATIONS

All forms of AV block may be persistent, and hence detected on resting ECG, or intermittent, necessitating the use of ambulatory ECGs. Sometimes the abnormalities may be so infrequent and elusive that implantable loop recorders are required to make the diagnosis.

In first-degree AV block, the PR is prolonged at >0.2 seconds. Every P-wave is followed by a QRS and the QRS is usually narrow, unless there is concomitant disease of the His–Purkinje system (see Figure 6.5).

Figure 6.5 ○ *First-degree AV block*

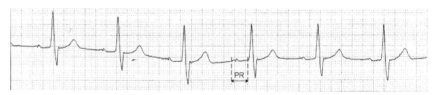

Note: Every P-wave is conducted, but the PR interval is >200 msec (actually ~300 msec).

In type I second-degree AV block, the ECG shows a progressive lengthening of the PR interval culminating in non-conducted P-wave. Again, the QRS is normally narrow unless there is concomitant His–Purkinje disease (see Figure 6.6).

168

Figure 6.6 ○ *Type I second-degree AV block*

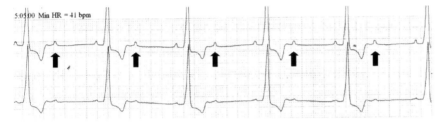

Note: Also known as Wenckebach, there is progressive PR prolongation culminating in a non-conducted beat (indicated by arrow).

In type II second-degree AV block, there are intermittent non-conducted P-waves, but the PR interval of the conducted beats is often normal (see Figure 6.7).

Figure 6.7 ○ *Type II second-degree AV block*

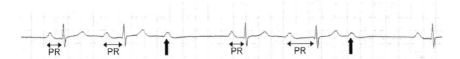

Note: In this ECG the conducted PR interval is normal, but every second P-wave is non-conducted (indicated by arrows). The QRS is also broad, indicating disease of the bundle branches as well.

In third-degree AV block, P-waves have no relation to QRS complexes (see Figure 6.8). When the block occurs in the AV node, the ventricular escape rhythm arises from the His bundle, resulting in a more reliable, narrow QRS escape rhythm with a rate of 40 to 60 b.p.m. When the block occurs at or below the His, the escape rhythm arises from the bundle branches, has a broad QRS and is generally slower and unreliable.

Figure 6.8 ○ *Third-degree AV block*

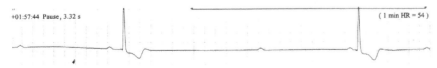

Note: Also known as complete heart block, the ECG shows no association between the P-waves and the QRS complexes.

MANAGEMENT AND PROGNOSIS

First-degree AV block in young people or athletes with no underlying heart disease is a normal phenomenon, is benign and requires no intervention.[4] Other presentations of first-degree AV block only very rarely require treatment, but may progress to higher levels of block.

The treatment of type II second-degree AV block is almost invariably insertion of a permanent pacemaker, unless there is an easily reversible cause, such as inferior myocardial infarction or drugs. Asymptomatic type I AV block in younger people with normal hearts requires no treatment.[5] However, type I second-degree AV block in older patients or those with structural heart disease is now thought to have a similar prognosis to type II block and is often treated by pacing.

In third-degree AV block, almost all patients require permanent pacing (usually dual chamber).[3] The exception to this is congenital AV block in which the indications to pace are more controversial.[3,6,7]

Patients who present with syncope/presyncope or whose ECGs suggest conduction system disease will often require ambulatory ECGs and referral to a specialist for assessment.

Tachyarrhythmias

There is a wide variety of tachyarrhythmias with differing prognoses and treatments, so establishing the correct diagnosis is crucial in the management of the arrhythmia. The arrhythmias can be further classified by their origin, as either supraventricular or ventricular.

Supraventricular tachycardias

These arrhythmias arise from the atria or the AV node and the ventricular activation is via the normal His–Purkinje system, resulting in normal (narrow) QRS complexes. The exception to this is when there is permanent or rate-related block in one of the bundle branches (aberrant conduction), or more rarely with certain arrhythmias seen in the Wolff–Parkinson–White (WPW) syndrome, when supraventricular tachycardias (SVTs) can present with broad QRS complexes. The most common SVTs are listed in Box 6.1.

Box 6.1 ○ *Supraventricular tachycardias*
▶ Sinus tachycardia.
▶ Atrial tachycardia.
▶ Atrial fibrillation.
▶ Atrial flutter.
▶ Atrioventricular nodal re-entrant tachycardia.
▶ Atrioventricular re-entrant tachycardia.

SINUS TACHYCARDIA

Sinus tachycardia is usually an appropriate, physiological response to a variety of stimuli, such as exercise, fever, pain, hypovolaemia, etc. As such it requires no treatment other than treating an underlying cause, if this is required. Chronic *inappropriate* sinus tachycardia is an uncommon condition where there is increased automaticity of the sinus node, probably due to abnormalities of either vagal or sympathetic tone, resulting in a persisting sinus tachycardia. Treatment options include BBs or CCBs, but can often prove ineffective.[8] If suspected, specialist referral is usually required.

Atrial tachycardia

PRESENTATION

Atrial tachycardia can be asymptomatic or present with symptoms typical of any SVT, namely palpitations, presyncope, dyspnoea, fatigue or anginal chest pain (even in the absence of coronary artery disease).

CAUSES

It is more common in older patients with structural heart disease, previous cardiac surgery or coronary artery disease, but may also be caused by digoxin toxicity. There can be a single ectopic atrial focus causing the tachycardia or there can be numerous different atrial foci.

ECG AND OTHER INVESTIGATIONS

Atrial tachycardias can sometimes be seen on a resting ECG if the arrhythmia is sustained, but usually ambulatory monitoring is required. They can resemble sinus tachycardia, but the P-wave morphology is normally different, reflecting the ectopic atrial focus.

Other investigations centre on the assessment or management of any underlying heart disease and the exclusion of digoxin toxicity in those receiving the drug.

MANAGEMENT AND PROGNOSIS

AV nodal blocking drugs (BBs, CCBs or digoxin) can be used to slow the ventricular response. If tachycardia persists then anti-arrhythmics such as flecainide or amiodarone may prove useful, if not contraindicated. In cases refractory to drug therapy, radiofrequency (RF) ablation can be considered, particularly if there is only one ectopic focus.[9] Accordingly, patients are best managed jointly with a cardiologist.

The prognosis of these arrhythmias is usually that of any underlying cardiac disease.

Atrial fibrillation

This arrhythmia is dealt with in Chapter 7.

Atrial flutter

Atrial flutter is a macro-reentrant arrhythmia, typically originating from the right atrium.[10] It is less common than AF, with an annual incidence of around 100 per 100,000, although the two arrhythmias often coexist.[11]

PRESENTATION

The presentation is that of any other SVT, with palpitations being common. Like AF, atrial flutter is associated with an increased risk of thromboembolism[12] and so may present with the consequences of such an event.

CAUSES

It usually occurs in the setting of structural heart disease, but can be idiopathic and, rarely, familial. Some of the predisposing conditions are listed in Box 6.2.

Box 6.2 ○ *Conditions predisposing to atrial flutter*

▶ Hypertension.

▶ Ischaemic heart disease.

▶ Valvular heart disease.

▶ Cardiomyopathy.

▶ COPD.

▶ Cardiac surgery.

▶ Congenital heart disease.

▶ Pericarditis.

▶ Thyrotoxicosis.

▶ Post-RF ablation.

▶ Alcohol.

▶ PE/pneumonia.

ECG AND OTHER INVESTIGATIONS

The atrial rate is around 300 b.p.m., although it is rarely conducted at this rate to the ventricles – there is usually 2:1 or more block, resulting in ventricular rates of around 150 or 100 (3:1). In typical atrial flutter the ECG shows the characteristic sawtooth flutter wave, best seen in the inferior leads (II, III or aVF; see Figure 6.9 on p. 174). Occasionally, these flutter waves may be hidden by the QRS and it may resemble other SVTs. In such cases transient slowing of the ventricular response with carotid sinus massage or adenosine will reveal the flutter waves. As with most arrhythmias, if symptoms are paroxysmal ambulatory ECG recording may be necessary.

Figure 6.9 ○ *Typical atrial flutter*

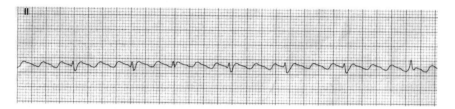

Note: Lead II shows the classical sawtooth pattern seen in atrial flutter.

Additional investigations are only required for the assessment of underlying cardiac disease or other predisposing conditions.

MANAGEMENT AND PROGNOSIS

The treatment of atrial flutter is similar to that of AF.[13] Unlike AF, though, atrial flutter responds readily to electrical cardioversion and relatively poorly to drugs. Control of the ventricular rate is normally the first-line treatment. This can be achieved by use of AV nodal blocking drugs such as BBs, CCBs or digoxin, alone or in combination. Anti-arrhythmic drugs such as flecainide or amiodarone have a role in chemical cardioversion, but are more often used in the prevention of recurrences. However, when used alone, without AV nodal blocking drugs, flecainide has the potential to slow the atrial flutter circuit just enough to allow 1:1 conduction to the ventricle at rates of over 200 b.p.m.

RF ablation for atrial flutter is a highly successful procedure and should be considered for the majority of patients with 'lone' atrial flutter[14] or those who have failed on medical treatment of their arrhythmia. Accordingly, such patients should be referred for investigation by a cardiologist.

Like those with AF, patients with atrial flutter should also be assessed for their thromboembolic risk and appropriate anticoagulation commenced.[12]

Atrioventricular nodal re-entrant tachycardia

PRESENTATION

Atrioventricular nodal re-entrant tachycardia (AVNRT) is a regular supraventricular tachycardia with sudden onset and termination, and ventricular rates between 150 and 250 b.p.m. The tachycardia is usually symptomatic, typically presenting in the third or fourth decade.[15] Symptoms are typical of other SVTs. Syncope or heart failure are rare unless there is underlying cardiac disease.

CAUSES

AVNRT is not caused by structural heart disease. The mechanisms of the arrhythmia are beyond the scope of this chapter, but patients who have AVNRT essentially are born with a minor variation on normal AV node electrophysiology that facilitates this tachycardia.

ECG AND OTHER INVESTIGATIONS

The resting ECG is usually normal. The ECG of AVNRT is characterised by a regular narrow QRS complex tachycardia with a rate between 150 and 250 b.p.m. (see Figure 6.10). P-waves are present, but usually hidden within the QRS. The ECG appearances can be difficult to distinguish from atrioventricular re-entrant tachycardia (AVRT). AVNRT is a paroxysmal arrhythmia and often requires ambulatory ECG monitoring to record it. As AVNRT is not associated with structural heart disease, other investigations are rarely indicated.

Figure 6.10 ○ *AVNRT*

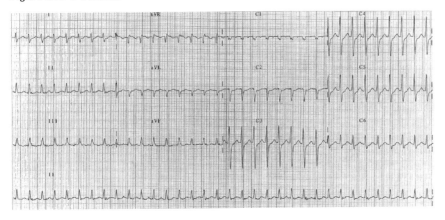

Note: This ECG shows a regular narrow complex tachycardia with a ventricular rate of 190 b.p.m. The ECGs of AVNRT and AVRT are often similar and very difficult to distinguish between.

MANAGEMENT AND PROGNOSIS

Patients should be reassured that the tachycardia is not dangerous and the prognosis is good in the absence of any heart disease. Prolonged episodes of AVNRT are often quite distressing for patients and they often present to the emergency room. Acute episodes can be terminated in a variety of ways: [13]

▷ vagal manoeuvres including carotid sinus massage and the Valsalva manoeuvres can be effective first-line treatments
▷ adenosine in doses of 6 to 18 mg by rapid IV bolus is highly effective, terminating AVNRT in over 90 per cent of cases, but should not be used in patients with asthma
▷ verapamil or beta-blockers can be used intravenously, with caution, if adenosine and vagal manoeuvres have failed
▷ DC cardioversion is also effective, but rarely needed.

When deciding on the best treatment for preventing recurrence of AVNRT, the frequency and severity of symptoms must be carefully evaluated with the patient. Infrequent attacks that are well tolerated may require reassurance but no treatment. If drug treatment is warranted, BBs or CCBs are used first line, with flecainide or sotalol used as second-line treatment.

RF ablation for AVNRT has a success rate of > 95 per cent for a cure and a low incidence of side effects.[16] As such it should be considered early in the management of AVNRT by referral to a cardiologist as it is preferable to long-term treatment with medication.

Atrioventricular re-entrant tachycardia

PRESENTATION

AVRT presents in a similar fashion to AVNRT. The heart rates in AVRT tend to be somewhat faster than AVNRT, but there is considerable overlap. In adults AVNRT is more common than AVRT.[17]

CAUSES

Like AVNRT, AVRT is not caused by structural heart disease. AVRT can only occur in the presence of an accessory pathway, which is a strand of myocardium bridging the groove between the atria and the ventricles, thereby bypassing the AV node. In AVRT the re-entry circuit is formed between the

AV node and the accessory pathway. These pathways can broadly be thought of as two types:

▷ 'concealed' accessory pathways – only conduct from ventricle to atrium and have a normal resting 12-lead ECG appearance
▷ pre-excited pathways – can conduct in both directions and consequently have a pre-excited ECG in sinus rhythm with a delta wave present in the QRS due to simultaneous activation of the ventricle via the AV node and the accessory pathway. When occurring with tachyarrhythmias, this is WPW syndrome (see below).

ECG AND OTHER INVESTIGATIONS

Unless the patient has WPW the resting ECG will be normal. The ECG during AVRT can be difficult to distinguish from that of AVNRT (see Figure 6.10 on p. 175). It is a regular narrow complex tachycardia around 170 to 250 b.p.m. AVRT is a paroxysmal arrhythmia and often requires ambulatory ECG monitoring to record it.

As AVRT is not associated with structural heart disease other investigations are rarely indicated.

MANAGEMENT AND PROGNOSIS

As with AVNRT, patients should be reassured that the tachycardia is not dangerous and the prognosis is good in the absence of any heart disease.

The treatment of acute AVRT is similar for AVNRT,[13] with vagal manoeuvres being first line, followed by adenosine. Prevention of recurrences is also similar to AVNRT with drug therapy escalating from BBs and CCBs to flecainide or sotalol.[13]

RF ablation has become the preferred treatment option for many patients with recurrent episodes of AVRT. It has high rates of cure, off all medications, and is low risk,[18] so all patients should be considered for this and referred accordingly.

Wolff–Parkinson–White syndrome

As mentioned above, WPW is the association of an AV conducting accessory pathway and tachycardias. The ECG incidence is about 1.5 per 1000,[13] with about 60 per cent having tachycardias, and it can present at almost any age. The majority of tachyarrhythmias occurring in WPW are AVRT as described above, but the ability of the pathway to conduct from atrium to ventricle enables other arrhythmias to occur. The resting ECG of ventricular pre-excitation shows a characteristic slurred beginning of the QRS complex, known as the delta wave (see Figure 6.11). This ECG appearance is due to activation of the ventricles via the accessory pathway as well as the normal His–Purkinje system.

Figure 6.11 ○ **Ventricular pre-excitation**

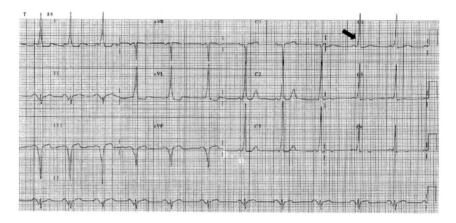

Note: This ECG shows a short PR interval with a slurred upstroke (delta wave, arrow) to the QRS, easily seen in the chest leads.

AF AND WPW

Patients with WPW also have an increased incidence of AF.[19] Unlike the AV node, the accessory pathway does not delay conduction between the atrium and ventricle, and some pathways are capable of very rapid conduction. During AF the atrial rate is often up to 600 b.p.m. and this can be conducted to the ventricles by the pathway resulting in ventricular rates higher than would normally be seen in AF without WPW. If the pathway is very rapidly conducting, there is a risk of ventricular fibrillation and sudden death. This is rare, with an estimated frequency of 0.1 per cent.[13]

TREATMENT OF WPW

Patients with pre-excitation on ECG but without symptoms of tachycardia may not require any treatment.[20] Acute AVRT in WPW should be treated as standard AVRT, but it should be noted that AF may occur after termination of AVRT, particularly if adenosine is used. It may have a rapid ventricular response, so full resuscitation facilities should be available. Acute treatment of AF in WPW can include flecainide and amiodarone, but AV nodal blocking drugs such as digoxin or verapamil must be avoided as they may facilitate rapid ventricular activation via the pathway. Often, electrical cardioversion is the *initial* treatment of AF in WPW.

RF ablation in WPW is highly successful and low risk, so should be considered for all patients with tachyarrhythmias in WPW.[20]

Ventricular tachycardias

VT is defined as the occurrence of three or more consecutive beats originating in the ventricle. *Sustained* VT refers to a VT that persists for 30 seconds or more, with shorter episodes being called *non-sustained* VT. Depending on the particular type of VT, rates can vary from 70 to 250 b.p.m. The QRS morphologies, the durations of which exceed 120 msec, may all be identical (monomorphic) or different (polymorphic).

PRESENTATION

The symptoms experienced during an episode of VT depend on the rate of the VT but also on the presence and extent of underlying heart disease. Slower episodes of sustained VT in normal hearts can be almost asymptomatic, whilst others may be haemodynamically unstable, resulting in circulatory collapse, or rapidly degenerate into ventricular fibrillation.

CAUSES

The commonest cause of VT in the Western world is ischaemic heart disease, both acutely due to myocardial ischaemia and chronically due to ventricular scar formation. There are a number of specific types of VT occurring in normal hearts or in the presence of ion channel abnormalities. The main causes and types of VT are shown in Table 6.3 (see p. 180), but the detailed discussion of many of these is beyond the scope of this chapter.

Table 6.3 ○ *Different types of VT*

Associated with structural heart disease	No overt structural heart disease
Acute myocardial ischaemia	Idiopathic VT (including RVOT VT)
Prior MI (scar VT)	Drug induced
Cardiomyopathy (dilated or hypertrophic)	Catecholaminergic polymorphic VT
ARVD	Brugada syndrome
Congenital heart disease (e.g. Fallot's tetralogy)	Fascicular VT
Myocarditis	Long QT syndrome

Notes: ARVD = arrhythmogenic right ventricular dysplasia; RVOT = right ventricular outflow tract.

ECG AND OTHER INVESTIGATIONS

The ECG of VT is that of a broad QRS complex tachycardia (see Figure 6.12). The rate may be regular or irregular and the QRS morphologies identical or different. The differentiation of VT from an SVT with aberrant conduction is often the source of much consternation for physicians of all grades, but it should be remembered that the commonest cause of a broad complex tachycardia is VT, even more so if there is a past history of ischaemic heart disease. Table 6.4 lists some of the ECG features that aid in the diagnosis.

Figure 6.12 ○ *Ventricular tachycardia*

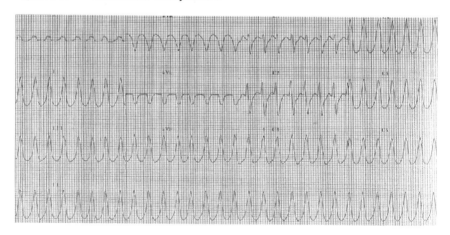

Note: ECG shows a broad, complex, regular tachycardia.

The ECG in sinus rhythm is also invaluable as it can provide other clues, such as the presence of a Brugada-type pattern, long QT interval or evidence of prior myocardial infarction.

Echocardiography is useful in the detection of structural heart disease, but also in the risk stratification and management of certain VTs. This is because a reduced left ventricular ejection fraction has been shown to be associated with a worse prognosis and is integral in all international guidelines on the use of implantable cardioverter defibrillators (ICDs).

Investigations to look for potential reversible triggers for the VT should also be undertaken, e.g. hypokalaemia or hypomagnesaemia, myocardial ischaemia or bradyarrhythmias, as well as stopping any arrhythmogenic drugs.

In certain cases electrophysiological testing may also be useful. This can aid the diagnostic process when there is doubt as to the nature of the arrhythmia, but can also be used to map the ectopic focus of the VT so that RF ablation can be considered, when indicated. The precise role of electrophysiological testing in the risk stratification of VT remains uncertain.

181

Table 6.4 ○ *Features differentiating VT from SVT with aberrancy*

Favours VT	Favours SVT
Fusion beats	Slowing with vagal manoeuvres
Capture beats	Termination with adenosine
AV dissociation	Onset with a premature P-wave

MANAGEMENT AND PROGNOSIS

As VT can be a malignant arrhythmia, acute VT is best managed in hospital. Chronic VT management is often complex, requiring joint care from the specialist and the GP.

Acute management[21]

Sustained VT with haemodynamic instability, heart failure or causing angina should be terminated urgently with synchronised DC cardioversion followed by measures to prevent recurrence. Stable, sustained VT can initially be treated pharmacologically with antiarrhythmics such as amiodarone or lignocaine. Lignocaine is significantly negatively inotropic and can convert stable VT to haemodynamically unstable VT, particularly in the setting of poor LV function. Amiodarone is effective with little impact on haemodynamics, but does not have a rapid onset of action. Any reversible factors should also be addressed to prevent recurrence.

Long-term management[21]

The goal of long-term treatment is to prevent sudden cardiac death and minimise the recurrence of symptomatic VT. Certain specific VTs in structurally normal hearts are associated with a good prognosis and if asymptomatic may require no treatment. However, as the majority occur in the context of underlying heart disease most VTs will require some treatment in the form of drugs, ICDs or both. Patients should ideally be managed by cardiac electrophysiologists.

DRUG TREATMENT

This includes beta-blockers and amiodarone as the main agents of choice. These can be used alone or in combination in patients with structural heart disease, and are given in preference to other agents. Class Ic drugs, such as flecainide, should be avoided in patients with structural heart disease due to their proarrhythmic effects.

ICDS

There have been numerous trials conducted into the use of ICDs for both primary and secondary prevention of VT and sudden cardiac death.[3] These studies generally concluded that ICD combined with medical therapy was better than medical therapy alone in patients with impaired left ventricular function, as it was this impaired function that was the strongest predictor of sudden cardiac death. The current guidelines from NICE on the use of ICDs are shown below:[22]

Primary prevention

Patients must have had a previous MI ≥4 weeks ago and:
> *either*

left ventricular ejection fraction (LVEF) <35 per cent with New York Heart Association (NYHA) class < IV
> *and*

non-sustained ventricular tachycardia (NSVT) on ambulatory monitoring
> *and*

inducible VT on electrophysiological testing

or

LVEF < 30 per cent with NYHA class < IV

and

QRS > 120 msec

Also, patients with a familial cardiac condition with a high risk of sudden death, including long QT syndrome, hypertrophic cardiomyopathy, Brugada syndrome or ARVD, or have undergone surgical repair of congenital heart disease qualify for ICD.

Secondary prevention

ICDs are indicated for patients who present with one of the following, provided no reversible cause is found:

▷ cardiac arrest due to VT or ventricular fibrillation (VF)
▷ spontaneous sustained VT with syncope/haemodynamic compromise
▷ sustained VT without syncope/arrest and LVEF < 35 per cent with NYHA class < IV.

In patients who have received an ICD and continue to have episodes of sustained VT, drug treatment is often used to try and suppress the arrhythmias and prevent defibrillation.

RF ablation for VT has good success rates for some VTs in structurally normal hearts, but does not perform as well in scar-related VT. However, with advanced techniques, the ablation of scar VT to reduce episodes and complement ICD therapy is being undertaken.[23]

The treatment of VTs and the use of ICDs require a multidisciplinary team approach, involving hospital specialists and arrhythmia nurses, as well as GPs and practice nurses, as the psychosocial impact of these potentially life-threatening arrhythmias can sometimes be overlooked.

Specific VTs

Idiopathic VT

This often arises from the RVOT with characteristic ECG appearance. It can be induced by exercise or stress, often in young people. However, it responds well to beta-blockers or RF ablation, and the prognosis is usually good.

Arrhythmogenic right ventricular dysplasia

This is cardiomyopathy involving the right ventricle, best detected with MRI. It is sometimes familial and can present in childhood or as an adult. VT is best treated with ICD, with or without drugs. Prognosis is usually poor if left untreated.

Brugada syndrome

Most cases of Brugada syndrome are due to sodium channel mutation and can run in families. Resting ECG can be diagnostic or may need flecainide challenge. The syndrome tends to present with VF, so the only effective treatment is ICD.

Conclusions

There is a wide variety of arrhythmias that can affect patients of all ages. In general, younger patients with no structural heart disease tend to have more benign arrhythmias, and older patients with known heart disease are more likely to have more concerning arrhythmias. Benign arrhythmias may still, however, be highly symptomatic and significantly impact an individual's lifestyle, whilst some potentially life-threatening VTs occur barely unnoticed by the patient.

Management of arrhythmias is often better done by joint care with a specialist and should not only focus on the diagnosis and treatment of the electrical abnormality, but also on educating the patient about his or her diagnosis, treatment options, likely long-term outcomes and providing reassurance where possible, as most arrhythmias produce high levels of anxiety in patients and their families.

Case-based discussion

> ### Box 6.3 ○ *Case scenario*
>
> A 70-year-old man presents to the surgery complaining of 'funny turns'. He describes several episodes over the past few weeks when he has suddenly felt light-headed and dizzy. He has not lost consciousness. He does not have any ear symptoms. He has felt tired recently and his daily walk to the local shop has felt like hard work. He has no chest pain or palpitations. Today, however, he has become more unwell, feeling dizzy for most of the day and getting breathless walking around the house. He is just on his way to pick up flowers to give his wife for their fiftieth wedding anniversary. He is keen to get back home as soon as he has seen you.
>
> He has a past medical history of myocardial infarction 10 years ago. His current medications are aspirin 75 mg o.d., simvastatin 40 mg nocte, bisoprolol 5 mg o.d. and perindopril 2 mg o.d. He lives at home with his wife and she is worried about what might be causing these funny turns. She relies on him for everything as she is housebound due to arthritis.
>
> On examination, he is alert with no pallor. Pulse rate is 45 b.p.m.; regular BP 105/75. His heart sounds normal, there are no murmurs and his chest is clear. There is no ankle swelling.

What are the issues in this case? What is the differential diagnosis? What investigations might you perform?

You explain to the patient that he has a low pulse rate and, whilst you understand he wants to get home to his wife, suggest he has an ECG done by the nurse first of all.

His ECG is shown below:

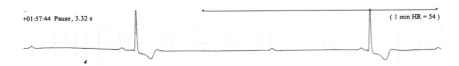

+01:57:44 Pause, 3.32 s   (1 min HR = 54)

What is the diagnosis? What is the appropriate next step?

The ECG shows complete heart block. The patient is admitted to the medical assessment unit of your local hospital by ambulance. His bisoprolol is stopped, a temporary pacing wire is inserted and he is referred urgently for permanent pacemaker insertion. He is discharged one week later and is able to return to his usual daily routine of walking to the local shops and caring for his wife.

Practising holistically

There are several issues raised by this case. This is an older man who is a carer for his wife. He was fit and well before the funny turns started. He is on appropriate secondary prevention following a myocardial infarction. He is bradycardic on examination but asymptomatic with an adequate blood pressure. Further investigations are warranted but the patient is keen to return home to his wife.

Data gathering and interpretation/Making a diagnosis/Making decisions

This patient has symptoms and signs of bradycardia. This may be due to the beta-blockers he takes but could also be due to ischaemic heart disease or idiopathic fibrosis. The ECG shows third-degree heart block.

Clinical management

This patient has a very low pulse rate with symptoms, so an urgent ECG is required. This shows complete heart block, which requires urgent treatment in secondary care. For patients presenting less acutely, in addition to an ECG, blood tests to exclude hypothyroidism and anaemia would also be helpful. In the first instance the beta-blocker should be stopped and referral for further management will depend on the ECG finding.

Managing medical complexity and promoting health

There are many reasons why older people may have dizziness or funny turns, so the differential is wide. Neurological and otological causes should also be considered. However, the history of presyncope in the presence of pre-existing ischaemic heart disease, rate-limiting medication and a low pulse rate should point to bradycardia as a probable cause of this patient's symptoms. The case is made more complex by the social dimension and the patient's desire to get back to his wife at home. This should be weighed up against the need for prompt investigation.

Working with colleagues and in teams

The nurse in the practice performed an ECG and blood tests. When the patient presented acutely unwell, the help of the ambulance service and acute medical team was required. Cardiologists were also involved to provide definitive treatment with insertion of a permanent pacemaker.

Community orientation

This patient is a carer for his wife. It is important that the healthcare system provides timely, definitive treatment to allow this patient to return home and continue his role as carer and prevent use of costly social services. This is in the interests of best using finite resources within the health and social care economy.

Maintaining an ethical approach

Do no harm ▶ appropriate emergency treatment was arranged when the patient presented acutely unwell to prevent further deterioration.

Autonomy ▶ this patient required appropriate investigation. With hindsight an ECG on the day of the initial consultation may have been helpful. However, the patient was adamant he needed to leave to get back to his wife at home.

Justice ▶ appropriate insertion of a pacemaker in this patient helped to return him to full health and continue his role as carer for his wife.

Beneficence ▶ the patient benefited from urgent transfer and pacemaker insertion to prevent further life-threatening complications such as asystole.

Fitness to practise

The doctor in this case put the patient as his first concern. He acted in a holistic manner to ensure the safe treatment of the patient and worked with colleagues to ensure a good outcome.

References

1 • Zipes DP, Garson A, Jr. 26th Bethesda conference: recommendations for determining eligibility for competition in athletes with cardiovascular abnormalities. Task Force 6: arrhythmias *Medicine and Science in Sports and Exercise* 1994; **26(10 Suppl)**: S276–83.

2 • Kennedy HL. Use of long-term (Holter) electrocardiographic recordings. In: DP Zipes, J Jalife (eds). *Cardiac Electrophysiology: from cell to bedside*. pp. 716–30. Philadelphia: WB Saunders, 2000.

3 • Epstein AE, Dimarco JP, Ellenbogen KA, *et al*. ACC/AHA/HRS 2008 guidelines for device-based therapy of cardiac rhythm abnormalities: executive summary *Heart Rhythm* 2008; **5(6)**: 934–55.

4 • Mymin D, Mathewson FA, Tate RB, *et al*. The natural history of primary first-degree atrioventricular heart block *New England Journal of Medicine* 1986; **315(19)**: 1183–7.

5 • Strasberg B, Amat YLF, Dhingra RC, *et al.* Natural history of chronic second-degree atrioventricular nodal block *Circulation* 1981; **63(5)**: 1043–9.

6 • Michaelsson M, Jonzon A, Riesenfeld T. Isolated congenital complete atrioventricular block in adult life. A prospective study *Circulation* 1995; **92(3)**: 442–9.

7 • Sholler GF, Walsh EP. Congenital complete heart block in patients without anatomic cardiac defects *American Heart Journal* 1989; **118(6)**: 1193–8.

8 • Olgin JE. Inappropriate sinus tachycardia and sinus node reentry. In: DP Zipes, J Jalife (eds). *Cardiac Electrophysiology: from cell to bedside.* pp. 459–68. Philadelphia: WB Saunders, 2000.

9 • Olgin JE, Miles W. Ablation of atrial tachycardias. In: I Singor, S Barold, A Camm (eds). *Nonpharmacological Therapy of Arrhythmias for the 21st Century: the state of the art.* pp. 197–217. Mount Kisco, NY: Futura; 1998.

10 • Kalman JM, Olgin JE, Saxon LA, *et al.* Activation and entrainment mapping defines the tricuspid annulus as the anterior barrier in typical atrial flutter *Circulation* 1996; **94(3)**: 398–406.

11 • Camm AJ, Obel OA. Epidemiology and mechanism of atrial fibrillation and atrial flutter *American Journal of Cardiology* 1996; **78(8A)**: 3–11.

12 • Lip GY, Kamath S. Thromboprophylaxis for atrial flutter *European Heart Journal* 2001; **22(12)**: 984–7.

13 • Blomstrom-Lundqvist C, Scheinman MM, Aliot EM, *et al.* ACC/AHA/ESC guidelines for the management of patients with supraventricular arrhythmias – executive summary. A report of the American College of Cardiology/American Heart Association Task Force on Practice Guidelines and the European Society of Cardiology Committee for Practice Guidelines (Writing Committee to Develop Guidelines for the Management of Patients with Supraventricular Arrhythmias) developed in collaboration with NASPE-Heart Rhythm Society *Journal of the American College of Cardiology* 2003; **42(8)**: 1493–531.

14 • Natale A, Newby KH, Pisano E, *et al.* Prospective randomized comparison of antiarrhythmic therapy versus first-line radiofrequency ablation in patients with atrial flutter *Journal of the American College of Cardiology* 2000; **35(7)**: 1898–904.

15 • Jazayeri MR, Hempe SL, Sra JS, *et al.* Selective transcatheter ablation of the fast and slow pathways using radiofrequency energy in patients with atrioventricular nodal reentrant tachycardia *Circulation* 1992; **85(4)**: 1318–28.

16 • Scheinman MM, Huang S. The 1998 NASPE prospective catheter ablation registry *Pacing and Clinical Electrophysiology* 2000; **23(6)**: 1020–8.

17 • Kwaku KF, Josephson ME. Typical AVNRT – an update on mechanisms and therapy *Cardiac Electrophysiology Review* 2002; **6(4)**: 414–21.

18 • Calkins H, Yong P, Miller JM, *et al.* Catheter ablation of accessory pathways, atrioventricular nodal reentrant tachycardia, and the atrioventricular junction: final results of a prospective, multicenter clinical trial. The Atakr Multicenter Investigators Group *Circulation* 1999; **99(2)**: 262–70.

19 • Sharma AD, Klein GJ, Guiraudon GM, *et al.* Atrial fibrillation in patients with Wolff–Parkinson–White syndrome: incidence after surgical ablation of the accessory pathway *Circulation* 1985; **72(1)**: 161–9.

20 • Tischenko A, Fox DJ, Yee R, *et al.* When should we recommend catheter ablation for patients with the Wolff–Parkinson–White syndrome? *Current Opinion in Cardiology* 2008; **23(1)**: 32–7.

21 • Zipes DP, Camm AJ, Borggrefe M, *et al*. ACC/AHA/ESC 2006 guidelines for management of patients with ventricular arrhythmias and the prevention of sudden cardiac death – executive summary: a report of the American College of Cardiology/ American Heart Association Task Force and the European Society of Cardiology Committee for Practice Guidelines (Writing Committee to Develop Guidelines for Management of Patients with Ventricular Arrhythmias and the Prevention of Sudden Cardiac Death) developed in collaboration with the European Heart Rhythm Association and the Heart Rhythm Society *European Heart Journal* 2006; **27(17)**: 2099–140.

22 • National Institute for Health and Clinical Excellence. *Implantable Cardioverter Defibrillators (ICDs) for arrhythmias* London: NICE, 2006, www.nice.org.uk/nicemedia/pdf/ TA095publicinfo.pdf [accessed September 2010].

23 • Aliot EM, Stevenson WG, Almendral-Garrote JM, *et al*. EHRA/HRS expert consensus on catheter ablation of ventricular arrhythmias: developed in a partnership with the European Heart Rhythm Association (EHRA), a registered branch of the European Society of Cardiology (ESC), and the Heart Rhythm Society (HRS); in collaboration with the American College of Cardiology (ACC) and the American Heart Association (AHA) *Heart Rhythm* 2009; **6(6)**: 886–933.

189

Atrial fibrillation

David Fitzmaurice, F.D. Richard Hobbs and Clare J. Taylor

7

Aims

The aim of this chapter is to discuss the epidemiology of atrial fibrillation (AF), the complications, in particular the risk of stroke, and the evidence for effective treatments in reducing stroke risk. We will also address the issue of rate versus rhythm control for patients with AF.

Key learning points

▶ AF is a common disorder that increases with age.
▶ Stroke risk is increased five-fold for patients with AF.
▶ Opportunistic pulse checks help to improve detection of AF in primary care.
▶ An electrocardiogram (ECG) interpreted by an appropriately trained individual should be used to confirm the diagnosis of AF.
▶ Rate- and rhythm-controlling medications can be used to reduce symptoms but are associated with side effects.
▶ Effective treatments such as warfarin exist to reduce stroke risk in patients with AF.
▶ Recent evidence shows warfarin use in stroke prevention is effective and safe in the over-75 age group.

Introduction

AF is a common arrhythmia that increases with age.[1] Patients are often asymptomatic but may present with symptoms such as palpitations, or an irregularly irregular pulse may be found during routine examination. AF is an important independent risk factor for thromboembolic disease – particularly stroke, where it indicates a five-fold increase in risk.[2] Rate- and rhythm-controlling medications can be used to manage symptoms, although these can have significant side effects. Anticoagulation can reduce the risk of stroke in moderate-to high-risk patients. The GP is well placed to identify patients with AF, ensure appropriate thromboprophylaxis and liaise with secondary care regarding rate or rhythm control where necessary.

Interestingly, it was a GP (called James MacKenzie) who was responsible for first describing an irregularly irregular pulse – which he named 'auricular fibrillation' – and the University of Birmingham (where all three authors of this chapter are based) was associated with the discovery of digoxin (see Box 7.1).

Box 7.1 ○ *A history of AF – discovery, treatments and the role of general practice research*

James MacKenzie was born in 1853 and trained as a pharmacist in Scotland before studying medicine. He moved to Burnley, Lancashire, in 1879 where he practised as a GP for 28 years. He found the lack of scientific explanation for patients' symptoms that existed at the time very troubling, and so began research in his practice population. He invented a machine called the polygraph that could record the waves of the venous pulsation and was a precursor to the electrocardiogram. In 1890, he identified extrasystoles and, in 1897, he described the irregularly irregular pulsations of auricular fibrillation (now called atrial fibrillation). He moved to London in 1907 as a visiting consultant and became a fellow of the Royal Society in 1915, then 4 years later moved to St Andrews to establish an institute for general practice research. He died in 1925, having suffered from angina for many years.

William Withering was born in Shropshire in 1741 and trained in Edinburgh before moving to Birmingham, establishing a medical practice in rural Shropshire and working at Birmingham General Hospital. He noted that patients with 'dropsy' (what is now known as heart failure) significantly improved when given foxglove extract by herbalists. The active ingredient was digitalis and Withering recognised the importance of dosage, identifying common side effects such as nausea, vomiting and yellow vision in patients receiving too much of the drug. Years later, MacKenzie developed a simple regime for prescribing digoxin to his patients that reduced the risk of overdose.

Further reading

□ Haslam DA. Who cares? The James MacKenzie Lecture 2006 *British Journal of General Practice* 2007; **57(545)**: 987–93.

□ Hobbs FDR. James MacKenzie lecture 2008: clinical burden and health service challenges of chronic heart failure *British Journal of General Practice* 2010; **60(57)**: 611–15.

□ Lee MR. William Withering (1741–1799): a Birmingham Lunatic *Proceedings of the Royal College of Physicians of Edinburgh* 2001; **31**: 77–83.

□ Roland M. Quality and efficiency: enemies or partners. The James MacKenzie Lecture 1998 *British Journal of General Practice* 1999; **49(439)**: 140–3.

Epidemiology of atrial fibrillation

Prevalence data for AF have been notoriously difficult to ascertain, with estimates of between 5 and 10 per cent in the population aged 65 and over. A review of four large community-based studies of AF suggested that the overall community prevalence in the US is 0.89 per cent.[3] In these studies, the prevalence increased sharply with age: 2.3 per cent of people aged 40 or over; 5.9 per cent of people aged over 65, and 10 per cent of those over 80. The vast majority (84 per cent) of people with AF are over the age of 65. The incidence of new cases of AF in people over the age of 65 is of the order of 1 per cent per annum.[4] The best UK data give a prevalence of 7.2 per cent for patients aged 65 and over.[5] AF is a particularly important risk factor for stroke in the elderly – while 15 per cent of all strokes are associated with the arrhythmia, it is associated with 36 per cent of strokes in people over the age of 80. The prevalence of AF is higher in men at all ages, although because of unequal death rates the overall number of patients with AF is approximately equal between the sexes. In overall terms, approximately 50 per cent of patients with AF are 75 or over, and over half of these are women.

Definitions of AF

AF can be considered in terms of duration and reversibility. There are three main categories in general use:[6]

▷ **paroxysmal AF** ▶ AF that spontaneously terminates in less than 7 days (most often less than 48 hours) and may be recurrent
▷ **persistent AF** ▶ AF that does not self-terminate and lasts >7 days or is present prior to cardioversion
▷ **permanent AF** ▶ AF that is not terminated by cardioversion or is terminated but relapses within 24 hours. Also can be longstanding AF (usually >1 year) where cardioversion has not been attempted.

AF and risk of stroke

The Framingham study identified atrial fibrillation as an independent risk factor for stroke, even in the absence of mitral valve disease (non-valvular atrial fibrillation).[2] This form of atrial fibrillation may be referred to as non-rheumatic atrial fibrillation (NRAF). In considering prophylaxis against stroke, the relative risk for stroke associated with NRAF must be of primary consideration, given that antithrombotic medication carries its own risks. The Whitehall study[7] and the British Heart Study[8] confirmed the increased risk of stroke associated with NRAF. However, the relative risks differed somewhat, as did the underlying rate of stroke within the control population (see Table 7.1 on p. 200).[9]

Table 7.1 ○ *Relative risk of stroke associated with NRAF*

| | Rate of stroke per 1000 person years | | | |
Cohort	No AF or rheumatic heart disease	NRAF (95% CI)	Excess rate (range) attributable to NRAF	Relative risk (95% CI)
Framingham	2.9	42 (25–64)	39 (23–61)	5.6 (3.4–8.4)
Whitehall	0.9	14 (5–23)	13 (4–23)	6.9 (3–13.5)
British Heart	1.6	3 (0.1–22)	2 (0–21)	2.3 (0.1–12.7)

Multivariate analysis[1] revealed the following as significant additional risk factors in prediction of stroke for patients with NRAF:

▷ **age** ▶ the annual risk of stroke in control patients younger than 65 with no other risk factors was 1.0 per cent. This increased to 8.1 per cent for patients older than 75 with one or more other risk factor. Warfarin reduced the risk of stroke in all subgroups except those less than 60 with no other risk factors in whom the incidence of stroke was < 1 per cent
▷ **history of hypertension** ▶ this gives a relative risk (RR) of stroke = 1.6 (95 per cent CI 1.3–2.8)
▷ **history of diabetes** ▶ RR = 1.7 (1.2–3.6)
▷ **history of prior stroke or transient ischaemic attack** ▶ RR = 2.5 (1.2–5.3).
▷ **history of myocardial infarction** ▶ RR = 1.7 (1.1–2.7)
▷ **history of congestive heart failure** ▶ RR = 1.7 (1.1–2.5).

Paroxysmal atrial fibrillation was found not to confer increased risk of stroke, although the number of patients who reverted from paroxysmal to persistent fibrillation could not be calculated. It is likely that the thrombotic risk of paroxysmal atrial fibrillation is related to the frequency and duration of paroxysms and the presence of associated factors such as structural heart disease or hypertension.[10] In clinical practice the risk of stroke is assumed to be constant between paroxysmal and persistent atrial fibrillation. The presence of angina was found within individual studies to be a risk factor. However, the significance of this factor was lost within the multivariate analysis and may be a coincidental finding due to the increasing prevalence of angina with age.

The use of effective antithrombotic agents in NRAF aims to prevent systemic embolism, particularly to the brain. The following sections provide data on: the case for screening for AF in the population over 65; which patients with NRAF would benefit from some form of prophylaxis against embolic stroke; the risk and benefits associated with antiplatelet therapy as opposed to oral anticoagulation therapy; and the optimal intensities of therapy for warfarin treatment.

Screening for atrial fibrillation

The elderly were until recently the most controversial population with regard to oral anticoagulant therapy. In the UK the Screening for Atrial Fibrillation in the Elderly (SAFE) study demonstrated a prevalence of 7.2 per cent in a population aged 65 and over, with a 10.3 per cent prevalence in those aged over 75.[5]

Screening for AF in the elderly fulfils many of the Wilson–Jungner criteria for a screening programme.[11] It is a common and important condition that can be diagnosed by means of a simple test (ECG), and the risk of serious sequelae such as stroke can be dramatically reduced by treatment.

Healthcare costs associated with atrial fibrillation

Approximately 5 per cent of total NHS expenditure can be attributed to stroke, and there would be expected to be about 1000 new cases of stroke per annum in a typical health authority with a half million population. Therefore, any programme that might lead to an important reduction in stroke incidence needs serious consideration, both because of the potential for health gain, and the potential for reduced overall NHS expenditure. Screening for AF might be one such programme since, in population terms, AF is an important risk factor for stroke (associated with 15 per cent of all strokes) and anticoagulation provides a highly effective treatment to reduce this risk. It has been estimated that optimal treatment of AF in the population might reduce the overall incidence of stroke by 10 per cent. However, before implementing screening programmes, unresolved questions over how the screening should be conducted must be answered.

Identifying cases of atrial fibrillation

The SAFE study aimed to elucidate both the epidemiology of AF and also the optimal screening strategy.[5] This large-scale, multicentred, randomised, controlled trial utilised fifty UK primary care centres, with random allocation to twenty-five intervention and twenty-five control practices. Intervention practice patients were randomly allocated to systematic or opportunistic screening. Opportunistic screening comprised pulse taking and ECG if the pulse was irregular. The principal outcome measure was screened AF detection rates compared with the detection rate in routine care. Screening took place for 12 months per practice between October 2001 and February 2003. The study included: 4936 controls; 4933 opportunistic screenings of patients; and 4933 systematic screenings of patients. In control practices the baseline prevalence of AF was 7.9 per cent compared with 6.9 per cent in intervention practices. The SAFE study identified the following:

▷ 47 new cases of AF (incidence 1.04 per cent/year) were identified in routine practice (control)

▷ 243 opportunistically screened patients had irregular pulse; 77 had ECG, yielding 31 new cases (0.69 per cent/year); 44 cases were detected outside screening (total 1.64 per cent/year)

▷ 2357 systematic patients had ECG, yielding 52 new cases (1.1 per cent/year); 22 further cases were detected outside screening (total 1.62 per cent/year).

The principal conclusion from the SAFE study was that active screening will identify an additional third of cases of AF. Opportunistic screening identified as many of these cases as systematic screening for considerably less effort, and should be promoted in primary care as long as a high level of coverage can be maintained.

Thromboprophylaxis for atrial fibrillation

Oral anticoagulants (predominantly warfarin in the UK) and antiplatelet agents are used to reduce the risk of stroke in patients with AF. The evidence for warfarin and aspirin in terms of safety and effectiveness in reducing stroke risk is discussed below. The decision regarding which treatment to choose ultimately depends on both clinician views and patient preferences. There are several stroke risk stratification algorithms and tools that can be used to assist in this decision.

Risk and benefits of warfarin

Eight randomised studies were published in the 1980s and 1990s [12-19] that informed the debate over the selection of patients for oral anticoagulation, the relative merits of anticoagulation versus antiplatelet agents, and the risk stratification for patients with AF with and without other risk factors for stroke. The relative risk reduction for warfarin compared with placebo is shown in Table 7.2.

Table 7.2 ○ **Relative risk reduction of thromboembolism from warfarin compared with placebo for patients with NRAF**

Study	Annual event rate (%)		Relative risk reduction of warfarin (%)
	Placebo	*Warfarin*	
AFASAK [12]	4.8	1.4	71
BAATAF [14]	2.9	0.4	86
SPAF I [13]	7.4	2.3	67
CAFA [15]	3.7	2.1	43
VETS [17]	4.3	0.9	79
EAFT [16]	17	8.0	53

These studies were all based in secondary care and caution is needed in extrapolating the data for primary care patients, particularly given the highly selected populations chosen for investigation.[20] Despite excluding up to 97 per cent of potentially eligible patients,[13] there remained a large percentage of patient withdrawals in all trials. The highest withdrawal rate occurred within the study that utilised a population most similar to that found in primary care.[12]

Interpreting the results of these studies is also problematic, as different levels of anticoagulant intensity were employed and actual levels of intensity achieved were either not stated or not subject to direct comparison (using prothrombin ratios rather than international normalised ratio, INR). Meta-analysis of the five primary prevention studies covered 1889 patient-years for those receiving warfarin and 1802 in the control group.[9] For the aspirin–placebo comparison there were 1132 patient-years receiving aspirin and 1133 receiving placebo. The primary endpoints were ischaemic stroke and major haemorrhage, as assessed by each study.

Patients within the control groups who gave no history of transient ischaemic attack (TIA) or stroke, hypertension or congestive heart failure, diabetes, angina or myocardial infarction had an annual incidence of stroke of 1.5 per cent.

Warfarin was found to be consistently effective for the prevention of ischaemic stroke, with a reduction in the incidence of all strokes of 68 per cent (95 per cent CI, 50 per cent to 79 per cent), representing an absolute annual reduction of 3.1 per cent ($p<0.001$). This risk reduction has to be viewed in the light of a reported low incidence of side effects, particularly haemorrhagic stroke, which may represent selection bias. The absolute reduction in risk, however, may have been underestimated as the analysis was performed on an intention-to-treat basis, when in fact eight of the twenty-seven patients in the warfarin group who had a stroke were not receiving warfarin at the time. Warfarin decreased the rate of death by 33 per cent (95 CI, 9 per cent to 51 per cent; $p=0.10$) and the rate of the combined outcome of stroke, systemic embolism, or death by 48 per cent (95 per cent CI, 34 per cent to 60 per cent; $p<0.001$).

Warfarin or aspirin for NRAF?

Four studies randomised patients to receive aspirin.[12,13,16,18] The Danish AFASAK trial,[12] using a 75 mg per day dose, showed a non-statistical reduction in stroke rate when compared with placebo. The SPAF study,[13] however, showed a reduction of 44 per cent (95 per cent CI, 7 per cent to 66 per cent) in the incidence of stroke at a dose of 325 mg per day. Meta-analysis of these studies[18] confirmed that oral anticoagulation is twice as effective as aspirin therapy for the prevention of ischaemic stroke in AF patients. Furthermore, the beneficial effects of aspirin do not appear to be dose related.[21]

The EAFT study[16] was a secondary prevention study and used aspirin at a dose of 300 mg per day compared with warfarin or placebo. No statistically significant reduction in thromboembolic disease was observed in the aspirin-treated group when compared with placebo, with warfarin achieving statistically significant improvement. Treatment with aspirin or other platelet inhibitors may have benefits in terms of safety, cost, and convenience (no need for regular blood tests), but from the current evidence aspirin alone is substantially less effective in stroke prevention for patients with AF when compared with warfarin.

In combination with warfarin, aspirin has little role to play in the prevention of stroke for patients with AF, as shown by the SPAF III study.[19] In this study, 1044 patients with AF and at least one other risk factor for thromboembolic disease were randomised to receive either warfarin to achieve a target INR of 2.0 to 3.0 or a fixed dose of warfarin to achieve an INR of 1.2 to 1.5 plus a fixed dose (325 mg) of aspirin. The study had to be discontinued after a mean follow-up period of 1.1 years because of the increased incidence of primary events (ischaemic stroke and systemic embolism) for patients given combination therapy. Furthermore, cost-effectiveness analysis using US data supports the view that warfarin is to be preferred to aspirin or no treatment in terms of quality-adjusted life years for all patients with NRAF.[22] Aspirin does appear to minimally increase the risk of haemorrhagic stroke. A meta-analysis of randomised, controlled trials using aspirin[23] found that, at a mean dose of 273 mg per day, there was an absolute risk increase in haemorrhagic stroke of twelve events per 10,000 people. This is incredibly small and must be weighed against the relative risk reductions of myocardial infarction (137 events per 10,000) and ischaemic stroke (39 events per 10,000).

Nevertheless, for patients with AF under 65 with no other risk factors, there is minimal benefit from warfarin as compared with no therapy, due to the low underlying risk of stroke. Treatment decisions ultimately depend on the patients' perception of the inconvenience and harm associated with taking warfarin.[22] Thus, whilst aspirin is an alternative to warfarin therapy it should be reserved only for those patients who genuinely cannot tolerate warfarin.

199

Stroke risk stratification

It is increasingly recognised that treatment decisions therefore need to be based on individual risk assessment. The NICE guideline in the UK includes a formal algorithm (see Figure 7.1 on p. 200), which is problematic in that the majority of patients are assessed as moderate risk and the recommendation is to use either oral anticoagulation or aspirin.[24] A more widely used assessment tool is the CHADS2 system, which gives a point each for congestive heart failure, hypertension, age greater than 75 and diabetes, and 2 points for a history of stroke or transient ischaemic attack, with risk of stroke increasing with the number of points acquired.[25] A CHADS2 score of 2 or more suggests warfarin is likely to be beneficial. While CHADS2 is simple to use, its predictive value is less than ideal and there are ongoing attempts to improve its efficacy. Patients should also be assessed for bleeding risk, which increases with CHADS2 score.

Thromboprophylaxis in the elderly

Until recently, the only area of major uncertainty over therapies was in patients over 75. There was concern that the bleeding risks with warfarin balanced out the benefits of treatment. This led to physician uncertainty over whether aspirin was a safer option in this population, though they

Figure 7.1 ○ *Stroke risk stratification algorithm*

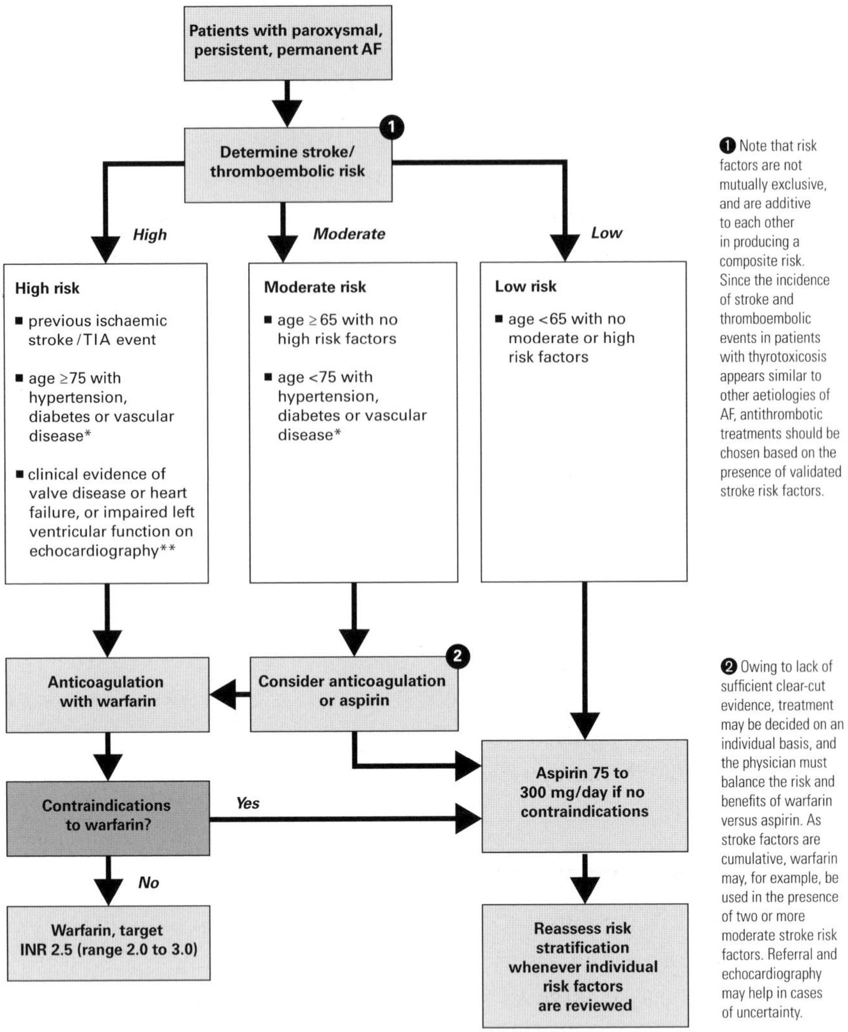

Source: National Institute for Health and Clinical Excellence. *Curriculum Guide 36, Atrial Fibrillation: the management of atrial fibrillation* London: NICE. Available from www.nice.org.uk/guidance/CG36. Quick reference guide. Reproduced with permission.[24]

Notes: *Coronary artery disease or peripheral artery disease. **An echocardiogram is not needed for routine assessment, but refines clinical risk stratification in the case of moderate or severe LV dysfunction and valve disease.

were perversely at greater risk of stroke, supported by a meta-analysis of *post-hoc* analyses of those over 75 from the warfarin versus aspirin trials.[26] Importantly, the BAFTA study has now also demonstrated that warfarin is 65 per cent more effective than aspirin in an elderly population (over-75s), with no difference in major haemorrhage rates.[27] These data make warfarin the single most effective therapeutic agent that we currently have for prophylaxis of stroke in AF.

The desired therapeutic range for oral anticoagulation in NRAF

The target level of anticoagulation (INR) in studies ranged between 1.2–1.5 and 2.8–4.2. It has been shown that the risk of stroke for patients with AF rises steeply below an INR of 2.0,[28] while the risk of haemorrhage increases rapidly at levels of INR greater than 4.0.[29] Interpretation of these data has been consistent with regard to the lower level of intensity recommended, with 2.0 being almost universally accepted.[30] The upper limit of intensity is more widely debated, ranging between 3.0 and 4.0. It may be argued that the aim is to keep INR below 4.0. However, this is unlikely to be successfully undertaken unless the *target* INR is set at 3.0, given the weaknesses associated with current models. Most guidelines now accept a target for INR of 2.5, giving a reasonable balance of efficacy and safety.[31]

Summary recommendations for thromboprophylaxis NRAF

As the evidence exists at present, all patients with AF should be considered for oral anticoagulation (with a target INR of 2.5), apart from those patients under 65 years of age with no other risk factors. Patients who cannot tolerate oral anticoagulation therapy should be considered for aspirin.

Future developments in anticoagulation

As the number of patients taking warfarin has increased the problems of regular monitoring and associated haemorrhagic events have led to the search for new agents targeted at more specific proteins in the coagulation cascade, such as Factor Xa and thrombin (Factor II). While none of these agents is currently licensed for use in AF, trial data is becoming available and is likely to lead to the licensing of new agents for thromboprophylaxis in AF for the first time in 60 years. For example, dabigatran, an oral direct thrombin inhibitor, has recently been investigated for use as thromboprophylaxis in patients with AF. The randomised evaluation of long-term anticoagulation therapy (RE-LY) study, which included over 18,000 patients, compared outcomes in patients with AF treated with warfarin (target INR 2.0–3.0), 110 mg dabigatran twice daily or 150 mg dabigatran twice daily. Patients in the higher dose of the dabigatran group had significantly lower rates of stroke and systemic embolism compared with the warfarin group. Rates of major haemorrhage were similar in the two groups. The lower dose of the dabigatran group had a lower rate of major haemorrhage compared with the warfarin group, but stroke and systemic embolism were similar in both groups.[31] At the time of writing, other clinical trials are underway to assess the effectiveness of other oral antithrombotic therapies. None of these agents is currently licensed for use in AF.

Rate versus rhythm control

Rate versus rhythm control in patients with atrial fibrillation is a subject of significant debate.[31] Conversion to sinus rhythm may be a reasonable therapeutic goal. However, rhythm control agents have significant side effects.[32] The latest guidance around rate and rhythm control treatments, as well as possible side effects and the role of cardioversion, is discussed below.

Rate control

The 2006 NICE guideline on AF recommends that patients over the age of 65 with coronary heart disease, contraindications to anti-arrhythmic drugs and those unsuitable for cardioversion are appropriate for treatment with rate-controlling medications. Beta-blockers or rate-limiting calcium channel blockers (CCBs) are first line with a treatment target of a heart rate less than 90 b.p.m. Digoxin can be added if rate control remains inadequate, and if this is ineffective then referral to secondary care for consideration of specialist pharmacological therapy or electrophysiological intervention may be appropriate.[24]

Beta-blockers have common side effects such as fatigue and are contraindicated in patients with asthma, bradycardia or uncontrolled heart failure. They can also worsen glycaemic control and mask hypoglycaemia in patients with diabetes.[33] CCBs may cause ankle swelling and cardiospecific CCBs such as verapamil can precipitate heart block if used with a beta-blocker.[34] Digoxin also has side effects including nausea, vomiting, yellow or blurred vision, and more rarely digoxin toxicity. Care should be taken in prescribing digoxin to patients with renal impairment.[35]

Rhythm control

Rhythm control is appropriate for patients who are younger, symptomatic, presenting for the first time with lone AF, where AF is secondary to a reversible precipitant or for those with heart failure.[34] Patients with persistent AF who are suitable for rhythm control may be considered for cardioversion. The evidence for the success of cardioversion is mixed and the role of car-

Table 7.3 ○ *Routine testing in patients receiving amiodarone*

Adverse effect	Test	Frequency
Arrhythmia	Electrocardiogram	At baseline Every 12 months
Hypo/hyperthyroidism	Thyroid function tests	At baseline Every 6 months
Hepatotoxicity	Liver function tests	At baseline Every 6 months
Pulmonary toxicity	Chest X-ray	At baseline Every 12 months
Ophthalmological disorders	Ophthalmological examination	At baseline if pre-existing visual impairment If symptoms occur

Source: Goldschlager N, Epstein AE, Naccarelli G, *et al*. Practical guidelines for clinicians who treat patients with amiodarone.[36]

dioversion in rhythm control is discussed in more detail in the next section. Anti-arrhythmic drugs may be used to maintain sinus rhythm after cardioversion or may be initiated to attempt to chemically cardiovert the patient. Standard beta-blockers can be used as first line. However, if this fails, different agents can be considered. Patients without structural heart disease can be offered a class 1c agent, such as flecainide or propafenone, or sotalol, which is a non-selective beta-blocker that also has class III anti-arrhythmic activity. Amiodarone may be considered for patients with structural heart disease but has significant potential side effects and is usually only initiated by a cardiologist.

Flecainide is now contraindicated in patients with structural heart disease as a result of the Cardiac Arrhythmia Suppression Trial (CAST) study, which found an increased mortality in patients with a history of myocardial infarction, and asymptomatic or mild ventricular arrhythmias in patients who were treated with flecainide.[37] Sotalol acts by slowing repolarisation leading to an increase in duration of the cardiac action potential, which can give rise to prolongation of the QT interval predisposing to ventricular arrhythmias.[38] Amiodarone is associated with several adverse events including pro-arrhythmic effects, thyroid disease, hepatotoxicity, pulmonary toxicity and ophthalmological disorders. Patients should be warned of these side effects before treatment is initiated and monitored regularly, as shown in Table 7.3.

Rhythm control in paroxysmal AF

Flecainide can also be used as 'pill-in-the-pocket' therapy for those with known paroxysmal AF. In this approach to treatment, patients with at least one episode of previous AF carry a dose of flecainide with them and take the medication at the onset of symptoms. This can be effective in terminating the arrhythmia.[39] Patients should have a resting heart rate above 70 b.p.m. and a systolic blood pressure above 100 mmHg, and should have a good understanding of how the drug should be used. If the patient is not suitable for the pill-in-the-pocket strategy, regular beta-blockers can be considered. If treatment fails, sotalol can be used for patients with coronary heart disease or flecainide for those without. If treatment then fails or the patient has heart failure, referral for consideration of electrophysiological treatment or amiodarone therapy may be appropriate.[34]

New developments

A new anti-arrhythmic drug to treat patients with AF called dronedarone has recently emerged. Dronedarone is structurally very similar to amiodarone but has less tissue accumulation and a shorter half-life. A recent randomised, controlled trial found that mortality and hospitalisation rates were less in patients receiving dronedarone than amiodarone. Adverse effects such as lung and thyroid disease were similar in both groups. However, there were significantly more reports of nausea, diarrhoea, bradycardia and prolonged QT syndrome in the dronedarone compared with the amiodarone group.[40]

Cardioversion – end of an era?

Direct electrical cardioversion has been a mainstay of therapy for the treatment of AF for many years. The theory underpinning its utilisation has some face validity, i.e. by restoring sinus rhythm any problems associated with AF will be ameliorated. This, however, does not take into account the underlying cause of the arrythmia, with the majority of AF caused by ischaemic heart disease. It is only relatively recently, however, that evidence for the ineffectiveness of cardioversion has begun to emerge. Paradoxically, this evidence has derived from trials designed to prove the effectiveness of the procedure.

The utility of cardioversion was originally explored in the AFFIRM study,[32] which recruited over 4000 patients aged 65 and over with atrial fibrillation and one additional risk factor for stroke. Patients were randomised to either rhythm control, using electrical cardioversion and medication as necessary, or to rate control using drugs such as beta-blockers or digoxin. To the surprise of the investigators the primary outcome, mortality, was worse in the rhythm control group, as were secondary outcomes such as hospitalisation and serious arrhythmias. Importantly, oral anticoagulation could be stopped at the clinician's discretion following cardioversion.

The AFFIRM investigators conducted a *post-hoc* treatment analysis that did show some survival advantage, if sinus rhythm was maintained.[41] The caveat to this was that use of anti-arrhythmic drugs was associated with increased mortality, and in fact the main predictor of survival was use of warfarin. This left even the AFFIRM investigators to conclude that any advantage from maintaining sinus rhythm through use of anti-arrhythmic agents was offset by their toxicity.

Despite the fact that these findings have been repeated in further studies,[42,43] and the problems associated with ensuring adequate oral anticoagulation prior to undertaking the intervention, cardioversion has remained a common intervention in patients with AF, particularly if there is associated co-morbidity such as heart failure. Roy and colleagues,[44] in trying to establish the efficacy of cardioversion for patients with AF and heart failure (defined as left ventricular ejection fraction of 35 per cent or less, or symptoms of congestive heart failure), recruited 1376 patients who were randomised to rhythm control, comprising cardioversion within 6 weeks of randomisation with additional cardioversions as necessary, or rate control with adjusted doses of beta-blockers with digoxin. There was no significant difference in primary outcome of death from cardiovascular causes, and no significant differences in secondary outcomes including death from any cause, stroke and worsening heart failure. The authors concluded that 'in patients with atrial fibrillation and congestive heart failure, a routine strategy of rhythm control does not reduce the rate of death from cardiovascular causes as compared with a rate-control strategy'.

Cardioversion therefore has no place in the routine treatment of AF, or in the treatment of high-risk patients. Cardioversion should no longer be offered routinely to patients with AF. The only clinical scenarios where it may be a useful intervention is for patients presenting acutely, within 24 hours of onset, or for patients who remain symptomatic despite medical therapy. Even in these instances, oral anticoagulation should be considered long term because of the high rate of recurrence.

Summary

AF is a common arrhythmia that is associated with an increased risk of stroke. Stroke risk assessment and appropriate thromboprophylaxis can reduce the risk of stroke. The choice of whether to use rate or rhythm-controlling medication should be made according to individual patient characteristics. Patients should be warned of potential adverse effects before initiating any medication. New drugs are emerging for the treatment of AF.

Self-assessment questions

1 ▷ A 76-year-old man with a history of hypertension attends the surgery for a routine blood pressure check. You struggle to get a blood pressure reading from the automated blood pressure machine. When you check his pulse you find it to be irregularly irregular. What would be your next course of action?

   a. Start warfarin.
   b. Start aspirin.
   c. Request an ECG and review the results.
   d. Reassure.
   e. Ask the patient to come back in a week's time.

2 ▷ An 80 year old diabetic woman with AF comes to see you after reading a newspaper article about the dangers of aspirin. She stopped her aspirin several weeks ago but wanted to check this was okay with you. Her notes show she had a possible TIA 10 years ago. She continues to take metformin and simvastatin. She lives alone and is very independent and mobile, enjoying long walks in the countryside. What would you advise her to do?

   a. Agree that this is no added benefit in taking the aspirin.
   b. Discuss the benefits and risks of warfarin therapy instead of aspirin.
   c. Prescribe warfarin.
   d. Advise she must restart aspirin.
   e. Prescribe clopidogrel instead of aspirin.

3 ▷ Which of the following is **not** an adverse effect commonly
   associated with amiodarone?

   a. Lung disease.
   b. Arrhythmia.
   c. Thyroid disease.
   d. Seizure.
   e. Prolonged QT interval.

4 ▷ Regarding stroke risk and atrial fibrillation, which of the following
   statements is **not** true?

   a. AF is associated with an overall five-fold increased risk of stroke.
   b. Hypertension increases stroke risk in patients with AF.
   c. The risks of warfarin outweigh the benefits in terms of reducing
      stroke risk in patients with AF over the age of 75.
   d. Stroke risk increases with age.
   e. Patients with diabetes and AF have a higher risk of stroke than
      patients with lone AF.

5 ▷ A 66-year-old man comes to see you for review. He recently had
   an ECG at a routine private medical that showed AF. This has been
   confirmed with an ECG in your practice. He has no symptoms and
   is otherwise fit and well. He has no significant past medical history
   of note. His pulse rate is 80 b.p.m. irregularly irregular, and BP
   120/80.
      Which of these actions would **not** be appropriate?

   a. Following discussion with the patient commence warfarin
      at 1 mg per day.
   b. Counsel the patient about possible triggers for AF.
   c. Prescribe aspirin.
   d. Initiate heparin to prevent acute stroke.
   e. Discuss the risks and benefits of warfarin and aspirin with
      the patient.

Answers

1 = c ▷ A formal diagnosis of AF should be made by ECG before any
treatment is initiated.

2 = b ▷ This patient is over age 75 and has diabetes and possible history
of TIA so should therefore be offered warfarin. The risks and benefits of
warfarin should be discussed with the patient.

3 = d ▷ Amiodarone is not commonly associated with seizures.

4 = c ▷ The BAFTA trial showed warfarin significantly reduces the risk of stroke compared with aspirin in patients over the age of 75 with AF.

5 = d ▷ This patient is age 66, has AF and is at moderate risk of stroke according to the NICE stroke risk stratification algorithm. There is no clear evidence whether warfarin or aspirin is most appropriate, therefore risks and benefits of either treatment should be weighed up in collaboration with the patient. The patient is likely to have had AF for a while so acute treatment with heparin is not necessary.

Acknowledgement

Some of the material in the anticoagulation section of this chapter has previously been published in the following review article: Fitzmaurice DA, Hobbs FDR. Anticoagulant management in patients with atrial fibrillation *Seminars in Thrombosis and Hemostasis* 2009; **35(6)**: 543–7.

References

1 • Atrial Fibrillation Investigators. Risk factors for stroke and efficacy of antithrombotic therapy in atrial fibrillation: analysis of pooled data from five randomised controlled trials *Archives of Internal Medicine* 1994; **154(13)**: 1449–57.

2 • Wolf PA, Abbott RD, Kannel WB. Atrial fibrillation as an independent risk factor for stroke: the Framingham Study *Stroke* 1991; **22(8)**: 983–8.

3 • Feinberg WM, Blackshear JL, Laupacis A, *et al.* Prevalence, age distribution, and gender of patients with atrial fibrillation *Archives of Internal Medicine* 1995; **155(5)**: 469–73.

4 • Wolf PA, Abbott RD, Kannel WB. Atrial fibrillation: a major contributor to stroke in the elderly – the Framingham study *Archives of Internal Medicine* 1987; **147(9)**: 1561–64.

5 • Fitzmaurice DA, Hobbs FDR, Jowett J, *et al.* Screening versus routine practice in detection of atrial fibrillation in patients aged 65 or over: cluster randomised controlled trial *British Medical Journal* 2007; **335(7616)**: 383–6, doi:10.1136/bmj.39280.660567.55.

6 • Levy S, Camm AJ, Saksena S, *et al.* International consensus on nomenclature and classification of atrial fibrillation *Europace* 2003; **5(2)**: 119–22.

7 • Reid DD, Brett GZ, Hamilton PJS, *et al.* Cardiorespiratory disease and diabetes among middle-aged male civil servants *Lancet* 1974; **1(7856)**: 469–73.

8 • Rose G, Baxter PJ, Reid DD, *et al.* Prevalence and prognosis of electrocardiographic findings in middle aged men *British Heart Journal* 1978; **40(6)**: 636–43.

9 • Flegel KM, Shipley MJ, Rose G. Risk of stroke in non-rheumatic atrial fibrillation *Lancet* 1987; **1(8532)**: 526–9.

10 • Lip GYH. Does paroxysmal atrial fibrillation confer a paroxysmal thromboembolic risk? *Lancet* 1997; **349(9065)**: 1565–6.

11 • Wilson JMG, Jungner G. *The Principles and Practice of Screening for Disease* (WHO Public Health Papers 34) Geneva: World Health Organization, 1968.

12 • Petersen P, Boysen G, Godtfredsen J, *et al.* Placebo-controlled, randomised trial of warfarin and aspirin for prevention of thromboembolic complications in chronic atrial fibrillation: the Copenhagen AFASAK study *Lancet* 1989; **1(8631)**: 175–9.

13 • Stroke Prevention in Atrial Fibrillation Investigators. Stroke Prevention in Atrial Fibrillation Study: final results *Circulation* 1991; **84(2)**: 527–39.

14 • The Boston Area Anticoagulation Trial for Atrial Fibrillation Investigators. The effect of low dose warfarin on the risk of stroke in patients with nonrheumatic atrial fibrillation *New England Journal of Medicine* 1990; **323(22)**: 1505–11.

15 • Connolly SJ, Laupacis A, Gent M, *et al.* Canadian Atrial Fibrillation Anticoagulation (CAFA) Study *Journal of the American College of Cardiology* 1991; **18(2)**: 349–55.

16 • European Atrial Fibrillation Study Group. Secondary prevention in non-rheumatic atrial fibrillation after transient ischaemic attack or minor stroke *Lancet* 1993; **342(8882)**: 1255–62.

17 • Ezekowitz ND, Bridgers SL, James KE, *et al.* Warfarin in the prevention of stroke associated with non-rheumatic atrial fibrillation *New England Journal of Medicine* 1992; **327(20)**: 1406–12.

18 • Warfarin versus aspirin for prevention of thromboembolism in atrial fibrillation: stroke prevention in atrial fibrillation II study *Lancet* 1994; **343(8899)**: 687–91.

19 • Stroke prevention in Atrial Fibrillation Investigators. Adjusted-dose warfarin versus low-intensity, fixed-dose warfarin plus aspirin for high-risk patients with atrial fibrillation: Stroke Prevention in Atrial Fibrillation III randomised clinical trial *Lancet* 1996; **348(9028)**: 633–8.

20 • Sweeney KG, Pereira Gray D, Steele R, *et al.* Use of warfarin in non-rheumatic atrial fibrillation: a commentary from general practice *British Journal of General Practice* 1995; **45(392)**: 153–8.

21 • Albers GW. Atrial fibrillation and stroke *Archives of Internal Medicine* 1994; **154(13)**: 1443–8.

22 • Gage BF, Cardinalli AB, Albers GW, *et al.* Cost-effectiveness of warfarin and aspirin for prophylaxis of stroke in patients with nonvalvular atrial fibrillation *Journal of the American Medical Association* 1995; **274(23)**: 1839–45.

23 • He J, Whelton PK, Vu B, *et al.* Aspirin and risk of haemorrhagic stroke *Journal of the American Medical Association* 1998; **280(22)**: 1930–5.

24 • National Institute for Health and Clinical Excellence. *Clinical Guideline 36, Atrial Fibrillation* London: NICE, 2006, www.nice.org.uk/Guidance/CG36 [accessed September 2010].

25 • Go AS, Hylek EM, Chang Y, *et al.* Anticoagulation therapy for stroke prevention in atrial fibrillation: how well do randomized trials translate into clinical practice? *Journal of the American Medical Association* 2003; **290(20)**: 2685.

26 • van Walraven C, Hart RG, Singer DE, *et al.* Oral anticoagulants vs aspirin in nonvalvular atrial fibrillation: an individual patient meta-analysis *Journal of the American Medical Association* 2002; **288(19)**: 2441–8.

27 • Mant J, Hobbs FDR, Fletcher K, *et al.* Warfarin versus aspirin for stroke prevention in an elderly population with atrial fibrillation (the Birmingham Atrial Fibrillation treatment of the Aged Study, BAFTA): a randomized controlled trial *Lancet* 2007; **370(9586)**: 493–503.

209

28 • Hylek EM, Skates SJ, Sheehan MA, *et al*. An analysis of the lowest effective intensity of prophylactic anticoagulation for patients with nonrheumatic atrial fibrillation *New England Journal of Medicine* 1996; **335(8)**: 540–6.

29 • Hylek EM, Singer DE. Risk factors for intracranial haemorrhage in outpatients taking warfarin *Annals of Internal Medicine* 1994: **120(11)**: 897–902.

30 • Lancaster T, Mant J, Singer DE. Stroke prevention in atrial fibrillation *British Medical Journal* 1997; **314(7094)**: 1563–4.

31 • Betts TR, Mitchell ARJ. Is rate more important than rhythm in treating atrial fibrillation *British Medical Journal* 2009; **339**: b3173.

32 • The Atrial Fibrillation Follow-up Investigation of Rhythm Management (AFFIRM) Investigators. A comparison of rate control and rhythm control in patients with atrial fibrillation *New England Journal of Medicine* 2002; **347(23)**: 1825–33.

33 • British National Formulary 58. Section 2.4 Beta-adrenoceptor blocking drugs.

34 • British National Formulary 58. Section 2.6.2 Calcium-channel blockers.

35 • British National Formulary 58. Section 2.1.1 Cardiac glycosides.

36 • Goldschlager N, Epstein AE, Naccarelli G, *et al*. Practical guidelines for clinicians who treat patients with amiodarone *Archives of Internal Medicine* 2000; **160(12)**: 1741–8.

37 • Task Force of the Working Group on Arrhythmias of the European Society of Cardiology. CAST and beyond. Implications of the Cardiac Arrhythmia Suppression Trial *European Heart Journal* 1990; **11(3)**: 194–9.

38 • Anderson JL, Prystowsky EN. Sotalol: an important new antiarrhythmic *American Heart Journal* 1999; **137(3)**: 388–409.

39 • Alboni P, Botto GL, Baldi N. Outpatient treatment of recent-onset atrial fibrillation with the 'pill-in-the-pocket' approach *New England Journal of Medicine* 2004; **351(123)**: 2384–91.

40 • Hohnloser SH, Crijns HJGM, van Eickels M, *et al*. Effect of dronedarone on cardiovascular events in atrial fibrillation *New England Journal of Medicine* 2009; **360(7)**: 668–78.

41 • The AFFIRM investigators. Relationships between sinus rhythm, treatment, and survival in the Atrial Fibrillation Follow-up Investigation of Rhythm Management (AFFIRM) study *Circulation* 2004; **109(12)**: 1509–13.

42 • Carlsson J, Miketic S, Windeler J, *et al*. Randomized trial of rate-control versus rhythm-control in persistent atrial fibrillation: the Strategies of Treatment of Atrial Fibrillation (STAF) study *Journal of the American College of Cardiology* 2003; **41(10)**: 1690–6.

43 • Opolski G, Torbicki A, Kosior DA, *et al*. Rate control vs rhythm control in patients with nonvalvular atrial fibrillation (HOT CAFE) *Chest* 2004; **126(2)**: 476–86.

44 • Roy D, Talajic M, Nattel S, *et al*. Rhythm control versus rate control for atrial fibrillation and heart failure *New England Journal of Medicine* 2008; **358(25)**: 2667–77.

Valvular and structural heart disease

8

Russell Davis and Edmond Walma

Aims

This chapter discusses the importance of recognising symptoms and signs of valvular or structural heart disease, and appropriate investigation and referral of patients presenting to primary care. The common valvular lesions are discussed in detail and the presentation of endocarditis and recent guidance around endocarditis prophylaxis is also reviewed. Features of cardiomyopathies and myocarditis are also discussed. Congenital heart disease in grownups is uncommon but it is important for GPs to have an understanding of these conditions to ensure safe management when these patients present to primary care.

Key learning points

▶ Valvular heart disease due to rheumatic fever has decreased in incidence. However, degenerative valvular disease is increasingly common as the population ages.

▶ Patients with symptoms and a murmur should be investigated using echocardiography.

▶ Patients should be appropriately referred for surgical assessment.

▶ Dental hygiene is crucial to prevent endocarditis in patients with valvular lesions; however, antibiotic prophylaxis prior to dental treatment is no longer routinely recommended.

▶ Hypertrophic cardiomyopathy (HCM) is the commonest cause of sudden death in the under-35 age group. All first-degree relatives of patients with HCM should be screened.

▶ Grown-up congenital heart disease is more commonly seen as surgical techniques and survival rates in childhood have improved. GPs should be aware of appropriate advice for these patients regarding issues such as pregnancy, contraception and exercise.

Valvular heart disease

Heart valve disease is common and more severe cases frequently require intervention. Despite this, and in contrast to other areas of cardiology practice, the evidence base for both pharmacological treatment of valve disease, and for percutaneous and operative intervention, is surprisingly thin, with particular paucity of randomised trial data.[1]

Over the past few years, there has been a change in the groups of patients suffering from heart valve disease. In Western countries, there has been a huge reduction in the incidence of acute rheumatic fever and this has led to relatively small numbers of patients with newly diagnosed rheumatic valvular disease in adult cardiology practice. However, those treating immigrant patients from Africa and South Asia do still need to be vigilant for new cases.

Whilst endocarditis remains a rare but important cause (and consequence) of valve disease, the dominant form of valve disease with the increasing age of the population in Western countries is now degenerative disease.[2] This principally causes calcific aortic stenosis and mitral regurgitation, while mitral stenosis and aortic regurgitation are much less commonly seen. In addition, many older valve disease patients have significant co-morbidities (coronary artery disease, chronic lung disease, renal impairment, etc.), which increase the risks of operative intervention and can make optimal decision-making complex.

A growing number of patients who have undergone surgery for valve disease will be seen in general practice over the coming years. While many will be followed up in specialist clinics, problems may arise in between specialist follow-ups, and more patients may solely be followed up in the community in the future. Primary care staff should therefore be vigilant for possible problems.

Valvular disease is a complex issue; however, several questions may arise in primary care:

Who needs an echocardiogram?

Diagnosis is now dominated by echocardiography, which has become the standard to evaluate valve structure and function. Echocardiography is indicated in all patients with a heart murmur where valvular disease is suspected. It is not essential in young and pregnant patients with asymptomatic soft mid-systolic murmurs.

How should a GP manage the patient who has undergone valve surgery?

▷ Good dental hygiene is essential. However, specific antibiotic prophylaxis for dental work is no longer recommended, according to the NICE recommendations.[3] These are discussed below in detail.

▷ Lifelong anticoagulation is essential for those with mechanical valve prostheses, and even temporary cessation of treatment, e.g. for non-cardiac surgical procedures, needs to be co-ordinated by specialists as patients will often need intravenous heparin. Detailed patient education on the importance of anticoagulation is essential.

▷ Atrial fibrillation has a high incidence in valve surgery patients and is associated with very high stroke risk in mitral valve disease. Therefore, many of those with mitral valve repair or biological prostheses will have a strong indication for anticoagulation.

▷ Heart failure may develop after valve surgery, which may be due to new left ventricular dilation and dysfunction, prosthetic or repaired valve dysfunction, disease in other heart valves, onset of atrial fibrillation, or myocardial ischaemia. Detailed reassessment of such patients including echocardiography is essential.

▷ Acute valve thrombosis is fortunately rare but is a medical emergency requiring hospitalisation and urgent specialist assessment. It should be suspected if there is a sudden onset of shortness of breath or new embolic event, especially if there has been recent inadequate anticoagulation.

213

Who will be appropriate to refer for surgery?

Treatment has not only developed through the continuing progress in prosthetic valve technology, but has also been improved by the development of conservative surgical approaches and the introduction of percutaneous interventional techniques. The decision regarding surgery is in the domain of the cardiologist, but it is important that the GP knows something about this. It may be appropriate to wait until symptoms develop; however, other criteria, primarily findings on an echocardiogram such as pressure gradients, may allow more timely intervention with better outcomes.[4] Several factors will need consideration including:

▷ age and co-morbidity
▷ the sort of valve lesion and the suitability for repair/replacement
▷ the risk of repair/replacement.

Specific valvular disease

Aortic stenosis

Calcific aortic stenosis is common in the elderly (2–7 per cent of the population aged >65). It is also found at a slightly younger age in those with congenitally bicuspid valves. Congenital aortic stenosis is relatively rare.

SYMPTOMS AND SIGNS

Worrying symptoms of aortic stenosis are syncope, angina and heart failure, which in the presence of severe echocardiographic aortic stenosis are very strong indications for valve surgery. Aortic stenosis causes an ejection systolic murmur usually heard loudest at the right second intercostal space, radiating to the carotids. A low blood pressure and a small pulse pressure are common. More severe cases may have a heaving apex beat, slow-rising pulse and quiet second heart sound. The loudness of the murmur is not a particularly good guide to severity, as in very severe cases the murmur may become quieter due to poor cardiac output.

INVESTIGATIONS

Doppler studies are essential for detailed echocardiographic assessment. They assess the peak transvalvular gradient and valve area, as well as left ventricular systolic function, presence of left ventricular hypertrophy, and any other associated disease. Exercise testing and stress echocardiography may be useful in specific circumstances. Most patients needing valve replacement will need to have invasive coronary angiography, to determine if bypass grafting is also needed – concomitant coronary artery disease being common. However, invasive transvalvular pressure measurement is no longer always needed, as it can cause embolic strokes, and echocardiography usually establishes the need for surgery.

TREATMENT

Symptomatic aortic stenosis is a strong indication for surgery; however, severe asymptomatic cases, usually with a transvalvular gradient above 64mmHg, may also be considered.[5] Balloon aortic valvuloplasty has unfortunately proven disappointing in the long term because of the risk of severe aortic regurgitation developing, and rapid restenosis frequently occurring. Valve replacement, either with mechanical or biological prostheses, is therefore the treatment of choice. In most cases, this will be by open-heart surgery. However, percutaneous valve replacement is now developing rapidly and may be an alternative in those with co-morbidities that make open surgery hazardous.

Aortic regurgitation

Aortic regurgitation (AR, also known as aortic incompetence, AI) may be the consequence of diverse aetiologies, the distribution of which has changed over time. The most frequent causes of AR are now not rheumatic or syphilitic disease but those related to aortic root disease (e.g. Marfan's syndrome) and congenitally bicuspid aortic valve. As a consequence, the ascending aorta is frequently involved.

SYMPTOMS AND SIGNS

The main symptoms of aortic regurgitation are those of heart failure, i.e. shortness of breath, fatigue and fluid retention. Physical signs include a collapsing pulse, wide pulse pressure with low diastolic blood pressure, displacement of the cardiac apex due to left ventricular enlargement, and a decrescendo early diastolic murmur heard parasternally. Classic signs of torrential aortic regurgitation found in textbooks are now very rarely seen in practice.

INVESTIGATION

Again, echocardiography is the key investigation of aortic regurgitation but quantification can require a lot of skill. Dimensions of the left ventricle and aorta are important also.

TREATMENT

Surgery is indicated for symptomatic aortic regurgitation. It is also indicated for severe asymptomatic aortic regurgitation once the left ventricle starts to dilate or function becomes impaired, as then the likelihood of onset of symptoms is very high.[6] Careful assessment of the aortic root and ascending aorta is needed to determine whether valve replacement alone will suffice or whether aortic root replacement is needed.

Mitral stenosis

With the decline of rheumatic heart disease in Western populations, there has been a great reduction in the prevalence of mitral stenosis. However, it remains a significant problem in developing countries.

Symptoms and signs

Again, the main symptoms are those of heart failure. Due to insidious onset of symptoms, some patients may not recognise their limitations. The onset of atrial fibrillation can frequently lead to a sudden deterioration of symptoms or even frank pulmonary oedema, and is associated with a very high risk of embolic stroke. Clinical features include: an irregular pulse in many cases; an undisplaced but 'tapping' cardiac apex beat (actually a palpable first heart sound); possibly an 'opening snap' audible in early diastole; and a rumbling mid- to late diastolic murmur heard at the apex. There may also be signs of heart failure.

Investigation

The severity of disease is best assessed by echocardiography, with mitral valve area calculated from two-dimensional images and also indirectly from Doppler flow studies. Valvular morphology (and thus suitability for balloon valvuloplasty) can be assessed, as well as the degree of concomitant mitral regurgitation and other valve disease, left atrial size, and an estimate of pulmonary artery pressure. Transoesophageal echocardiography (where the echo probe is incorporated in a special upper-GI endoscope) and invasive cardiac catheterisation may also be helpful in some cases.

Treatment

Percutaneous approaches have replaced surgical valvotomy in modern healthcare systems; however, heavily calcified or significantly regurgitant valves may be unsuitable and will frequently need surgical valve replacement.[7] Generally, valvular intervention is reserved for those with symptoms and a valve area of less than 1.5 cm^2, as measured by echocardiogram.

Mitral regurgitation

Minor degrees of mitral regurgitation are extremely common; more severe disease is the second most common form of valvular disease (after aortic stenosis) requiring intervention. Advances in mitral valve repair since the 1990s have significantly affected its treatment. Mitral regurgitation may be structural, in which leaflet abnormalities are the primary cause, or ischaemic or functional, when the regurgitation is secondary to left ventricular disease. Degenerative, ischaemic and functional mitral regurgitation are now much more common than rheumatic.

Symptoms and signs

The symptoms of mitral regurgitation are those of heart failure, which may be of slow onset or occur suddenly, e.g. with papilliary muscle rupture. As with mitral stenosis, onset of atrial fibrillation may cause acute deterioration and is associated with high embolic stroke risk.

Clinical features are of an apical pan-systolic murmur radiating to the axilla. Serious concomitant features include an irregular pulse, a displaced, thrusting cardiac apex (where there is left ventricular volume overload), light ventricular heave (with pulmonary hypertension) and signs of heart failure.

Investigation

Echocardiography is the principal examination and should include an estimation of severity, mechanisms and potential repairability, as well as consequences (left ventricular volume overload, left atrial size, pulmonary pressures, etc.). While transthoracic studies have become increasingly sophisticated, transoesophageal studies and invasive catheterisation are frequently needed when valve repair or replacement are being contemplated.

In patients with few overt symptoms, exercise testing to establish true exercise tolerance may be helpful in determining the need for surgery. Symptomatic severe mitral regurgitation is a strong indication for surgery and, in asymptomatic patients, it may be considered when left ventricular dilation or systolic dysfunction, or pulmonary hypertension, develop.[8]

Treatment

Treatment has been revolutionised by the advent of successful mitral repair surgery in many cases; this preserves the mitral valve apparatus and left ventricular architecture, and is now frequently performed earlier in the natural history of the disease than valve replacement. Although there are few direct comparisons, registry data have shown lower perioperative mortality for repair surgery, better long-term survival, better preservation of left ventricular function, and lower long-term morbidity.

Medical therapy does not affect mitral regurgitation *per se*, but, in cases of heart failure, diuretics and vasodilators improve symptoms. In cases with left ventricular systolic dysfunction, conventional therapy including ACE inhibitors, beta-blockers and spironolactone in more severe cases is indicated. Anticoagulation with warfarin is very strongly indicated in cases of atrial fibrillation (both paroxysmal and persistent permanent) and either mitral stenosis or regurgitation – this will reduce the very high stroke risk by two thirds.

Endocarditis

Endocarditis is a, fortunately rare (incidence less than 1 in 10,000 per year), condition of infection of the endocardium of the heart, usually by bacteria. The inflammation may spread to the heart valves, causing destruction and valvular dysfunction. If untreated, infective endocarditis (IE) is a fatal disease. Major diagnostic (primarily echocardiography) and therapeutic progress (mainly improved ability to perform surgery successfully during active IE) have contributed to some prognostic improvement during the last decades.

If the diagnosis is delayed or appropriate therapeutic measures postponed, mortality is still high. In this respect, it is of utmost importance that 1) IE is considered early in every patient with fever or septicaemia and cardiac murmurs; 2) echocardiography is applied without delay in suspected IE; 3) cardiologists, microbiologists and cardiac surgeons co-operate closely if IE is suspected or definite.[9]

Criteria that should raise suspicion of IE in primary care include:

▷ new murmur
▷ known prosthetic material in the heart
▷ persistent fever of unknown origin
▷ embolic event of unknown origin.

Recent NICE guidance has given a clear indication of patients who should receive endocarditis prophylaxis as shown in Box 8.1 (see p. 220).

Healthcare professionals should regard people with the following cardiac conditions as being at risk of developing IE:

▷ acquired valvular heart disease with stenosis or regurgitation
▷ valve replacement
▷ structural congenital heart disease, including surgically corrected or palliated structural conditions, but excluding isolated atrial

septal defect, fully repaired ventricular septal defect or fully repaired patent ductus arteriosus, and closure devices that are judged to be endothelialised
▷ previous IE
▷ hypertrophic cardiomyopathy.

Patient advice

Healthcare professionals should offer people at risk of IE clear and consistent information about prevention, including:

▷ the benefits and risks of antibiotic prophylaxis, and an explanation of why antibiotic prophylaxis is no longer routinely recommended (see below)
▷ the importance of maintaining good oral health
▷ symptoms that may indicate IE and when to seek expert advice
▷ the risks of undergoing invasive procedures, including non-medical procedures such as body piercing or tattooing.

Prophylaxis against IE

Antibiotic prophylaxis against IE is not recommended:

▷ for people undergoing dental procedures
▷ for people undergoing non-dental procedures at the following sites:
  ☐ upper and lower gastrointestinal tract
  ☐ genitourinary tract; this includes urological, gynaecological and obstetric procedures, and childbirth
  ☐ upper and lower respiratory tract; this includes ear, nose and throat procedures and bronchoscopy.

Box 8.1 ○ *Summary of NICE guidance on endocarditis prophylaxis: adults and children with structural cardiac defects at risk of developing infective endocarditis*[3]

Chlorhexidine mouthwash should not be offered as prophylaxis against infective endocarditis to people at risk of infective endocarditis undergoing dental procedures.

Infection

▶ Any episodes of infection in people at risk of IE should be investigated and treated promptly to reduce the risk of endocarditis developing.

▶ If a person at risk of IE is receiving antimicrobial therapy because he or she is undergoing a gastrointestinal or genitourinary procedure at a site where there is a suspected infection, the person should receive an antibiotic that covers organisms that cause infective endocarditis.

Note: This NICE guideline is in line with other recent guidelines on endocarditis prophylaxis. Its publication has caused considerable controversy in the cardiology and dental communities; in particular, a lack of evidence for treatment does not equate to evidence that the treatment is not effective. Like other long-held beliefs in medicine that have been taught to generations of students and doctors, e.g. beta-blockers should be avoided in heart failure, or that exercise should be avoided in patients with ischaemic heart disease, it may take some time for the guidance not to use antibiotic prophylaxis to be universally accepted. This is likely to apply even more to patients (who have been told that antibiotic prophylaxis is essential for years) than their doctors and dentists. Some healthcare professionals may elect to continue to recommend antibiotic prophylaxis for particularly high-risk patients, e.g. those who have already had endocarditis and those with prosthetic valves.

The NICE implementation tool suggests telling patients:

The causal link between a recent dental (or non-dental) procedure and the development of infective endocarditis has not been proved. The effectiveness of antibiotic prophylaxis in preventing infective endocarditis has also not been proved and routinely prescribing antibiotic prophylaxis for patients at risk of infective endocarditis increases the likelihood that antibiotic resistance will emerge. Routine antibiotic prophylaxis may even lead to more deaths because of the risk of anaphylaxis with amoxicillin-based regimens.
   A key piece of recent research evidence that led the guideline development group to recommend that antibiotics should not be used prophylactically is that everyday activities, such as chewing and brushing teeth, cause bacteraemia (bacteria in the blood) far more frequently than dental procedures. Therefore these everyday activities almost certainly present a far greater risk of infective endocarditis than that from having a dental procedure.[3]

The British Heart Foundation (BHF) has produced a leaflet for patients on IE, which can be freely downloaded from www.bhf.org.uk. This sensibly advises that if those at high risk of endocarditis have flu-like symptoms with a high temperature lasting longer than a week, they should see a specialist. The BHF also produces an endocarditis warning card, available via their Heart HelpLine on 08450 708070 or Orderline on 0870 600 6566.

Myocarditis

Myocarditis is clinically and pathologically defined as 'inflammation of the myocardium'. Despite this apparently clear-cut definition, the classification, diagnosis, and treatment of myocarditis are still controversial.[10] The more routine use of endomyocardial biopsy has helped to better define the natural history of human myocarditis and to clarify clinicopathological correlations, although biopsy results may not affect treatment. Viral causes include Coxsackie's, CMV and influenza virus.

Symptoms and signs

Clinically, myocarditis can present with non-specific systemic symptoms (fever, myalgia, palpitations, or shortness of breath on exertion) or even fulminant haemodynamic collapse and sudden death. Clinical features include those of acute viral illness, e.g. fever, lymphadenopathy, etc., along with tachycardia, heart murmurs, pericardial rub if there is associated pericarditis, and clinical evidence of heart failure.

Investigation

An ECG may show arrhythmias including atrial fibrillation and ventricular ectopics, heart block, repolarisation changes, and bundle branch blocks. Blood tests will show leucocytosis and elevated inflammatory indices (ESR, CRP); chest radiography may show cardiomegaly and congestion, and echocardiography is important to document left ventricular size and function, along with associated pericardial and valve disease.

The great variation in presentations, and the possibility that there are a great number of mild, undiagnosed cases, makes the true incidence of myocarditis difficult to determine. Post-mortem data have implicated myocarditis in sudden cardiac death of young adults at rates of 8.6 per cent to 12 per cent. Furthermore, it has been identified as a cause of dilated cardiomyopathy in up to 10 per cent of cases. Molecular techniques have facilitated new insights into inflammatory autoimmune processes that affect the myocardium and ultimately result in acute or chronic dilated cardiomyopathy.

Cardiomyopathy

Hypertrophic cardiomyopathy

Hypertrophic cardiomyopathy (HCM) (also known as hypertrophic obstructive cardiomyopathy or HOCM where there is dynamic obstruction of blood flow leaving the heart) is a primary cardiac muscle disorder, characterised by hypertrophy, usually of the left ventricle and especially of the septum. This is in the absence of a cause, such as hypertension or aortic stenosis. It was formerly thought to be a rare and frequently fatal condition; however, more recent studies suggest that there are many milder, previously undiagnosed cases and the population prevalence may be as high as 0.2 per cent.[11]

Over ten genetic abnormalities in cardiac muscle proteins that are causative in HCM have been identified already, and further advances are being made. Where there are living affected family members, screening is possible if the genetic defect is known.

Fabry's disease, a lysosomal storage disorder, can mimic hypertrophic cardiomyopathy and also cause renal failure and other problems. This is a rare (less than 1 in 100,000 births) X-linked recessive genetic condition; identification is important as it is treatable by galactosidase enzyme replacement treatment.

RECOGNITION

HCM is an autosomal dominant genetic condition with variable penetrance. Many cases are due to new mutations so patients may not give a clear family history. It is recommended that all first-degree relatives of an affected individual be clinically screened for HCM, including a physical examination, an ECG and an echocardiogram. The best interval between repeat screens is debatable, but every 3–5 years seems appropriate in adults, and more frequently in adolescents, especially where there is a strong family history of sudden death.

SYMPTOMS AND SIGNS

HCM is the commonest cause of sudden death in those under 35 years, including sudden death during sport activities, and sudden death may be the first disease presentation. Symptoms are often non-specific, such as chest pains, palpitations, exertional shortness of breath, and dizzy spells or blackouts. There may be a jerky carotid pulse, heaving cardiac apex and basal systolic murmur and fourth heart sound.

INVESTIGATION

Diagnosis is made with ECG and echocardiography. The ECG may show very high voltages, repolarisation changes (e.g. lateral ST depression and T-wave inversion) or bundle branch block. Echocardiography 'classically' shows asymmetric septal hypertrophy, dynamic left ventricular outflow tract obstruction due to the septum bulging into the outflow tract, and systolic anterior motion of the anterior mitral valve leaflet. However, other areas of the myocardium may be affected including the left ventricular apex and even the right ventricle. Cardiac biopsy is rarely needed.

TREATMENT

Management includes advice to avoid competitive sports, and treatment with beta-blockers or the rate-limiting calcium antagonist, verapamil. Occasionally patients may benefit from surgical myomectomy, septal ablation with alcohol (causing a localised myocardial infarct of the basal septum), or multisite pacing, but these treatments should only be considered by super-specialists in the condition.

A great treatment advance has been use of implantable cardioverter defibrillators (ICDs), to treat potentially fatal arrhythmias. These should be particularly considered in those at very high risk of sudden arrhythmic death, i.e. those with septal thickness of over 30 mm, those with a family history of sudden death at a young age from the condition, and those with previously documented ventricular arrhythmias (especially those who have survived resuscitated ventricular tachycardia and fibrillation).

Dilated cardiomyopathy

Dilated cardiomyopathy is a primary disorder of cardiac muscle, characterised by dilatation, thinning and dysfunction of the left and sometimes right ventricles. The term is frequently used to describe any cases of systolic dysfunction not secondary to coronary artery disease; thus some cases may follow myocarditis (which may have been undiagnosed at the time), some may be from 'burned out' hypertension, and some from toxicity, e.g. from alcohol.

About a third of cases of completely 'idiopathic' dilated cardiomyopathy may have a family history, with variable genetic inheritance – not all autosomal dominant, as with hypertrophic cardiomyopathy. It may present in the late stages of pregnancy or postpartum; some cases of peripartum cardiomyopathy deteriorate rapidly and may need to be considered for urgent ventricular assist devices and transplantation.

SYMPTOMS AND SIGNS

The clinical presentation is with systolic heart failure, as discussed in Chapter 9.

INVESTIGATION

The ECG is usually abnormal, with arrhythmias including atrial fibrillation and ventricular ectopics, axis deviation, repolarisation changes and left bundle branch block being common. Pathological Q-waves are less common than in ischaemic heart failure cases. Echocardiography shows a dilated, thinned and frequently globally hypokinetic left ventricle, although some cases may show a more regional pattern of hypokinesia or dyskinesia.

Coronary angiography may help establish aetiology. However, if there is relatively mild coronary artery disease and severe left ventricular dysfunction it can still be difficult to say for certain if the left ventricular dysfunction is of ischaemic origin or due to cardiomyopathy.

TREATMENT

Treatment of dilated cardiomyopathy is detailed as for heart failure due to systolic dysfunction (see Chapter 9).

Grown-up congenital heart disease

The population of patients with congenital heart disease who survive to adulthood has expanded greatly over the past three decades, due to improved medical and surgical care in childhood.[12] Prior to the advent of successful surgery, fewer than 20 per cent of children with significant congenital heart disease survived to adult life; however, most deaths from congenital heart disease now occur in adults, and the population of patients with congenital heart disease over the age of 16 is now starting to exceed that under 16. This major change has led to the establishment of grown-up congenital heart disease (GUCH) units in major population centres; however, those living in rural areas may have a long distance to travel and care may be shared between GPs, more local general adult cardiologists and GUCH specialists in the regional centre.

Prevalence and causes

It is estimated that congenital heart disease affects 0.6–0.8 per cent of new-borns, i.e. about 5000 a year in the UK, of whom about a third have serious or complex disease.[13] There are many and varied forms of congenital heart disease, which are considered in detail in specialised textbooks. In general terms, disease can be divided into cyanotic and non-cyanotic; non-invasive pulse oximetry makes this easy to assess.

Cyanotic diseases include transposition of the great vessels and Fallot's tetralogy (ventricular septal defect, over-riding aorta, right ventricular outflow tract obstruction and right ventricular hypertrophy). Cyanosis may develop after the Fontan operation (a common method of surgical correction) or in cases of septal defects where pulmonary hypertension develops and there is shunt reversal, e.g. with a ventricular septal defect, right ventricular pressure becomes higher than left ventricular pressure and there is flow of deoxygenated blood from the right to left ventricles.

Common acyanotic forms of congenital heart disease seen in adults include atrial and ventricular septal defects, pulmonary stenosis, left ventricular outflow tract obstruction, aortic coarctation, and anomalous pulmonary drainage.

Symptoms and signs

Worrying symptoms, especially if they are new or worsening, of congenital heart disease include shortness of breath, reducing exercise tolerance, orthopnoea, chest pain, dizziness and blackouts, and palpitations. History taking should include family history of congenital disease, prolonged childhood illnesses, and any previous hospitalisations, interventions and surgery. Names of consultants involved and places may be invaluable in finding more details where patients are uncertain what has been going on. Clinical features on examination of relevance include features of congenital syndromes, e.g. Down's; anaemia, polycythaemia, jaundice and cyanosis; clubbing; pyrexia (especially in the acutely unwell); and evidence of poor dental hygiene. There may be previous surgical scars, elevated jugular venous pressure, abnormal apex beat, thrills and heaves, and a wide variety of murmurs according to the condition.

Investigation and management

Echocardiography is the most useful investigation for those with suspected congenital heart disease and to monitor progress and response to treatment.

225

Chest radiology and ECG may be required serially; exercise testing and MRI are also frequently useful in avoiding invasive investigation. Increasingly, invasive cardiac catheterisation is being used only as a prelude to facilitate catheter-based procedures, e.g. septal defect occlusion device insertion.

In general terms, congenital heart disease patients should see a specialist to determine the diagnosis and for education on the specific condition and formulation of a management plan. Complex patients will often need lifelong specialist follow-up; simpler disease may be followed up by less specialised staff so long as rapid reassessment by specialists is available if there is clinical deterioration.

Some specific considerations in general practice

DENTAL WORK

Dental hygiene is important in view of the high risk of endocarditis. All patients with haemodynamically significant lesions should see a dentist regularly. However, routine use of antibiotic prophylaxis for dental and surgical procedures is no longer recommended. Body piercings are also best avoided.

PREGNANCY

Many patients with congenital heart disease are able to have successful pregnancies; however, pre-pregnancy counselling and detailed assessment (including echocardiography and often exercise testing to assess exercise capacity) is very strongly advised. Genetic counselling, especially where there is a strong family history of congenital disease, may help inform decision making, and medications may need to be reviewed, e.g. ACE inhibitors are potentially toxic to a fetus. Very high-risk patients include those with poor left ventricular systolic function, pulmonary hypertension, cyanosis, aortic and mitral stenosis, coarctation of the aorta and Eisenmenger's syndrome patients.

CONTRACEPTION

Contraception advice is very important for GUCH patients; specialist advice on the optimal type will frequently be needed. Barrier methods are safe, but carry higher risk of unwanted pregnancy, which could be disastrous in high-risk patients; however, the thrombogenic properties of the combined oral contraceptive pill lead to risks in those with pulmonary hypertension, shunts, and atrial fibrillation. Progesterone depots and progesterone-only pills may lead to fluid retention. Intrauterine devices may have a small endocarditis risk, but this should be weighed up against the risk of pregnancy. Surgical sterilisation seems a good option in those who are certain they do not want any more children.

Anaesthetics for non-cardiac surgery in patients with GUCH can frequently be given safely but should be done in consultation with a specialist in the condition and by an anaesthetist familiar with the patient's physiology who has experience of monitoring such patients perioperatively. In particular, the risks of hypotension, hypovolaemia, hypoxia, arrhythmia and embolisation need to be appreciated.

EXERCISE

Exercise is generally to be encouraged, although those with particularly severe and complex disease may have significant limitations and ideally should get detailed advice from experts in the condition and from exercise physiologists, and cardiac rehabilitation. Formal exercise testing and derivation of a target heart rate may be ideal to tailor activities to capacity. Dehydration is a potential concern of excessive exercise and patients should keep well hydrated.

WORK

Many with GUCH are able to do normal jobs and have a good quality of life. However, unemployment and long-term disability rates in those with GUCH are high, and sensitive counselling from experts should ideally be available. Those with cyanotic disease and cerebral infarctions may have intellectual difficulties, and clearly many with associated Down's syndrome and other disorders will have major learning disabilities. Good social worker support, especially for such patients with complex diseases who may have ageing parents, should ideally be available; GPs may be important patient advocates in this respect.

Summary

Valvular and structural heart disease may be encountered less commonly than other cardiovascular conditions in general practice; however, it is important to recognise the symptoms and signs, arrange appropriate investigation and refer to specialists as required to ensure safe management of these patients. After investigation and/or intervention many of these patients will be managed in primary care. Recognising signs of deterioration, appropriate anticoagulation or advice regarding issues such as dental hygiene may be expected from the primary care team.

Case-based discussion

Box 8.2 ○ *Case scenario*

Patient KL is a 70-year-old woman with diabetes, hypertension and osteoarthritis. She lives alone independently in a first floor flat. She is a non-smoker and only drinks the occasional glass of sherry at Christmas time. She is an only child and her parents both lived well into their eighties. Her current medications are aspirin 75 mg once daily, metformin 500 mg three times daily, ramipril 5 mg once daily, bendrofluazide 2.5 mg once daily, simvastatin 40 mg once daily and co-codamol 8/500 two tablets four times a day as needed. She has started to become increasingly breathless and is now struggling to get up the stairs to her first floor flat. She also gets some chest pain and feels lightheaded when she gets to the top of the stairs. Her symptoms have been present for several months but have been getting worse over recent weeks, and she is now struggling to manage. Her examination findings are: pulse 82 regular, blood pressure 195/75 mmHg; a loud ejection systolic murmur was heard at the right sternal edge radiating to the carotids and inspiratory crepitations bilaterally at the lung bases; and pitting oedema of both ankles.

What would be your differential diagnosis? What investigations would be helpful? What would you do next?

You should send an urgent referral to cardiology and advise the patient to stop the ramipril in the mean time. You receive a letter from the cardiologist a week later, which details an echocardiogram done in clinic that shows aortic stenosis with a transvalvular gradient of 65 mmHg with left ventricular hypertrophy and moderate left ventricular function. It was advised that surgical intervention would be appropriate after a multidisciplinary team meeting with cardiac surgeons. An angiogram has been planned for 3 weeks' time to identify any coronary artery disease that may benefit from bypass grafting at the time of surgery. The patient returns to see you to discuss what the hospital doctors had said. What would you discuss with her?

Patient's perspective

This patient is an independent lady who doesn't like to bother the doctor. She attends for her annual diabetic check, follows instruction about diet and always takes her medications. She was not very sure what was causing her symptoms but suspected it may be something to do with her heart. She was tolerating the symptoms at first but they are now having a significant impact on her life and she fears one day she will not be able to get up the stairs to her flat. She has lived in this flat for 15 years since her husband died and she has very good neighbours. She does not want to have to move. She does not like the idea of an operation; however, she realises her symptoms will severely limit what she is able to do and may get worse over time if she is not treated.

The following discussion is in the format of a case-based discussion that demonstrates the core competencies required by a GP.

Practising holistically

There were several issues raised by the case. Patient KL has symptoms consistent with significant valvular disease. She also has other cardiovascular risk factors and co-morbidities. Her main concern is being able to continue to live independently in her flat.

Data gathering and making a diagnosis

The most likely diagnosis in this patient is aortic stenosis. She may also have concomitant coronary artery disease given her history of diabetes and hypertension. She also has features consistent with heart failure that could be secondary to valvular disease, ischaemic heart disease or both.

Clinical management

Her blood pressure is low, which may represent critical aortic stenosis. The antihypertensives she is taking should be reduced. ACE inhibitors reduce peripheral vascular resistance, which can lead to significant hypotension in patients with severe aortic stenosis due a compromised cardiac output so it is appropriate to stop ramipril. An urgent referral to cardiology is appropriate to facilitate investigation of symptoms suggestive of aortic stenosis, ischaemic heart disease and possibly heart failure to allow timely definitive treatment.

Managing medical complexity

This patient has multiple co-morbidities but manages to live alone independently in a first-floor flat. The operative risks must be weighed against the benefits of surgery for this patient. The patient's wishes must be taken into account. It is not the decision of the GP whether or not this patient should have surgery, but as her trusted family doctor it is appropriate to discuss the surgery in a broad sense and address any concerns she may have specifically as appropriate within the knowledge base of a generalist. Any specific technical questions and estimation of operative risk should be addressed by the cardiac surgeon or anaesthetist.

Primary care administration

Optimal management of this patient is best achieved with careful documentation in the medical record and clear letters of communication between primary and secondary care.

Working with colleagues

Timely intervention by cardiology and discussion with cardiac surgery was required to appropriately manage this patient.

Community orientation

This patient currently lives independently in her own home and is a minimal cost to society. Cardiac surgery has associated healthcare costs; however, correction of the valvular abnormality, allowing this patient to continue living a full and independent life for many years, may result in savings in health and social care costs in the longer term.

Maintaining an ethical approach

The autonomy of this patient should be considered. She has a right to choose whether or not she would like to have surgery and should be given the most accurate information in a way she can understand in order to make an informed decision. The implications for this patient and wider society of going ahead with surgery or not have been discussed and the balance of risk versus harm should be carefully considered.

Fitness to practise

This patient was the first concern of her GP and treated in a timely, holistic manner to ensure high-quality, safe, effective clinical care. If the patient did decide to have surgery, effective communication between primary and secondary care will be required prior to admission and on discharge. This ensures continuity of care is maintained for the patient as she moves through the healthcare system.

Self-assessment questions

1 ▷ The most common cause of valvular heart disease in the UK is:

    a. Degenerative.
    b. Congenital.
    c. Rheumatic.
    d. Infection.
    e. None of the above.

2 ▷ Aortic stenosis is associated with:

    a. Pan-systolic murmur.
    b. Young age of presentation.
    c. Syncope, chest pain and/or breathlessness.
    d. Irregular pulse.
    e. Wide pulse pressure.

3 ▷ Regarding endocarditis prophylaxis:

    a. Antibiotic therapy should be routinely prescribed for patients with valvular lesions undergoing dental procedures.
    b. There is a strong evidence base for use of antibiotics in endocarditis prophylaxis.
    c. Antibiotics are no longer routinely recommended for patients with valvular lesions undergoing dental procedures.
    d. Body piercing is safe in patients with valvular lesions.
    e. Infective endocarditis is common if antibiotics are not used during dental procedures.

4 ▷ Regarding hypertrophic cardiomyopathy (HCM):

a. It is the leading cause of death in patients under age 45.
b. The whole family of patients with HCM should be screened for the disease.
c. It is an autosomal recessive condition.
d. All first-degree relatives of patients with HCM should be screened.
e. It is a benign condition.

5 ▷ Which statement is true for grown-up congenital heart disease patients?

a. Pregnancy is contraindicated.
b. Grown-up congenital heart disease has increased since survival rates for infant cardiac surgery have improved.
c. Will often need a sick note as they are generally unable to work
d. Should not exercise.
e. All of the above.

Answers

1 = a ▷ Degenerative disease is the biggest cause of valvular abnormalities in the UK. However, rheumatic heart disease is still a major cause of morbidity in the developing world.

2 = c ▷ Syncope, chest pain and/or breathlessness are typical symptoms of aortic stenosis. However, patients are often asymptomatic.

3 = c ▷ Recent NICE guidance[3] has suggested it is no longer necessary to prescribe routine antibiotic prophylaxis to patients with valvular heart disease.

4 = d ▷ HCM is associated with specific genetic mutations that are often autosomal dominantly inherited so first-degree relatives should be screened.

5 = b ▷ Significant advances in paediatric cardiac surgery have resulted in many children with congenital heart disease now surviving into adulthood.

References

1 • Vahanian A, Baumgartner H, Bax J, *et al.* Guidelines on the management of valvular heart disease: the Task Force on the Management of Valvular Heart Disease of the European Society of Cardiology *European Heart Journal* 2007; **28(2)**: 230–68.

2 • Soler-Soler J, Galve E. Worldwide perspective of valve disease *Heart* 2000; **83(6)**: 721–5.

3 • National Institute for Health and Clinical Excellence. *Clinical Guideline 64, Prophylaxis against Infective Endocarditis: antimicrobial prophylaxis against infective endocarditis in adults and children undergoing interventional procedures* London: NICE, 2008, http://guidance.nice.org.uk/CG64 [accessed September 2010].

4 • Ambler G, Omar RZ, Royston P, *et al.* Generic, simple risk stratification model for heart valve surgery *Circulation* 2005; **112(2)**: 224–31.

5 • Rosenhek R, Binder T, Porenta G, *et al.* Predictors of outcome in severe, asymptomatic aortic stenosis *New England Journal of Medicine* 2000; **343(9)**: 611–17.

6 • Borer JS, Hochreiter C, Herrold EM, *et al.* Prediction of indications for valve replacement among asymptomatic or minimally symptomatic patients with chronic aortic regurgitation and normal left ventricular performance *Circulation* 1998; **97(6)**: 525–34.

7 • Iung B, Garbarz E, Michaud P, *et al.* Late results of percutaneous mitral commissurotomy in a series of 1024 patients. Analysis of late clinical deterioration: frequency, anatomic findings, and predictive factors *Circulation* 1999; **99(25)**: 3272–8.

8 • Rosenhek R, Rader F, Klaar U, *et al.* Outcome of watchful waiting in asymptomatic severe mitral regurgitation *Circulation* 2006; **113(18)**: 2238–44.

9 • Horstkotte D, Follath F, Gutschik E, *et al.* Guidelines on prevention, diagnosis and treatment of infective endocarditis executive summary; the task force on infective endocarditis of the European society of cardiology *European Heart Journal* 2004; **25(3)**: 267–76.

10 • Magnani JW, Dec GW. Myocarditis: current trends in diagnosis and treatment *Circulation* 2006; **113(6)**: 876–90.

11 • Semsarian C; CSANZ Cardiovascular Genetics Working Group. Guidelines for the diagnosis and management of hypertrophic cardiomyopathy *Heart, Lung and Circulation* 2007; **16(1)**: 16–18.

12 • Deanfield J, Thaulow E, Warnes C, *et al.* Management of grown up congenital heart disease *European Heart Journal* 2003; **24(11)**: 1035–84.

13 • Wren C, O'Sullivan JJ. Survival with congenital heart disease and need for follow up in adult life *Heart* 2001; **85(4)**: 438–43.

Heart failure

9

F. D. Richard Hobbs

Aims

This chapter highlights the epidemiological importance of heart failure as a clinical syndrome and its relation to other cardiovascular diseases. We discuss the most common causes of heart failure, the symptoms, signs and appropriate investigations required to establish the diagnosis and the evidence-based treatments available to reduce morbidity and mortality. The impact of the disease is demonstrated with a case-based discussion that highlights the need for a patient-centred, holistic, multidisciplinary approach to provide optimal care.

Key learning points

▶ Heart failure is linked to substantial morbidity and mortality, high treatment costs, and is predicted to rise in prevalence in many countries.
▶ The commonest cause of heart failure is left ventricular systolic dysfunction (LVSD).
▶ LVSD is found in 1.8 per cent of the population over 45 years; borderline left ventricular dysfunction in a further 3.5 per cent; and heart failure (left ventricular ejection fraction (LVEF) <40 per cent) in 2.3 per cent.
▶ Diagnosis requires the presence of symptoms such as breathlessness, fatigue and oedema plus objective evidence of cardiac dysfunction.
▶ Criteria for diagnosing heart failure may be relaxed in the future to use an LVEF cut-off of <50 per cent rather than 40 per cent.
▶ Prevalence rises rapidly from 65 onwards, so heart failure is likely to become a more significant problem as the population ages and there is improved survival of patients post-myocardial infarction, the principal aetiology of heart failure.

Introduction

Heart failure and LVSD are increasingly important chronic diseases, or more accurately disease syndromes, associated with a poor prognosis, very poor quality of life for patients and resulting in some of the highest healthcare costs for a single condition.[1,2] Estimates suggest it is the second or third most expensive condition to treat in the NHS, this being a reflection of high admission and re-admission rates. Annual mortality in severe heart failure is around 60 per cent.[3] In the general population, where all grades of heart failure are represented, 5-year mortality is around 42 per cent,[4] but where the diagnosis is established during a hospital admission 5-year mortality is between 50–75 per cent.[5,6]

Prevalence and incidence of heart failure

Studies examining the prevalence of LVSD, utilising objective assessment of LV function such as echocardiography,[7,8] indicate a prevalence of LVSD of 2.9 per cent in patients under 75 and up to 7.5 per cent in 75–84-year-olds. However, limitations of some of these studies include not screening all adult age groups, with data particularly lacking in the elderly in whom LVSD is more common, or not examining representative populations. Overcoming these limitations, the largest recent prospective evaluation of heart failure in the community (ECHOES), LVSD was found in 1.8 per cent (95 per cent CI 1.4–2.3) of the population over 45 years; borderline LV dysfunction (LVEF 40–50 per cent) in a further 3.5 per cent; definite heart failure in 2.3 per cent (95 per cent CI 1.9–2.8) of the population (with LVEF <40 per cent in 41 per cent of cases); and using an LVEF cut-off of <50 rather than 40, 3.1 per cent (95 per cent CI 2.6–3.7) of people aged 45 or over had heart failure.[9]

Estimates on heart failure incidence are less available, and vary from 0.9[10] to 2.2 cases per 1000 population per annum in females aged 45–74 years and 1.6 to 4.6 cases per 1000 population per annum in men aged 45–74 years.[10] Incidence rises rapidly in the elderly, however, with 1 per cent of men per year developing heart failure after 75 and almost 2 per cent per year in the over-85s.

Prognosis of heart failure

Mortality rates in heart failure are high. Annual mortality rates in the placebo arms of recent trials, against the background of ACE inhibitors, have ranged from 7 per cent[11] in mild heart failure (NYHA II), 11 per cent[12] to 13 per cent in moderate cases (NYHA III), and 20 per cent, 23 per cent,[13] or 28 per cent[14] in severe heart failure. By comparison, the Framingham cohort showed an overall 1-year heart failure (defined initially on ECG criteria, but latterly on echocardiography) mortality rate of 17 per cent, 2-year mortality rate of 30 per cent, and a 10-year mortality rate of 78 per cent.[15] The National Health and Nutrition Examination Survey (NHANES) study, conducted from 1971–86 in the US, revealed 10-year mortality rates of 43 per cent in patients who self-reported heart failure and 38 per cent in patients who had heart failure defined by a clinical score.[16]

Mortality data from more recent epidemiological studies provide more reliable case definitions, but mainly report on only LVSD heart failure, younger patients only,[17] or patients presenting to hospital, usually with incident symptomatic heart failure.[18, 19] In the latter studies, mortality is particularly high with 50 per cent 2-year mortality, probably indicating late presentations, rates which equate to the prognosis of newly diagnosed color-ectal cancer in men or ovarian cancer in women.

Probably the most reliable contemporary estimate of prognosis of preva-lent heart failure, across all ages and stages, is available from follow-up of the ECHOES cohort.[4] Five-year survival rate of the general population was 93 per cent compared with 58 per cent of those with a prevalent diagnosis of LVSD and 58 per cent with prevalent definite heart failure. Median survival time of definite heart failure was 7 years and 7 months. Those with a prior diag-nostic label of heart failure had the lowest survival compared with the gen-eral population and survival improved significantly with increasing ejection fraction. Importantly, significantly worse mortality rates were seen amongst patients with 'borderline' ejection fraction levels of between 40–50 per cent. Indeed, people identified with this degree of 'minor' systolic impairment suf-fered mortality rates over 1.5 times higher than people with ejection fractions over 50 per cent. Those persons with multiple causes of heart failure had the poorest survival. The ECHOES mortality data provide recent confirmation on the poor prognosis of patients suffering heart failure across the community, providing a generalisable mortality risk estimate of 8–9 per cent per year. Importantly, outcomes in heart failure are improving, presumed to be due to better initiation and maintenance of evidence-based therapies.[20]

Burden of heart failure on patients: morbidity and quality of life

Morbidity in heart failure is considerable, whether measured by symptom severity, quality of life, need for consultation, treatment and hospital admis-sion. Studies with comparative normative data are few and suggest that heart failure worsens quality of life more than other chronic diseases[21] (although heart failure diagnosis in this study was not determined on the basis of objective tests), and that women may suffer worse impairment.[22]

Other studies have shown heart failure is associated with depressive illness,[23] and further that this is then linked to a worse prognosis.[24] Those with heart failure had significant impairment of all the measured aspects of physical and mental health, not only physical functioning. Significantly worse impairment was found in those with more severe heart failure by NYHA class. Patients with asymptomatic left ventricular dysfunction and patients rendered asymptomatic by treatment had similar scores to the random population sample. Those with heart failure reported more severe impairment of quality of life than people giving a history of chronic lung disease or arthritis, with a similar impact to patients reporting depression.

Burden of heart failure on healthcare costs

Chronic heart failure remains one of the most costly conditions to manage in many health systems. This is principally because the syndrome is common and it frequently results in hospital admission (which is the disproportionate driver of healthcare expenditure). Mean admissions are prolonged (averaging 11 days in Europe), and readmission is frequent (nearly 25 per cent of patients are readmitted within 12 weeks of discharge).[25] In the UK, 4.9 per cent of admissions to one hospital were for heart failure, extrapolating to up to 120,000 admissions per year nationally.[26] Admissions continue to rise.[27,28]

As a consequence, heart failure accounts for at least 2 per cent of total healthcare expenditure,[29] namely €26m per million population in the UK, €37m per million population in Germany, €39m per million population in France and €70m per million population in the US. The average cost per hospital admission in Europe is €10,000. The burden of heart failure is expected to rise as prevalence rises, presumed to be due to improved survival of patients post-myocardial infarction and better treatment of heart failure once developed.[30]

Diagnostic issues in heart failure

The evaluation of patients with suspected heart failure entails determining whether the syndrome is present, plus identification of underlying cardiac abnormalities. Guidelines for the evaluation and management of heart failure are established in both the US (ACC/AHA and Consensus Recommendations)[31] and Europe (ESC).[20] These state that the diagnosis of heart failure is justified when there are typical signs and symptoms of heart failure and myocardial dysfunction, confirmed by the objective evidence of cardiac dysfunction at rest. In case of diagnostic uncertainty, a clinical response to treatment directed at heart failure is helpful in establishing the diagnosis. Simple and reliable diagnostic procedures are essential for primary care physicians, who are responsible for the early diagnosis of heart failure and implementation of adequate therapy.

CURRENT UK GUIDANCE

The current NICE guideline recommends that patients with suspected heart failure should have an ECG and/or natriuretic peptides performed.[32] If both are normal, then heart failure is unlikely, and an alternative diagnosis to explain the symptoms should be considered. If either is abnormal, then the patient should have an echocardiograph. This guidance was based on the high sensitivity of BNP (B-type natriuretic peptide) and ECG (electrocardiogram), and the result of a health economic analysis that demonstrated that the cost per life year gained through echocardiography is dependent upon the proportion of patients referred for echocardiography in whom the diagnosis of heart failure is confirmed.

However, current diagnosis of heart failure in primary care is often inaccurate. In one recent UK study, only 34 per cent of patients with an existing clinical label of heart failure in routine general practice records had this diagnosis confirmed at echocardiography and review.[33] The Healthcare Commission found only 1 in 5 patients with a diagnosis of heart failure had had an echocardiogram, where the average wait was 67 days.[34] There have been seven recent systematic reviews relevant to the diagnosis of heart failure. Three covered all symptoms, signs and diagnostic tests, two concerned BNP, and one a review of the accuracy of 12-lead ECG.

SYMPTOMS AND SIGNS

Individual symptoms (such as breathlessness, fatigue, exercise intolerance and fluid retention) and signs (such as resting tachycardia, raised jugular venous pressure, displaced apex beat, third heart sound) are generally weak predictors of heart failure, and they have poor reliability, with little agreement between clinicians on their presence.

In the most recent systematic review, a number of symptoms were reasonably specific, including history of myocardial infarction (89 per cent), orthopnoea (89 per cent), cardiomegaly (85 per cent), added heart sounds (99 per cent), lung crepitations (81 per cent), and hepatomegaly (97 per cent) (see Box 9.1 and Table 9.1 on p. 240).[35] However, in primary care, the most useful symptoms/signs in diagnosis have high sensitivity, since this might enable the clinician to rule out heart failure if the symptom/sign was absent, without the need to refer for further investigation. Dyspnoea is the only reasonably reliable clinical feature with a sensitivity of 87 per cent. In practice this symptom is present in the majority of patients in whom heart failure is suspected, with a frequency as high as 95 per cent in one of the data-sets. Nevertheless, a sensitivity of 87 per cent is not high enough on its own to rule out heart failure if dyspnoea is absent.

Box 9.1 ○ **NICE guidance on diagnosing heart failure**

In all patients with suspected heart failure, a 12-lead ECG and/or a BNP or NT-proBNP test should be performed to exclude heart failure, and only those patients with a positive ECG or BNP should proceed to echocardiography.

Table 9.1 ○ **Overall accuracy of investigations for heart failure**

	Number of patients (studies)	Sensitivity (%)	Specificity (%)	Youden index*
ECG	4702 (11)	89	56	45
CXR: any abnormality	2323 (5)	68	83	51
CXR: increased cardiothoracic ratio	2797 (6)	67	76	43
BNP	4744 (20)	93	74	67
NT-proBNP	4229 (16)	93	65	58

* Youden index = sensitivity % + specificity % –100%. This is a measure of the overall diagnostic accuracy of the test.

The New York Heart Association (NYHA) Functional Classification provides a method to describe symptoms in relation to the effect they have on the patient's daily activities:[36]

▷ **class I** ▶ no limitation of activities; patient has no symptoms from ordinary activities
▷ **class II** ▶ mild limitation of activity; patient is comfortable at rest or with mild exertion
▷ **class III** ▶ marked limitation of activity; patient is comfortable only at rest
▷ **class IV** ▶ has symptoms even at rest.

INVESTIGATIONS

Both ECG [37,38] and BNP assays have high sensitivity for heart failure, and so are good tests at ruling out the diagnosis (see Table 9.1). UK-based studies restricted to use of ECG in primary care, however, give a more mixed picture on the value of ECG, with sensitivity in one study as low as 73 per cent. This may relate to both differences in population characteristics, and to the skill of the practitioner interpreting the ECG. While the chest X-ray may show evidence of heart failure (e.g. cardiomegaly, pulmonary vascular congestion), it is not a good independent predictor, and is of most value in identifying alternative causes of symptoms of heart failure.

Four studies have evaluated the diagnostic accuracy of ECG in the specific context of referral from primary care to echocardiography.[39] They found that sensitivity in these studies varied from 73 per cent to 91 per cent, and concluded therefore that the ECG was an inadequate screening tool. A study reviewed the diagnostic accuracy of natriuretic peptides and ECG in the diagnosis of LVSD, and found similar diagnostic accuracy between ECG, BNP and NT-proBNP, and no value from combining BNP with ECG.[40] A recent systematic review confirmed that adding ECG to clinical features plus BNP result did not improve accuracy of diagnosis.

It is likely that BNP is a more accurate test for heart failure than it is for LVSD. Indeed, a recent systematic review of BNP studies concluded that, while BNP is useful for excluding heart failure, it is more limited for ruling out systolic dysfunction, with an AUC of 0.93 for heart failure but only 0.75 for systolic dysfunction.[41] There is no evidence of any significant differences in test performance between BNP and NT-proBNP.[42] Other recent reviews of BNP have confirmed its value as a 'rule out' test for heart failure.[43,44] For example, both NT-proBNP and BNP assays, set at cut-offs to achieve a sensitivity of 100 per cent, showed a specificity of 70 per cent, a positive predictive value of 7 per cent, a negative predictive value of 100 per cent, and an area under receiver operator characteristic (ROC) curve of 0.92 (95 per cent CI 0.82–1.0) for diagnosing heart failure in the general population.[34] These data indicate that a normal level of natriuretic peptides excludes heart failure, but that confirmatory echocardiography is needed in patients with elevated peptides to confirm the diagnosis. The cost-effectiveness of natriuretic peptides versus standard diagnostic triage is not established.

Echocardiography is the 'gold standard' investigation for LVSD and valve disease. Indirect measures of diastolic dysfunction can be made on echocardiography, but the interpretation of the findings may be difficult, particularly in the elderly and in patients with atrial fibrillation (up to 30 per cent of new cases of heart failure in most series). In practice today, 'diastolic' (or 'non-systolic') heart failure remains a diagnosis of exclusion. The reality of availability of echocardiography services in the NHS means that referral of all patients straight to echocardiography is problematic. In this context, echocardiography after a BNP test has been performed is an attractive option, though appropriate cut points for BNP (or NT-proBNP) are then needed.

CLINICAL DECISION RULES

There are several well-developed heart failure prognostic tools that combine the results of different symptoms/signs and tests. Mosterd applied criteria from six established HF scores including Framingham, Walma and Boston to a sample of 54 participants in the Rotterdam study. Most showed high sensitivity to detect definite heart failure with Areas Under the ROC Curve (AUC) ranging between 0.89 and 0.96. However, use of these would be impractical in primary care because of the substantial number of variables in several scores, and also because many of the clinical signs have considerable inter-observer variation even amongst specialists (raised JVP, third heart sound, hepatojugular reflux). Furthermore, four of the scores include specific chest X-ray parameters difficult to apply in general practice.

A recent meta-analysis using individual patient data [36] identified a simple diagnostic score that awaits empirical testing. This rule suggests that, in a patient presenting with symptoms such as breathlessness in whom heart failure is suspected, if the patient has any one of 1) history of MI or 2) basal crepitations or 3) is a male with ankle oedema, then refer straight for echocardiography. Otherwise carry out a BNP test, and refer to echocardiography depending on the results of the BNP.

COMPLEXITIES OF THE EVIDENCE BASE

There is no single ideal reference standard for heart failure, since there is no single cardiac disorder that accounts for the syndrome. The underlying cardiac disorders can be classified in different ways. The standard approach is to divide heart failure into low ejection fraction and normal ejection fraction heart failure. Echocardiography is a suitable reference standard for low ejection fraction heart failure, but not for normal ejection fraction heart failure. The definitive tests to diagnose normal ejection fraction heart failure are often not carried out, so the diagnosis usually relies upon clinical judgement and supportive evidence. The NICE guidance on diagnosing heart failure is shown in Box 9.1 (see p. 240).

Studies that have tested the value of the ECG in the diagnosis of heart failure have used different criteria with which to define abnormality, and there
has been variation in the experience and expertise of the person reading the
ECG. Many GPs are unable to interpret ECGs accurately.[45]

The cut-off level for BNP and NT-proBNP is an important consideration
when assessing the probability of a patient with a 'raised' natriuretic peptide
having heart failure. If the cut-off point is low, a patient with a result below
this level is very unlikely to have heart failure; however, a large proportion of
patients will have a result above the threshold value but will not have heart
failure. The converse is true for a high cut-off point. The probabilities of heart
failure for different values of natriuretic peptide are shown in Figure 9.1.

Figure 9.1 ○ **_Cut-off levels for natriuretic peptides and probability of heart
failure_**

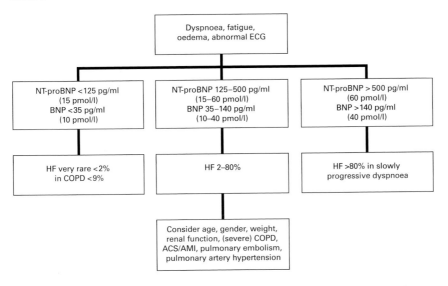

For natriuretic peptides, most of the existing research has been done
on secondary care populations, or in the context of screening studies that
identify prevalent cases of heart failure, or include patients with existing
diagnoses of heart failure. This may introduce significant spectrum bias
and affect whether the cut-off values are reliable for the target population,
namely symptomatic patients presenting in primary care.

DIAGNOSTIC PERFORMANCE IN GENERAL PRACTICE

Unfortunately, primary care physicians in Europe have variable and often delayed access to echocardiography. As a consequence, doctors rely on symptoms alone or on alternative tests such as ECG or chest X-ray to diagnose most cases of heart failure, as shown by the IMPROVEMENT study.[46] It is therefore not surprising that studies exploring the validity of a clinical diagnosis of heart failure in primary care report high rates of misdiagnosis when patients are assessed against objective criteria (rates of 25–50 per cent accuracy reported in different series).[47,48] Furthermore, under-diagnosis of heart failure is not confined to the primary care physician,[49] with only 31 per cent of patients being offered echocardiography by hospital physicians following referral with possible heart failure in one study.[50] The sensitivity and specificity of tests commonly used in the diagnosis of heart failure are shown in Table 9.1 (see p. 240).

Management of heart failure: mortality and morbidity

The evidence base for treatment strategies in heart failure continues to expand with primary indications for the use of ACE inhibitors and beta-blockers in mild to moderate heart failure and evidence for aldosterone antagonists in severe heart failure. The largest evidence base to date relates to the use of ACE inhibitors. There are also important drug classes to avoid or withdraw in heart failure, especially NSAIDs and glitazones, because of their fluid-retaining characteristics that worsen heart failure.

Loop diuretics, such as frusemide, have an important role in heart failure where there is evidence of fluid retention such as peripheral oedema or lung crepitations. They are critical and urgent therapy in patients who have decompensated heart failure with oedema of the lungs, who require initial doses parenterally. They provide rapid relief of symptoms of breathlessness. There are no trial data for diuretics but their use alongside therapies that have been shown to alter prognosis remains important. The co-administration of evidence-based therapies has, however, substantially reduced the escalating diuretic dose requirements that used to be common practice.

Angiotensin-converting enzyme (ACE) inhibitors improve both morbidity and mortality in all grades of symptomatic heart failure due to LVSD, and, in patients with asymptomatic LVSD, can delay or prevent progression to symptomatic heart failure.[51] The evidence base for ACE inhibitors is huge. A systematic review of thirty-two trials showed the pooled-odds ratio for mortality was 0.77 (95 per cent CI 0.66–0.88) in mortality and 0.65 (95 per cent CI 0.57–0.84) in mortality or hospitalisation.[52]

More recent data have demonstrated the utility of some angiotensin receptor blockers, namely candesartan 32 mg daily, for all types of heart failure, and valsartan 160 mg daily or b.d., for LVSD post-infarction. The CHARM studies showed candesartan provided overall mortality benefits in patients intolerant of ACE inhibitors or as 'triple therapy', in addition to ACE inhibitors and beta-blockers, in people with impaired LV function.[53]

Certain beta-blockers in heart failure due to LVSD have also been demonstrated to improve prognosis and reduce admission rates,[54,55] although these agents have to be introduced slowly and are associated with a slight initial worsening of symptoms in a proportion of patients. The only beta-blockers licensed for heart failure are:

▷ carvedilol
  □ initially 3.125 mg twice daily (with food)
  □ dose increased at intervals of at least 2 weeks to 6.25 mg twice daily, then to 12.5 mg twice daily, then to 25 mg twice daily
  □ increase to highest dose tolerated, max. 25 mg twice daily in patients with severe heart failure or body weight less than 85 kg, and 50 mg twice daily in patients over 85 kg
▷ bisoprolol fumarate
  □ initially 1.25 mg once daily (in the morning) for 1 week then, if well tolerated, increased to 2.5 mg once daily for 1 week, then 3.75 mg once daily for 1 week, then 5 mg once daily for 4 weeks, then 7.5 mg once daily for 4 weeks, then 10 mg once daily
  □ max. 10 mg daily
▷ nebivolol
  □ in stable mild to moderate heart failure in those over 70, initially 1.25 mg once daily, then if tolerated increased at intervals of 1–2 weeks to 2.5 mg once daily, then to 5 mg once daily, then to max. 10 mg once daily.

The aldosterone blockers reduce hospitalisation and reduce mortality in severely symptomatic (NYHA class III and IV) patients[13] using spironolactone, but at 12.5–25 mg daily, or in post-MI LVSD patients[56] using eplerenone 25 mg daily. The latter is better tolerated with fewer side effects, such as avoiding gynaecomastia and reduced electrolyte disturbance. Care is needed with these agents, though, in the elderly community since they may be associated with raising mortality if not used carefully in routine practice.[57] This is particularly a risk with spironolactone, which should only be used in low doses (well below the typical antihypertensive doses of 50 or 100 mg) and withdrawn during periods of illness, especially when dehydration is a risk.

Digoxin has a limited role in heart failure. There are no data to support its initiation in heart failure, though its withdrawal in patients appears to increase hospitalisation rates.[12] Guidelines therefore relegate digoxin for use only in patients with heart failure and atrial fibrillation. This is a relatively common co-morbidity, where there is an indication to seek rhythm or rate control and the preferred therapy in this indication, beta-blockers, is contraindicated or ineligible. However, in patients already stabilised on digoxin, the drug should not be withdrawn. The critical additional therapy in patients with heart failure and atrial fibrillation is thrombo-prophylaxis for stroke prevention, where warfarin should be the treatment of choice above aspirin in all patients wherever possible.

The same recommendations apply to statins. There is no evidence that adding a statin will benefit patients who develop heart failure; however, these drugs are safe to use in patients with heart failure and they should be withdrawn if a patient with heart failure is already on a statin.[58]

Other approaches to consider in primary care are more intensive treatment of blood pressure, although hypotension is a more common problem in heart failure, or worsening angina. If calcium channel blockers are used, verapamil and diltiazem should be avoided, and amlodipine used in preference.

Consideration of other agents or revascularisation should be made by a heart failure specialist. Referral may also be necessary for the minority of heart failure patients where cardiac resynchronisation devices may improve prognosis and symptoms in patients with LVSD and ejection fractions below 35 per cent, refractory symptoms on maximal therapy, and prolonged QRS interval of >120ms. Implantable cardiac defibrillators (ICDs) may also be considered in some at-risk patients, such as those with episodes of symptomatic ventricular tachycardia (VT).

Careful and regular follow-up of patients with heart failure is essential, with evidence that this can be effectively and safely performed by nurses, pharmacists, specialists or GPs. Probably the most important components to such structured follow-up are regular weighing (rising weight may indicate increased fluid retention), stressing the importance of staying on therapy, and discussion about warning signs (increased symptoms, increased weight) with patients and their carers. The most important monitoring tests are serum electrolytes on a 6-monthly basis, during intercurrent illness, and when up-titrating therapies.

MANAGEMENT OF HEART FAILURE: QUALITY OF LIFE

ACE inhibitors[51] and beta-blockers[59] have been shown to improve exercise tolerance and symptoms (as assessed by the NYHA functional class) in patients with heart failure due to LVSD, as well as significantly prolonging survival and reducing hospitalisation rates. These drugs have also been shown to improve global quality of life in sufferers,[60,61] as have other interventions producing symptom gains, such as exercise training[62] and intensive nurse-led discharge and outreach programmes.[63]

UNDER-MANAGEMENT OF HEART FAILURE

Despite the rich evidence base, heart failure remains suboptimally diagnosed and treated in many countries,[50,64] due at least in part to many patients with suspected heart failure not receiving formal assessment of LV function. Another factor in this under-management is concerns over treatment risk: a small qualitative survey of GPs in one UK town did not indicate lack of knowledge of ACE benefit but showed exaggerated concerns over the risks of ACE inhibitors in heart failure.[65] Support for the findings of this small study emerged from the larger Euro HF survey of primary care practitioners' practice across six European countires.[6] In this study a vast majority of practitioners were aware that ACE inhibitor therapy reduced mortality in patients with heart failure. However, there were significant concerns expressed by the doctors that such treatment also posed significant risks to patients. Half to two thirds of doctors perceived ACE therapy as having significant risks. These risks were reported as fear of first-dose hypotension and possible renal damage, although both sets of adverse risks are rare and usually avoidable if patients are selected and initiated on therapy appropriately and subsequently monitored. On the basis of these data, it would appear that, when balancing the risks and benefits of treatment, primary care physicians were more driven by perceptions of risk than perceptions of benefit.

The Quality and Outcomes Framework is a voluntary annual reward and incentive programme available to all GPs in England to encourage best practice since 2004. There are currently four heart failure indicators, as shown in Box 9.2 (see p. 248).[66,67] The percentages achieved for each of these indicators relates to payment. The thresholds for payment and number of indicators can change over time.

Improving management in primary care is therefore partially dependent on improving primary care access to heart failure diagnostic tests and more structured care in initiating and up-titrating therapies. Emerging data

---

Box 9.2 ○ *Current Quality and Outcomes Framework indicators for heart failure*

▶ Indicator HF1: the practice can produce a register of patients with heart failure.

▶ Indicator HF2: the percentage of patients with a diagnosis of heart failure that has been confirmed on echocardiogram or the GP's specialist assessment.

▶ Indicator HF3: the percentage of patients with a current diagnosis of heart failure due to LVSD who are currently treated with an ACE inhibitor or ARB.

▶ Indicator HF4: the percentage of patients with a current diagnosis of heart failure due to LVSD who are currently treated with an ACE inhibitor or angiotensin receptor blocker, who are additionally treated with a beta-blocker licensed for heart failure, or recorded as intolerant to or having a contraindication to beta-blockers.

---

suggest that the use of natriuretic peptide assays may have an important role in guiding therapy, at least in specialist settings,[68] on the basis of small follow-up studies. If these data are confirmed in primary care then this may improve triage to therapies.

Summary

Heart failure is therefore a common disorder, especially in the elderly, with major and increasing significance for patients and healthcare systems. We need better identification of patients and more intensive attempts to introduce and maintain the large evidence base for therapies. However, given the burden of disease, prevention of heart failure is a priority, and this requires formalised programmes of cardiovascular disease prevention.

Case-based discussion

Box 9.3 ○ **Case scenario**

Patient AB, a 65-year-old male, was seen by the nurse for a new patient check at 5.45 p.m. He mentioned he had nearly 'run out of tablets' so the nurse booked an appointment for AB to see the doctor in evening surgery. He lived in Cornwall but was staying with his son following a recent admission to a local hospital with heart failure. He had run out of medication a week before his admission and become increasingly breathless even at rest, with swollen ankles and a large abdomen. He had a history of four myocardial infarctions and atrial fibrillation, and had been told his heart was not pumping properly and things were 'touch and go', so he was staying with his son. He lived in a small flat on the fifteenth floor of a tower block and was out at work all day. The patient stated he 'didn't really know what was wrong with him'. On further discussion he also admitted to a previous problem with alcohol but had not been drinking for over 2 weeks. He also had a swollen toe caused by gout and took occasional diclofenac.

The patient brought a discharge summary that detailed his current medications, which included aspirin 75 mg o.d., simvastatin 20 mg nocte, digoxin 125 mcg o.d., furosemide 120 mg a.m. and 80 mg p.m., perindopril 4 mg o.d., bisoprolol 5 mg o.d. and spironolactone 25 mg o.d. He had been hyponatraemic while receiving intravenous diuretics; however, his renal function was normal prior to discharge. Echocardiogram had shown severely impaired systolic function with an ejection fraction of 20 per cent. Follow-up was arranged for 3 months' time in cardiology clinic.

On review today, he said he was still breathless when he walked, but his legs were less swollen than before he was admitted to hospital. On examination he was comfortable at rest, pulse 80 beats per minute, irregularly irregular, JVP was not visible, normal heart sounds, a few inspiratory crepitations at the bases of the lungs and pitting oedema to the knees bilaterally.

Patient's perspective

This patient is an older gentleman who lives alone in Cornwall but found himself in an unfamiliar part of the country visiting his son when he was taken ill. He had become very unwell because he had run out of medication and required an emergency hospital admission. This raises issues around patient empowerment and encouraging responsibility for managing his own chronic disease, while also recognising the significant medication burden this patient has to manage. He seemed frightened by the experience and by what he had been told, so frightened in fact that he was reluctant to return home to Cornwall. He did not really understand what was causing his symptoms and the importance of taking his medication regularly. He had been a heavy drinker for years and acknowledged this was a problem: he was taking the doctor's advice of not drinking, but with recent stresses was finding this very difficult. He had significant pain from gout when his toe swelled up and found diclofenac did provide some relief.

Questions

Think about this case in the style of a case-based discussion. Consider the following questions:

1 ▷ What issues does this case highlight in terms of practising holistically?
2 ▷ From the data above, what NYHA class does this patient fall into?
3 ▷ What is the appropriate clinical management at this stage?
4 ▷ What factors make this case more complex?
5 ▷ Which colleagues may you involve?
6 ▷ What are the ethical implications of this case?

The following discussion is in the format of a case-based discussion, which demonstrates the core competencies required by a GP.

Practising holistically

There were several issues raised by the case. AB is a new patient to the practice with no previous records other than the discharge summary he brought from the hospital. Running out of medication precipitated the hospital admission and a similar scenario was possible if he ran out of medication again. He did not have an understanding of the diagnosis of heart failure or the prognosis, and was frightened he may die so was staying with his daughter, fearing going back home to Cornwall alone. He did not appreciate the importance of medications in managing his condition. He also had a history of alcoholism and gout that may have been precipitated by medication. Use of non-steroidal anti-inflammatories may worsen fluid retention in heart failure and affect renal function, and should be stopped if at all possible.

Data gathering and making a diagnosis

Full history and examination is presented in the case. This patient describes NYHA class IV prior to admission but improvement to class III symptoms on discharge. He has heart failure with severe LVSD.

Clinical management

An explanation of the diagnosis of heart failure and importance of regular medication was necessary. A discussion around long-term outlook is also necessary at an appropriate time. This patient needed repeat medications to ensure he did not require readmission to hospital with decompensated heart failure. He is taking appropriate evidence-based treatments; however, the dose of bisoprolol and perindopril should possibly be titrated upwards if possible. Close monitoring of renal function is required. He should also have a lipid profile and up-titration of his statin if he has a cholesterol above 4 or LDL above 2 to ensure adequate secondary prevention given his prior history of four myocardial infarctions. This patient also required regular follow-up by a specialist heart failure clinic. Self-monitoring by daily weighing can be helpful to highlight any worsening of heart failure early. A weight gain of 2 to 3 kg over a few days should prompt a visit to the doctor.

Managing medical complexity

This patient has severe heart failure but also had alcoholism and gout. The medication for heart failure such as frusemide will worsen the gout; however, non-steroidals such as diclofenac can increase fluid retention and worsen heart failure. Diclofenac was stopped and changed to co-codamol. The patient also had a history of alcoholism and, although he had not drunk any alcohol for 2 weeks, was at risk of relapse given the current stresses he was under. He was referred to the local alcohol service for follow-up and support.

Primary care administration

Urgent request for transfer of previous records was needed to gain background medical information.

Working with colleagues

The heart failure lead nurse was contacted the next morning to arrange appropriate follow-up of this patient in the community. He was seen 2 days later.

Community orientation

It is in the interests of wider society to prevent further hospital admissions in this patient to reduce healthcare costs. It is also appropriate to optimise this patient's treatments to ensure he can continue an independent life for as long as possible to allow his son to go out to work.

Maintaining an ethical approach

The four medical ethical principles of beneficence, non-maleficence, autonomy and justice are well demonstrated in this case. This patient needed a script for repeat medications during this consultation to avoid worsening heart failure and readmission, so a timely consultation was necessary to avoid harm. The patient needed appropriate information about his diagnosis and long-term outlook in order to both appreciate the importance of medications and also to plan his future. He needed involving in decision making around further care and regular follow-up to address the questions he had, to ensure he was able to make informed decisions such as where he should live in the longer term. By avoiding an emergency readmission, healthcare costs were reduced for the wider community. Appropriate patient education, a script for medication and arranging timely specialist follow-up will all benefit this patient.

Fitness to practise

It was important for the doctor to put this patient as his first concern and ensure patient safety by arranging close follow-up and support. A multidisciplinary-team approach was appropriate to optimise patient care.

Self-assessment questions

1 ▷ A 78-year-old patient with a history of previous myocardial infarction attends for annual review. He comments that recently he is becoming breathless when he goes up the stairs. He does not have any chest pain. He is a non-smoker. On examination, his ankles are swollen and he has crepitations at both lung bases. What is the single best investigation to diagnose heart failure?

   a. ECG.
   b. Chest X-ray.
   c. BNP.
   d. Echocardiogram.
   e. CT scan.

2 ▷ An 80-year-old patient with heart failure has been seen by the cardiologist and her dose of ramipril has been increased from 2.5 to 5 mg. Her previous renal function tests were normal. When would it be appropriate to do another blood test?

   a. As previous blood tests were fine this is not required.
   b. Check renal function in 24 hours.
   c. Check renal function in 1–2 weeks after dose change.
   d. Check renal function when next blood pressure reading is done.
   e. Check renal function in 3 months.

3 ▷ Which treatment does not have an evidence base for improving prognosis in heart failure?

    a. Frusemide.
    b. Candesartan.
    c. Bisoprolol.
    d. Ramipril.
    e. Spironolactone.

4 ▷ What proportion of patients with suspected heart failure will have a normal ECG?

    a. Less than 1 per cent.
    b. Around 5 per cent.
    c. Around 10–15 per cent.
    d. Around 25 per cent.
    e. More than 25 per cent.

5 ▷ Which of the following statements is **false**?

    a. Heart failure is a chronic disorder.
    b. Angiotensin receptor blockers are effective in treating heart failure when ACE inhibitors are contraindicated.
    c. The prognosis of heart failure is worse than many cancers.
    d. Spironolactone can be beneficial in patients with NYHA class II–IV heart failure.
    e. Palliative care is not appropriate for patients with heart failure and should be reserved for cancer patients primarily.

Answers

1 = d ▷ Echocardiography is the most commonly used definitive test for diagnosis in the presence of symptoms and signs of heart failure.

2 = c ▷ The NICE guidelines suggest checking renal function at baseline, then 1–2 weeks after each dose adjustment.

3 = a ▷ Frusemide may help to improve symptoms of fluid overload but has not been shown to have a prognostic benefit. All the other treatments listed have evidence to support their effectiveness in reducing mortality from randomised controlled trials.

4 = c ▷ Approximately 90 per cent of ECGs in patients with heart failure are abnormal.

5 = e ▷ Heart failure has a poor prognosis and palliative care can be an important aspect of care for patients with severe heart failure.

References

1 • Gillum RF. Epidemiology of heart failure in the United States *American Heart Journal* 1993; **126(4)**: 1042–7.

2 • O'Connell JB, Bristow MR. Economic impact of heart failure in the United States: time for a different approach *Journal of Heart and Lung Transplantation* 1994; **13(Suppl 4)**: S107–12.

3 • The CONSENSUS Trial Study Group. Effects of enalapril on mortality in severe congestive heart failure *New England Journal of Medicine* 1987; **316(23)**: 1429–35.

4 • Hobbs FDR, Roalfe AK, Davis RC, *et al*. Prognosis of all-cause heart failure and borderline left ventricular systolic dysfunction: 5 year mortality follow-up of the Echocardiographic Heart of England Screening Study (ECHOES) *European Heart Journal* 2007; **28(9)**: 1128–34.

5 • McKee PA, Castelli WP, McNamara PM, *et al*. The natural history of heart failure: the Framingham study *New England Journal of Medicine* 1971; **285(26)**: 1441–6.

6 • Ho KKL, Pinsky JL, Kannel WB. The epidemiology of heart failure: the Framingham study *Journal of the American College of Cardiology* 1993; **22(Suppl A)**: 6A–13A.

7 • McDonagh TA, Morrison CE, Lawrence A, *et al*. Symptomatic and asymptomatic left-ventricular systolic dysfunction in an urban population *Lancet* 1997; **350(9081)**: 829–33.

8 • Morgan S, Smith H, Simpson I, *et al*. Prevalence and clinical characteristics of left ventricular dysfunction among elderly patients in general practice setting: cross sectional survey *British Medical Journal* 1999; **318(7180)**: 368–72.

9 • Davies MK, Hobbs FDR, Davis RC, *et al*. Prevalence of left ventricular systolic dysfunction and heart failure in the general population: main findings from the ECHOES (Echocardiographic Heart of England Screening) Study *Lancet* 2001; **358(9280)**: 439–45.

10 • Cowie MR, Wood DA, Coats A, *et al*. Incidence and aetiology of heart failure: a population-based study *European Heart Journal* 1999; **20(6)**: 421–8.

11 • MERIT-HF Study Group. Effect of metoprolol CR/XL in chronic heart failure: metoprolol CR/XL Randomised Intervention Trial in Congestive Heart Failure (MERIT-HF) *Lancet* 1999; **353(9169)**: 2001–7.

12 • Digitalis Investigation Group. The effect of digoxin on mortality and morbidity in patients with heart failure *New England Journal of Medicine* 1997; **336(8)**: 525–33.

13 • RALES Investigators. Effectiveness of spironolactone added to an angiotensin-converting enzyme inhibitor and a loop diuretic for severe chronic congestive heart failure (the Randomized Aldactone Evaluation Study [RALES]) *American Journal of Cardiology* 1996; **78(8)**: 902–7.

14 • Domanski MJ. Beta-Blocker Evaluation of Survival Trial (BEST) *Journal of the American College of Cardiology* 2000; **35(Suppl A)**: 202A.

15 • Ho KKL, Anderson KM, Kannel WB, *et al*. Survival after the onset of congestive heart failure in Framingham Heart Study subjects *Circulation* 1993; **88(1)**: 107–15.

16 • Schocken DD, Arrieta MI, Leaverton PE, *et al*. Prevalence and mortality rate of congestive heart failure in the United States *Journal of the American College of Cardiology* 1992; **20(2)**: 301–6.

17 • McDonagh TA, Cunningham AD, Morrison CE, *et al*. Left ventricular dysfunction, natriuretic peptides, and mortality in an urban population *Heart* 2001; **86(1)**: 21–6.

18 • Cleland JGF, Gemmell, I, Khand A, *et al*. Is the prognosis of heart failure improving? *European Journal of Heart Failure* 1999; **1(3)**: 229–41.

19 • Stewart S, MacIntyre K, Hole DJ, *et al*. More 'malignant' than cancer? Five-year survival following a first admission for heart failure *European Journal of Heart Failure* 2001; **3(3)**: 315–22.

20 • Swedberg K, Cleland J, Dargie H, *et al*.; Task Force for the Diagnosis and Treatment of Chronic Heart Failure of the European Society of Cardiology. Guidelines for the diagnosis and treatment of chronic heart failure: executive summary (update 2005): the Task Force of the Diagnosis and Treatment of Chronic Heart Failure of the European Society of Cardiology *European Heart Journal* 2005; **26(11)**: 1115–40.

21 • Stewart AL, Greenfield S, Hays RD, *et al*. Functional status and well-being of patients with chronic conditions. Results from the medical outcomes study *Journal of the American Medical Association* 1989; **262(7)**: 907–13.

22 • Cline CM, Willenheimer RB, Erhardt LR, *et al*. Health related quality of life in elderly patients with heart failure *Scandinavian Cardiovascular Journal* 1999; **33(5)**: 278–85.

23 • Havranek EP, Ware MG, Lowes BD. Prevalence of depression in congestive heart failure *American Journal of Cardiology* 1999; **84(3)**: 348–50.

24 • Murberg TA, Bru E, Svebak S, *et al*. Depressed mood and subjective health symptoms as predictors of mortality in patients with congestive heart failure: a two-years follow-up study *International Journal of Psychiatry in Medicine* 1999; **29(3)**: 311–26.

25 • Cleland JGF, Swedberg K, Follath F, *et al*. The EuroHeart Failure survey programme: a survey on the quality of care among patients with heart failure in Europe Part 1: patient characteristics and diagnosis *European Heart Journal* 2003: **24(5)**; 442–63.

26 • Sutton GC. Epidemiological aspects of heart failure *American Heart Journal* 1990; **120(6 pt 2)**: 1538–40.

27 • McMurray J, McDonagh T, Morrison CE, *et al*. Trends in hospitalisation for heart failure in Scotland 1980–1990 *European Heart Journal* 1993; **14(9)**: 1158–62.

28 • Eriksson H. Heart failure: a growing public health problem *Journal of Internal Medicine* 1995; **237(2)**: 135–41.

29 • Bundkirchen A, Schwinger RHG. Epidemiology and economic burden of chronic heart failure *European Heart Journal* 2004; **6(Suppl D)**: D57–60.

30 • Owan TE, Hodge DO, Herges RM, *et al*. Trends in prevalence and outcome of heart failure with preserved ejection fraction *New England Journal of Medicine* 2006; **355(3)**: 251–9.

31 • Hunt SA, Abraham WT, Chin MH, *et al*. ACC/AHA 2005 guideline update for the diagnosis and management of chronic heart failure in the adult: a report of the American College of Cardiology/American Heart Association Task Force on Practice Guidelines (Writing Committee to Update the 2001 Guidelines for the Evaluation and Management of Heart Failure): developed in collaboration with the American College of Chest Physicians and the International Society for Heart and Lung Transplantation: endorsed by the Heart Rhythm Society *Circulation* 2005; **112(12)**: e154–235.

32 • Royal College of Physicians. *NICE Clinical Guideline 108, Chronic Heart Failure: national clinical guideline for diagnosis and management in primary and secondary care conditions* London: RCP, 2003, http://guidance.nice.org.uk/CG108/Guidance/pdf/English [accessed September 2010].

33 • Hobbs FDR, Davis RC, Roalfe AK, *et al*. Reliability of N-terminal pro-brain natriuretic peptide assay in diagnosis of heart failure: cohort study in representative and high risk community populations *British Medical Journal* 2002; **324(7352)**: 1498–503.

34 • Healthcare Commission. *Getting to the Heart of It: coronary heart disease in England: a review of progress towards the national standards* London: Commission for Healthcare Audit and Inspection, 2005.

35 • Mant J, Doust J, Roalfe A, *et al*. Systematic review and individual patient data meta-analysis of diagnosis of heart failure, with modelling of implications of different diagnostic strategies in primary care *Health Technology Assessment* 2009; **13(32)**: 1–207.

36 • Hurst JW, Morris DC, Alexander RW. The use of the New York Heart Association's classification of cardiovascular disease as part of the patient's complete Problem List *Clinical Cardiology* 1999; **22(6)**: 385–90.

37 • Davie AP, Francis CM, Love MP, *et al*. Value of an electrocardiogram in identifying heart failure due to left ventricular systolic dysfunction *British Medical Journal* 1996; **312(7025)**: 222.

38 • The NETWORK Investigators. Clinical outcome with enalapril in symptomatic chronic heart failure; a dose comparison *European Heart Journal* 1998; **19(3)**: 481–9.

39 • Khunti K, Squire I, Abrams KR, *et al*. Accuracy of a 12-lead electrocardiogram in screening patients with suspected heart failure for open access echocardiography: a systematic review and meta-analysis *European Journal of Heart Failure* 2004; **6(5)**: 571–6.

40 • Davenport C, Cheng EYL, Kwok YTT, *et al*. Assessing the diagnostic test accuracy of natriuretic peptides and ECG in the diagnosis of left ventricular systolic dysfunction: a systematic review and meta-analysis *British Journal of General Practice* 2006; **56(522)**: 48–56.

41 • Latour-Perez J, Coves-Orts FJ, Abad-Terrado C, *et al*. Accuracy of B-type natriuretic peptide levels in the diagnosis of left ventricular dysfunction and heart failure: a systematic review *European Journal of Heart Failure* 2006; **8(4)**: 390–9.

42 • Clerico A, Fontana M, Zyw L, *et al*. Comparison of the diagnostic accuracy of BNP and NTproBNP in chronic and acute heart failure: a systematic review *Clinical Chemistry* 2007; **53(5)**: 813–22.

43 • Cardarelli R, Lumicao TG. B type natriuretic peptide: a review of its diagnostic, prognostic, and therapeutic monitoring value in heart failure for primary care physicians *Journal of the American Board of Family Practice* 2003; **16(4)**: 327–33.

44 • Korenstein D, Wisnivesky JP, Wyer P, *et al*. The utility of B type natriuretic peptide in the diagnosis of heart failure in the emergency department: a systematic review *BMC Emergency Medicine* 2007; **7**: 6.

45 • Mant J, Hobbs FDR, Fletcher K, *et al*. Warfarin versus aspirin for stroke prevention in an elderly community population with atrial fibrillation (the Birmingham Atrial Fibrillation Treatment of the Aged Study, BAFTA): a randomised controlled trial *Lancet* 2007; **370(9586)**: 493–503.

46 • Cleland JGF, Cohen-Solal A, Cosin Aguilar J, *et al*. Management of heart failure in primary care (the IMPROVEMENT of Heart Failure Programme): an international survey *Lancet* 2003; **360(9346)**: 1631–9.

47 • Wheeldon NM, MacDonald TM, Flucker CJ, *et al*. Echocardiography in chronic heart failure in the community *Quarterly Journal of Medicine* 1993; **86(1)**: 17–20.

48 • Remes J, Miettinen H, Reunanen A, *et al*. Validity of clinical diagnosis of heart failure in primary health care *European Heart Journal* 1991; **12(3)**: 315–21.

49 • Anonymous. Failure to treat heart failure (editorial) *Lancet* 1992; **339(8788)**: 278–9.

50 • Clarke KW, Gray D, Hampton JR. Evidence of inadequate investigation and treatment of patients with heart failure *British Heart Journal* 1994; **71(6)**: 584–7.

51 • Pfeffer MA, Braunwald E, Moye LA, *et al*. for the SAVE Investigators. Effect of captopril on mortality and morbidity in patients with left ventricular dysfunction after myocardial infarction: results of the Survival and Ventricular Enlargement Trial *New England Journal of Medicine* 1992; **327(10)**: 669–77.

52 • Garg R, Yusuf S, for the Collaborative Group on ACE Inhibitor Trials. Overview of randomized trials of angiotensin-converting enzyme inhibitors on mortality and morbidity in patients with heart failure *Journal of the American Medical Association* 1995; **273(18)**: 1450–6.

53 • Pfeffer MA, Swedberg K, Granger CB, *et al*., for the CHARM Investigators and Committees. Effects of candesartan on mortality and morbidity in patients with chronic heart failure: the CHARM-Overall programme *Lancet* 2003; **362(9386)**: 759–66.

54 • CIBIS-II Investigators and Committees. The Cardiac Insufficiency Bisoprolol Study II *Lancet* 1999; **353(9146)**: 9–13.

55 • American College of Cardiology/American Heart Association. Guidelines for the evaluation and management of heart failure. Report of the American College of Cardiology/American Heart Association Task Force on Practice Guidelines (Committee on Evaluation and Management of Heart Failure) *Circulation* 1995; **92(9)**: 2764–84.

56 • Pitt B, White H, Nicolau J, *et al*.; EPHESUS Investigators. Eplerenone reduces mortality 30 days after randomization following acute myocardial infarction in patients with left ventricular systolic dysfunction and heart failure *Journal of the American College of Cardiology* 2005; **46(3)**: 425–31.

57 • Juurlink DN, Mamdani MM, Lee DS, *et al*. Rates of hyperkalemia after publication of the Randomized Aldactone Evaluation Study *New England Journal of Medicine* 2004; **351(6)**: 543–51.

58 • Kjekshus J, Apetrei E, Barrios V, *et al*. Rosuvastatin in older patients with systolic heart failure *New England Journal of Medicine* 2007; **357(22)**: 2248–61.

59 • Lechat P, Packer M, Chalon S, *et al*. Beta-blockers in heart failure: meta-analysis of randomized trials *Circulation* 1998; **98(12)**: 1184–91.

60 • SOLVD Investigators. Effect of enalapril on survival in patients with reduced left ventricular ejection fractions and congestive heart failure *New England Journal of Medicine* 1991; **325(5)**: 293–302.

61 • SOLVD Investigators. Effect of enalapril on mortality and the development of heart failure in asymptomatic patients with reduced left ventricular ejection fractions *New England Journal of Medicine* 1992; **327(10)**: 685–91.

62 • Willenheimer R, Erhardt L, Cline C, *et al*. Exercise training in heart failure improves quality of life and exercise capacity *European Heart Journal* 1998; **19(5)**: 774–81.

63 • Rich MW, Beckham V, Wittenberg C, *et al*. A multidisciplinary intervention to prevent the readmission of elderly patients with congestive heart failure *New England Journal of Medicine* 1995; **333(18)**: 1190–5.

64 • Hobbs FDR, Jones MI, Allan TS, *et al*. European survey of primary care physician perceptions and practice in heart failure diagnosis and management (Euro-HF study) *European Heart Journal* 2000; **21(22)**: 1877–87.

65 • Houghton AR, Cowley AJ. Why are angiotensin converting enzyme inhibitors underutilised in the treatment of heart failure by general practitioners? *International Journal of Cardiology* 1997; **59(1)**: 7–10.

66 • Department of Health. *New GMS Contract QOF Implementation: heart failure indicator set* London: DoH, 2006.

67 • British Medical Association. *QOF Changes and New Indicators for 2009/10* London: BMA, www.bma.org.uk/images/QOFchanges200910_tcm41-178932.pdf [accessed September 2010].

68 • Troughton R, Frampton C, Yandle T, *et al.* Treatment of heart failure guided by plasma aminoterminal brain natriuretic peptide (N-BNP) concentrations *Lancet* 2000; **355(9210)**: 1126–30.

Venous thromboembolism and varicose veins

10

David Fitzmaurice

Aims

This chapter discusses the importance of prevention, clinical recognition, appropriate investigation and short- and long-term management of venous thromboembolism (VTE) including deep-vein thrombosis (DVT) and pulmonary embolism (PE). The epidemiology and main risk factors for VTE are also discussed. The second part of the chapter focuses on varicose veins and the management of common complications in primary care.

Key learning points

- ▶ VTE is an important cause of morbidity and mortality, and prevention of VTE during hospital admission is important for patient safety.
- ▶ DVT may present with symptoms of leg swelling and pain.
- ▶ Doppler ultrasound is the most commonly used investigation for definitive diagnosis of DVT. D-dimer can be used as a screening tool to rule out DVT.
- ▶ PE is a medical emergency and may present with chest pain, breathlessness and tachycardia.
- ▶ Anticoagulation is the mainstay of treatment for VTE and duration of treatment depends on several factors.
- ▶ Varicose veins are common.
- ▶ Patients likely to benefit from surgery, such as those with significant symptoms or skin changes, should be referred to vascular surgery.
- ▶ Complications such as venous ulceration can be managed by the multidisciplinary team in primary care.

Introduction

Venous thromboembolic disease is usually clinically differentiated into DVT and PE, although these two entities are essentially different presentations of the same disease process. DVT is a radiologically confirmed partial or total thrombotic occlusion of the deep venous system of the legs, sufficient to produce symptoms of pain or swelling. The term 'proximal DVT' refers to thrombosis affecting the veins above the knee (popliteal, superficial femoral, common femoral, and iliac veins). Isolated calf DVT is confined to the deep veins of the calf and does not affect the veins above the knee. Pulmonary embolism is radiologically confirmed partial or total thromboembolic occlusion of pulmonary arteries, sufficient to cause symptoms of breathlessness, chest pain, or both. Post-thrombotic syndrome is a long-term complication of DVT resulting in oedema, ulceration, and impaired viability of the subcutaneous tissues of the leg DVT.[1] In contrast, the principal manifestation of arterial thromboembolism is stroke, although arterial thrombosis and emboli can occur throughout the arterial tree.

The challenge for primary care lies in diagnosis, although more recently there have been developments in preventive strategies, especially in relation to venous thromboembolism associated with hospital admission.

This chapter looks at the diagnosis and management of venous thromboembolic disease from a primary care perspective. Arterial embolism is discussed in Chapters 4 and 5.

Venous thromboembolic disease

VTE is a major cause of morbidity and mortality worldwide, although routine data collection for these conditions is unreliable. It has been estimated that VTE occurs in up to 2 per cent of the UK population annually, while US data suggest that there are around 250,000 hospital admissions, with around 50,000 deaths, for either DVT or PE per year.[2] The fatality rate from acute PE of approximately 10 per cent appears not to have altered since the 1970s.[3]

Deep-vein thrombosis

The classical presentation of DVT is as an acutely painful, swollen, red calf. DVT is associated with pregnancy, contraceptive pill use, immobility, surgery, malignancy, advancing age, smoking and certain clotting disorders.[4] Both proximal and isolated calf vein thromboses can cause post-thrombotic syndrome, recurrent venous thrombosis and pulmonary embolus, with associated morbidity and mortality.

Anticoagulation, in terms of early intervention with heparin and warfarin, with prolonged warfarin treatment, has been demonstrated to reduce sequelae associated with DVT, particularly PE.[5] Since anticoagulation therapy carries a risk of haemorrhagic complications, it is important that a diagnosis of DVT is objectively confirmed before commencement of treatment. The treatment of below-knee DVT remains controversial but there is evidence to suggest that, where calf thrombi are symptomatic, anticoagulation treatment is of benefit and reduces the risk of extension.[6,7]

DIAGNOSIS AND INVESTIGATION

Clinical diagnosis of DVT is made on the basis of pain, swelling and venous distension, but is notoriously unreliable.[8,9] The clinical sign of pain on forced dorsiflexion of the foot (Homan's sign) has fallen out of favour and is no longer recommended due to risk of proximal embolism.[9] The differential diagnosis of DVT includes musculoskeletal pain and popliteal inflammatory cysts (Baker's cysts).[8]

The gold standard for diagnosis remains venography, but this is an invasive test that is inconvenient, painful and can be associated with allergic and other side effects.[9] The most widespread diagnostic procedure in the UK is ultrasound. The reliability of this modality is very user dependent and it is not very useful, even in the best hands, for diagnosing below-knee DVT. Light-reflection rheography is also an effective non-invasive technique for screening patients with suspected DVT,[10] while D-dimer tests can be used as a pre-screening tool before ultrasound. The sensitivity and specificity of ultrasound have been reported as 78 per cent and 98 per cent respectively.[9] D-dimer tests indicate active fibrinolysis and hence provide a screening technique for DVT. While not specific to DVT, D-dimer has a high (>95 per cent) negative predictive value and is a reliable method for the exclusion of DVT in symptomatic patients.[11]

PREVENTION

One of the most useful advances in the area of thromboembolic disease has been preventive therapy, particularly for hospital in-patients, with medical patients increasingly recognised as being at risk of developing venous thrombosis. For medical patients who are at high risk, or for high-risk surgical patients, there are a variety of options to reduce the incidence of DVT. These include formal anticoagulation, use of compression stockings, intra-operative pressure devices, and use of chemical agents such as low molecular weight heparin (LMWH). Newer agents such as oral thrombin inhibitors and oral factor Xa inhibitors are now also licensed in Europe for thrombo-prophylaxis of high-risk surgical patients, particularly patients undergoing orthopaedic procedures.

The prevention of venous thromboembolism in adult in-patients was described as the number-one patient safety issue by the Agency for Health-care Research and Quality in the US,[12] while in the UK a Health Select Committee report in 2005 estimated that venous thromboembolism caused in excess of 25,000 potentially preventable deaths per annum, with around half due to hospital admission.[13] Overall deaths from venous thromboem-bolism in the UK are five times greater than the combined total deaths from breast cancer, AIDS and road traffic accidents. Indeed a revised estimate, based on an epidemiological model using extrapolation from European data, has suggested a figure of approximately 60,000 annual venous thromboem-bolism deaths in the UK.[14] Post-mortem data suggest that about 10 per cent of deaths occurring in hospital are due to pulmonary embolism.[15] While risks to surgical patients, in particular those undergoing orthopaedic proce-dures, are well known, the majority of people who develop venous throm-boembolism while in hospital are medical patients. There is a large body of evidence showing that pharmacological thromboprophylaxis can reduce the rate of venous thromboembolism by 60–65 per cent.[16–18]

The 2005 Health Select Committee report stated that thromboprophy-laxis was not being effectively implemented in the UK, with rates as low as 20 per cent of eligible patients receiving appropriate prevention.[13] The main recommendations following this report were that the National Insti-tute for Health and Clinical Excellence (NICE) should produce guidelines for venous thromboembolism for surgical procedures more quickly than planned and that an independent venous thromboembolism expert work-ing group (EWG) should be set up to report to the Chief Medical Officer (CMO) on how current best practice and guidance could be promoted and implemented, and on what resources might be needed to support delivery of any strategy through existing structures.

The EWG report and the CMO's response have been published.[19] The first recommendation of the EWG was that all hospitalised adults should have a documented mandatory venous thromboembolism risk assessment on admission. It also recommended that this risk assessment be embedded within the Clinical Negligence Scheme for Trusts (CNST). They also recom-mended that core standards be set by the Department of Health to ensure that ultimately there is 100 per cent compliance with risk assessment for thromboprophylaxis. Importantly the report states that aspirin should not be used for thromboprophylaxis due to a relative lack of effectiveness compared with other agents such as LMWH.

A NICE guideline for surgical patients has also been published, recommending that aspirin should not be used, but retained the emphasis on mechanical rather than chemical means of thromboprophylaxis. It classed patients aged over 60 as high risk rather than those aged over 40.[20] Prevention of thrombosis for patients admitted to hospital is an area that will continue to evolve and will increasingly involve primary care.

RISK FACTORS FOR VTE

Exogenous female hormones, either as hormone replacement therapy (HRT) or as oral contraception, contribute to the development of VTE. The absolute increased risk is very small, however, and, particularly in the case of oral contraception, the overall health risk of not taking therapy is outweighed by the risk of taking it. The absolute risk of venous thrombosis in healthy young women is around 1 per 10,000 person years, rising to 3 to 4 per 10,000 person years during the time oral contraceptives are being used.[21] Pregnancy, however, is itself a risk factor for DVT. Pregnant patients at high risk or with a previous history of thrombosis should be treated with LMWH. Warfarin is contraindicated in pregnancy as it is teratogenic.

There are various conditions that may predispose to a clotting tendency. These are generally congenital (e.g. Factor V Leiden, protein C deficiency) but may be acquired (e.g. lupus anticoagulant). These are not usually problematic and are only investigated if a patient presents with an unusual thrombotic history.

An increasing problem encountered in primary care is what to do with patients who have a history of thrombosis and who wish to travel by air. The risk of thrombosis appears to be greatest when there is travel of over 6 hours where the patient is confined to a particular position (usually sitting). Traveller's thrombosis has been reported from air, car and bus travel. If there is any suggestion of an association between long-distance travel and thrombosis, or there is a strong family history of thrombosis, then specialist referral is indicated. The risk of prolonged travel, either by air or other means, is probably overstated, with patients suffering an event being predisposed to thromboembolism anyway.[22] The principal risk factor for traveller's thrombosis appears to be previous history of a clot. The main preventive measures are the use of full-length graduated compression stockings, or prophylactic LMWH.[23]

263

TREATMENT

Goals of treatment of DVT are prevention of pulmonary embolism with the restoration of venous patency and valvular function.[24,25] The principles of management for these patients have remained essentially unchanged over several years; however, there has been a shift in terms of admission to hospital. The main initial management is to arrange for diagnostic confirmation, which is usually organised through secondary care.

The American College of Chest Physicians (ACCP) guidelines recommend that initial treatment for patients with VTE should be a once- or twice-daily therapeutic subcutaneous dose of LMWH, while also starting an oral vitamin K antagonist, most commonly warfarin.[26] However, for at least the first 3 months of long-term treatment of either DVT or PE in patients with cancer, a recent systematic review has shown that there are improved outcomes in terms of recurrence and/or bleeding when LMWH is used throughout instead of warfarin.[27]

Patients should also be advised to stop smoking, to lose excess weight and to stop taking any combined hormonal contraceptives.

Women who are pregnant or in the puerperium and diagnosed with VTE should be managed according to guidelines published by the Royal College of Obstetricians and Gynaecologists.[28]

Treatment with anticoagulation historically involved a hospital in-patient stay of around 7 days for intravenous heparin administration with daily partial thromboplastin time (PTT) estimation, together with warfarin for approximately 3 months (with monitoring).[8] More recently, however, subcutaneous administration of LMWH has been demonstrated to be as safe and effective as traditional intravenous therapy with fewer complications, and the advantage that PTT monitoring is not required.[29] Dosing schedules for LMWH are based solely on body weight. Secondary care data suggest that LMWH can be cost-effective due to the reduced cost of monitoring and reduced hospital stay.[30] These studies also highlight the possibility of home treatment, with patients either self-dosing or receiving injections from a nurse or a relative.[31]

While oral anticoagulation is established in the treatment of patients with DVT, the duration of therapy remains debatable. Two prospective randomised studies for treatment of proximal DVT, comparing 4 weeks with 3 months[32] and 6 weeks with 6 months warfarin therapy,[33] have gone some way to resolving the issue. While there are problems in comparing studies due to difficulties in standardising diagnostic criteria, these studies showed recurrence rates after two years of 8.6 per cent in the 4-week group compared with 0.9 per cent in the 3-month group (OR = 10.1, 95 per cent CI 1.3–81.4), and 18.1 per cent in the 6-week group compared with 9.5 per cent in the 6-month group (OR = 2.1, 95 per cent CI 1.4–3.1).

Whatever the proposed duration of treatment, once a patient with a VTE reaches the end of the planned treatment period of anticoagulant therapy, the patient needs to be reviewed as to whether he or she is at a higher risk of recurrence and hence needs longer than normal treatment. Medical conditions, such as cancer, inflammatory conditions or nephrotic syndrome, put patients at increased risk of recurrence, as does an initial VTE where no cause was found for it. Men are at higher risk than women for recurrence, as are those who continue to smoke or have an increased BMI. Although currently largely a research tool, a raised D-dimer level at the end of treatment also suggests an increased risk of recurrence.[34] This is also a good opportunity to check that the patient is wearing the appropriate graduated compression stockings (if the patient presented initially with a DVT) to ensure that his or her risk of developing post-thrombotic syndrome is reduced. Post-thrombotic syndrome is oedema, ulceration, and impaired viability of the subcutaneous tissues of the leg occurring after DVT.

If one or more of the risk factors are present, the risk of recurrence should be discussed with the patient, as well as the possibility of continuing anticoagulant therapy. However, this risk needs to be balanced with the increased risk of bleeding while on anticoagulant therapy, and how the patient feels about the implications of being on long-term anticoagulant therapy (in terms of regular monitoring and anticoagulant medication interaction with other medications).

Debate continues over the treatment of distal DVT where thrombus is limited to the calf veins only. However, evidence for treatment is strong. Untreated symptomatic calf vein thrombosis in non-surgical patients has a recurrence rate of over 25 per cent, with an attendant risk of proximal extension and pulmonary embolisation. This risk is reduced to 7.6 per cent with treatment aiming for an international normalised ratio (INR) of 2.0–3.0 for 3 months, which compares with rates of 12.4 per cent with 4 weeks, 11.8 per cent with 6 weeks, and 5.8 per cent with 6 months of oral anticoagulant therapy.[34]

RECOMMENDATIONS FOR DEEP-VEIN THROMBOSIS

Treatment of idiopathic proximal DVT should be continued for 6 months. For patients with isolated DVT without continuing risk factors, 6 weeks of oral anticoagulation therapy is sufficient. The evidence for patients with idiopathic symptomatic isolated distal calf vein thrombosis is for treatment aimed at a target INR of 2.5 for 3 months. For post-operative calf vein thrombosis, however, 6 weeks' therapy is as effective as treatment for 3 months.

The guidelines for recurrent thrombosis while off treatment recommend lifelong therapy, and for recurrence while on treatment lifelong therapy at a higher therapeutic intensity.[35]

Pulmonary embolism

Pulmonary emboli usually arise from veins in the pelvis and leg. The risk factors are the same as for DVT. Up to 50 per cent of those with fatal PE have no warning signs. The clinical presentation depends upon the size of the emboli, with small emboli remaining asymptomatic. Large non-fatal emboli cause acute pleuritic chest pain associated with shortness of breath, tachycardia and pyrexia. Associated features include haemoptysis, pleural effusion, hypotension, cyanosis and shock. All cases of suspected pulmonary embolism need to be treated as acute medical emergencies with admission to hospital arranged if possible. The mainstay of diagnosis remains the ventilation/perfusion scan, although spiral CT scan is now regarded as the preferred test due to its high negative predictive value for clinically relevant pulmonary embolism.[36]

TREATMENT

The traditional management of PE has been to stabilise the patient medically and then anticoagulate in exactly the same manner as for DVT. This remains essentially the same today; however, advances in the use of LMWH for DVT has seen investigation into the use of LMWH for the home management of PE.[37] While this may be suitable for a small number of stable patients, the main priority from a primary care perspective is to arrange for hospital admission for assessment, stabilisation and confirmation of diagnosis.

No studies have looked specifically at the intensity of oral anticoagulation therapy for the treatment of pulmonary embolus. The current UK recommendation for patients diagnosed with a first pulmonary embolus is to aim for an INR of 2.5. These recommendations are based on results of studies primarily investigating the treatment of proximal DVT where the occurrence of a pulmonary embolus was taken as an endpoint in interventional studies.

Data are available which show that fatal recurrence of PE following DVT is extremely rare when treated, with heparin initially, followed by a longer period of warfarin therapy.[38] The range of INR between 2.0 and 3.0 was chosen as it gives the lowest recurrence and bleeding rates in treatment of proximal DVT.[39]

RECOMMENDATIONS FOR PULMONARY EMBOLUS

The clinical decision as to whether or not to anticoagulate patients with suspected PE will be dependent upon the strength of the clinical suspicion (pretest probability) combined with the results of ventilation perfusion scanning.[40] Patients with a normal or low probability scan should not be treated.[41]

Varicose veins

The term 'varicose' means dilated and tortuous. Varicose veins may be found in several anatomical sites: anal canal (haemorrhoids); testicles (varicocoele); oesophagus (associated with portal hypertension); trunk (telangiectasia). This section, however, deals with varicose veins and the associated problems of the lower limbs. These are, in part, a price we have to pay for upright posture.

INCIDENCE AND PREVALENCE

The prevalence of lower-limb varicosities in the UK is around 10 per cent for men and 20 per cent for women between the ages of 35 and 70. The prevalence increases with age and maintains a female gender bias, although interestingly trunk varicosities remain fairly equally distributed between the sexes.[42] While the incidence is not well defined, the Framingham study described an annual incidence of around 2 per cent for men and 2.5 per cent for women, although the exact case mix and age-specific distribution were not defined. These figures do seem high compared with UK practice, where the consultation rate for new presentations of varicose veins in primary care is around 0.5 per 1000 population. This will obviously vary dependent on the age and sex mix of the practice population.

AETIOLOGY

Blood returning to the heart from the lower limbs passes through the deep venous system. This is fed from the skin and subcutaneous tissues through the superficial (or perforating) veins. The blood flow is uni-directional because of the presence of valves within the superficial system that prevent back-flow. Traditional surgical teaching was that damage to the valves of the superficial veins meant that blood could leak back into the superficial system from the deep system instead of flowing into the inferior vena cava. This in turn creates more pressure on the remaining veins until the superficial system becomes a reservoir of venous blood leading to distortion and dilatation of the vessel walls. The theory of reflux and dilatation has more recently been replaced by the idea that the principal pathological process is weakness of the vessel wall with dilatation preceding valvular damage. Thus it is observed that initial dilatation is actually distal to the valve (whereas it should be proximal if the primary abnormality was valve damage).

The majority (around 80 per cent) of varicose veins are primary (or idiopathic). There is often a family history, although there does not appear to be a genetic predisposition. Females are more affected than males, and they may be exacerbated by pregnancy either as a direct result of fetal pressure or in combination with smooth-muscle relaxation from raised levels of progesterone. Secondary causes include: DVT; pelvic tumours (including pregnancy); occupations requiring long periods of standing. The other principal risk factor is age. Smoking and social class do not appear to affect the incidence, while obesity only seems to be a risk factor for women.

SYMPTOMS

The majority of patients with varicose veins have little in the way of symptoms. The commonest presenting complaint is that of 'unsightliness' or worries about appearance. Alongside this patients can complain of heaviness in the legs, itching, occasional bleeding from large varices, a lump in the groin, leg swelling, lower leg ulceration, and a rash around the garter area ('varicose eczema').

DIAGNOSIS

The diagnosis is principally clinical, based on the appearance of distended veins. One needs to be careful, however, as the visual appearance can be influenced by ambient temperature and hormonal status (in women), while obesity can hide the natural appearance. Occasionally, superficial venous flaring can mask underlying venous insufficiency, which may be unmasked with colour duplex scanning. Abdominal palpation is suggested to exclude secondary causes of varicose veins. Vascular surgeons may recommend routine duplex venous scanning for all patients with suspected varicose veins; however, this is costly, probably unnecessary and will not be available in many countries. It may be useful in recurrence to exclude DVT. It has been suggested that hand-held Doppler assessment of reflux at the sapheno-femoral junction is a useful aid in diagnosis with sensitivity of 97 per cent and specificity of 73 per cent compared with colour duplex scanning.[43]

Once the connection between the superficial and deep venous system has been compromised, the increase in pressure results in the development of venules around the ankle (particularly the medial malleolus). The development of venules is a warning sign for the development of ulcers. Similarly, varices tend to be largest at the junctions between the superficial and deep system, with the commonest manifestation being the saphena varix. This is seen as a lump in the groin where the long saphenous vein joins the femoral vein. Its importance is really as a differential diagnosis of a lump in the groin and it is usually fairly obviously associated with lower-limb varicosities.

TREATMENT

Around 50 per cent of patients presenting for the first time in primary care will require no treatment. Patients are usually happy to be reassured that there is no gross underlying pathology and that simple measures such as keeping the feet elevated at rest, wearing some form of elasticated stocking and trying to avoid long spells of standing will keep things under control.

Patients with either gross varicosities or evidence of complications (such as varicose eczema) will benefit from some form of intervention. The decisions from a primary care perspective are when to refer, who to refer to, and what to request. Referral will be dictated by the patient with some patients having a low threshold for cosmetic appearance and others tolerating quite disfiguring varices. Once there is evidence of skin changes, however, it is likely that the patient would benefit from surgical intervention. Referral should preferably be to a vascular surgeon with a specific interest in this problem. One of the issues for primary care in recent years has been the relatively high recurrence rates following surgical intervention. These appear to be much lower if a specialist surgeon is responsible for patient care. It is usual to request a surgical opinion; however, it is not unreasonable to actually request a specific intervention such as venous stripping, following discussion with the patient.

CONSERVATIVE MANAGEMENT

For patients whose main symptoms are aching, oedema and itching with no skin changes, or where the diagnosis is in doubt, a trial of compression hosiery may help. It must be pointed out, however, that a successful response to compression hosiery suggests that surgery would be beneficial.

SURGICAL MANAGEMENT

There are basically two options for surgical management, injection sclero-therapy and venous disconnection – stripping and avulsion.

Injections are generally only used now for varices that remain after for-mal surgery. This is due to skin staining and high recurrence rates (up to 65 per cent).

The exact nature of surgical intervention will depend upon the nature of the lesions. The classical surgical procedure is the Trendelenburg pro-cedure. This describes the disconnection of the saphenous vein from the femoral vein with the terminal branches of the saphenous vein individually ligated and divided. This is classically described as the treatment of choice for an incompetent sapheno-femoral junction. Other incompetencies can be identified by using a tourniquet and applying it to the leg and thigh at various levels while the patient is lying down. If upon standing there is no filling of the superficial venous system, the problem can be controlled by disconnection at this point. If there is filling there are further leaks distal to where the tourniquet has been applied. By identifying the individual incompetencies these can be marked prior to operation and individually ligated and divided.

An alternative to this rather drawn-out procedure is to strip the vein completely. This involves introducing a flexible wire vein stripper into the saphenous vein in front of the medial malleolus. The wire is passed up into the groin where the saphenous vein has been disconnected from the femo-ral vein. The wire is pulled proximally, disconnecting the tributaries of the main saphenous system.

Most surgery can be undertaken as a day case with patients able to resume driving after around 1 week and returning to work within 3 weeks. Serious complications such as pulmonary embolism occur in less than 1 per cent of patients, although minor problems such as bleeding or neuralgia may occur in up to 17 per cent of cases.[44]

Complications of varicose veins

HAEMORRHAGE

This is inevitably the result of trauma to a varix. Treatment is simple with pres-sure and elevation followed by the application of a pressure bandage. Unless there is some associated illness such as haemophilia, this is all that is required.

THROMBOPHLEBITIS

This describes inflammation of the superficial veins. It is not an infective condition and does not require antibiotic treatment. Generally this will require simple treatment with oral non-steroidal anti-inflammatory agents, elevation if practical, compression hosiery and possibly aspirin. If there is any suspicion that thrombus has extended into the deep venous system or symptoms are not resolving after 72 hours, referral for investigation should be undertaken. This is rare.

VARICOSE ECZEMA (LIPODERMATOSCLEROSIS)

At the onset of skin changes the patient should be considered for referral. Skin changes often result from a combination of venous and arterial insufficiency and may be associated with DVT. Paradoxically, if the deep venous system of valves remains intact, surgical intervention in terms of dislocation and ligation of the superficial venous system will be of benefit. Conversely, if the deep venous system is damaged, surgery will have little role to play, with treatment combining compression stockings and topical steroids.

ULCERATION

Ulceration is most likely to occur around the malleoli and is predominantly associated with varicose eczema and DVT. Chronic venous ulceration is a huge problem in the many countries consuming large amounts of money and large amounts of nursing (particularly community nursing) time. Treatment is problematic and has been the subject of many reviews. Obesity is a risk factor and arterial disease is present in around 20 per cent of cases. This is an important consideration in assessment in order to prevent unnecessary damage occurring from compression treatment.

Early hospital specialist vascular assessment of leg ulcers (including duplex scanning of the arterial and venous systems) offers potential clinical benefit (in terms of prevention of chronic ulceration) with associated cost savings.[45]

Compression is useful for the treatment of ulcers as long as this does not compromise arterial supply. The exact nature of the compression remains controversial with two-layer, three-layer and four-layer compression being compared, as well as intermittent pneumatic compression and Class 3 support stockings having been evaluated. Generally the studies have been poor quality. It is clear that compression is important and it is suggested that layered compression appears to be better than simple support stockings. In the absence of any better data it can be concluded therefore that it is safe to use three-layer compression and elevation.

It may be that specialist nursing care can improve outcomes; however, drug treatment such as stanazol and zinc sulphate have no beneficial effect, while ultrasound, laser therapy and electrical stimulation have not been sufficiently investigated.

Summary

Venous disorders are an important cause of morbidity and mortality. It is important to identify VTE in patients with characteristic clinical features, as effective treatment with anticoagulants can be life saving. Varicose veins are common and can be unsightly; however, they are not life-threatening. Only those likely to benefit from surgery should be referred.

Self-assessment questions

1 ▷ Which of the following statements regarding DVT is **not** correct?

    a. DVT is a common reversible cause of death in hospitalised patients.
    b. It is reduced by prophylactic heparin.
    c. It is more common in smokers.
    d. It is less common in women taking the oral contraceptive pill.
    e. Can be asymptomatic.

2 ▷ Which of the following statements about warfarin is **not** correct?

    a. Warfarin is the anticoagulant of choice in pregnancy.
    b. The action of warfarin can be affected by other medication.
    c. Warfarin can be used in older patients.
    d. Has been shown to reduce recurrence of DVT.
    e. Inhibits vitamin K metabolism.

3 ▷ The INR target range for a patient with a first diagnosis of proximal DVT is:

a. 1.0–2.0.
b. 2.0–3.0.
c. 2.5–3.5.
d. 1.5–2.5.
e. 4.0–5.0.

4 ▷ Pulmonary embolism:

a. Is a medical emergency.
b. Is usually caused by trauma to the chest.
c. Is mainly treated in primary care.
d. Is always symptomatic.
e. Can be treated effectively with aspirin.

5 ▷ Varicose veins are:

a. Often a marker of underlying malignancy.
b. Most commonly idiopathic.
c. Best treated by early surgical intervention.
d. Less common in pregnancy.
e. Often caused by DVT.

Answers

1 = d ▷ DVT is more common in women taking the oral contraceptive pill.

2 = a ▷ Warfarin is potentially teratogenic so heparin is more commonly used, although warfarin may be considered in some circumstances.

3 = b ▷ Studies have shown a reduction in recurrence of DVT in patients treated with warfarin with an INR of 2.0–3.0.

4 = a ▷ Pulmonary embolism can be life threatening and should be managed as a medical emergency.

5 = b ▷ Are most commonly idiopathic.

References

1 • http://clinicalevidence.bmj.com/ceweb/conditions/cvd/0208/0208_keypoints.jsp [accessed September 2010].

2 • Anderson FA Jr, Wheeler HB, Goldberg RJ, *et al.* A population-based perspective of the hospital incidence and case-fatality rates of deep vein thrombosis and pulmonary embolism: the Worcester DVT study *Archives of Internal Medicine* 1991; **151(5)**: 933–8.

3 • Rubinstein I, Murray D, Hoffstein V. Fatal pulmonary emboli in hospitalized patients: an autopsy study *Archives of Internal Medicine* 1988; **148(6)**: 1425–6.

4 • Hirsh J, Hoak J. Management of deep vein thrombosis and pulmonary embolism *Circulation* 1996; **93(12)**: 2212–45.

5 • Lensing AWA, Prandoni P, Prins MH, *et al.* Deep-vein thrombosis *Lancet* 1999; **353(9151)**: 479–85.

6 • Lagerstedt C, Olsson C, Fagher B, *et al.* Need for long-term anticoagulant treatment in symptomatic calf-vein thrombosis *Lancet* 1985; **2(8454)**: 515–18.

7 • Giannoukas AD, Labropoulos N, Burke P, *et al.* Calf deep venous thrombosis: a review of the literature *European Journal of Vascular and Endovascular Surgery* 1995; **10(4)**: 398–404.

8 • Weinmann EE, Salzman EW. Deep-vein thrombosis *New England Journal of Medicine* 1994; **331(24)**: 1630–44.

9 • Wells PS, Hirsh J, Anderson DR, *et al.* Accuracy of clinical assessment of deep-vein thrombosis *Lancet* 1995; **345(8961)**: 1326–30.

10 • Thomas PRS, Butler CM, Bowman J, *et al.* Light reflection rheography: an effective non-invasive technique for screening patients with suspected deep venous thrombosis *British Journal of Surgery* 1991: **78(2)**: 207–9.

11 • Turkstra F, van Beek JR, ten Cate JW, *et al.* Reliable rapid blood test for the exclusion of venous thromboembolism in symptomatic outpatients *Thrombosis and Haemostasis* 1996; **76(1)**: 9–11.

12 • www.ahrq.gov/clinic/ptsafety/summary.htm [accessed September 2010].

13 • House of Commons Health Committee. *The Prevention of Venous Thromboembolism in Hospitalised Patients: second report of session 2004–05* London: The Stationery Office, 2005, www.parliament.the-stationery-office.co.uk/pa/cm200405/cmselect/cmhealth/99/99.pdf [accessed September 2010].

14 • Cohen AT, Kakkar AK. Venous thromboembolic disease in cancer patients in Europe: an opportunity for improved prevention. The VITAE thrombosis study *European Journal of Cancer* 2005; **3(Suppl 2)**: 155.

15 • Sandler DA, Martin JF. Autopsy proven pulmonary embolism in hospital patients: are we detecting enough deep vein thromboses? *Journal of the Royal Society of Medicine* 1989; **82(4)**: 203–5.

16 • Collins R, Scrimgeor A, Yusuk S, *et al.* Reduction in fatal pulmonary embolism and venous thrombosis by perioperative administration of subcutaneous heparin. Overview of results of randomised trials in general, orthopaedic, and urologic surgery *New England Journal of Medicine* 1988; **318(18)**: 1162–73.

17 • Mismetti P, Laporte S, Darmon JY, *et al.* Meta-analysis of low molecular weight heparin in the prevention of venous thromboembolism in general surgery *British Journal of Surgery* 2001; **88(7)**: 913–30.

18 • Cohen AT, Davidson BL, Gallus AS, *et al*. Efficacy and safety of fondaparinux for the prevention of venous thromboembolism in older acute medical patients: randomised placebo controlled trial *British Medical Journal* 2006; **332(7537)**: 325–9.

19 • Department of Health; Donaldson L. *Recommendations of the Expert Working Group on the Prevention of Thromboembolism (VTE) in Hospitalised Patients* London: DoH, 2007, www.dh.gov.uk/en/Publicationsandstatistics/Lettersandcirculars/Dearcolleagueletters/DH_073957 [accessed September 2010].

20 • National Institute for Health and Clinical Excellence. *Clinical Guideline 92, Venous Thromboembolism: reducing the risk* London: NICE, 2010, www.nice.org.uk/nicemedia/live/12695/47195/47195.pdf [accessed September 2010].

21 • Vandenbroucke JP, Rosing J, Blomenkamp KWM, *et al*. Oral contraceptives and risk of venous thrombosis *New England Journal of Medicine* 2001; **344(20)**: 1527–35.

22 • Department for Transport. *Air Travel and Deep Vein Thrombosis* London: DfT, n.d., www.dft.gov.uk/pgr/inclusion/dvt/airtravelanddeepveinthrombosis [accessed September 2010].

23 • Scurr JH, Machin SJ, Bailey-King S, *et al*. Frequency and prevention of symptomless deep-vein thrombosis in long-haul flights: a randomised trial *Lancet* 2001; **357(9267)**: 1485–9.

24 • Lagerstedt CI, Olsson CG, Fagher BO, *et al*. Need for long-term anticoagulant treatment in symptomatic calf-vein thrombosis *Lancet* 1985; **2(8454)**: 515–18.

25 • Kakkar VV, Howe CT, Flanc C, *et al*. Natural history of postoperative deep-vein thrombosis *Lancet* 1969; **2(7614)**: 230–2.

26 • Hirsh J, Guyatt G, Albers GW, *et al*. Antithrombotic and thrombolytic therapy *Chest* 2008; **133(Suppl 6)**: 110S–112S.

27 • Akl EA, Barba M, Rohilla S, *et al*. Anticoagulation for the long term treatment of venous thromboembolism in patients with cancer *Cochrane Database of Systematic Reviews* 2008; **2**: CD006650.

28 • www.guideline.gov/summary/summary.aspx?doc_id=11385&nbr=005922&string=venous [accessed September 2010].

29 • Hull R, Raskob GE, Pineo GF, *et al*. Subcutaneous low-molecular-weight heparin compared with continuous intravenous heparin in the treatment of proximal-vein thrombosis *New England Journal of Medicine* 1992; **326(15)**: 975–82.

30 • Gould MK, Dembitzer AD, Sanders GD, *et al*. Low-molecular-weight heparins compared with unfractionated heparin for treatment of acute deep venous thrombosis. A cost-effectiveness analysis *Annals of Internal Medicine* 1999; **130(10)**: 789–99.

31 • Wells PS, Kovacs MJ, Bormanis J, *et al*. Expanding eligibility for outpatient treatment of deep venous thrombosis and pulmonary embolism with low-molecular-weight heparin: a comparison of patient self-injection with homecare injection *Archives of Internal Medicine* 1998; **158(16)**: 1809–12.

32 • Levine MN, Hirsh J, Gent M, *et al*. Optimal duration of oral anticoagulant therapy: a randomized trial comparing four weeks with three months of warfarin in patients with proximal deep vein thrombosis *Thrombosis and Haemostasis* 1995; **74(2)**: 606–11.

33 • Schulman S, Rhedin A, Lindmarker P, *et al*. A comparison of six weeks with six months of oral anticoagulant therapy after a first episode of venous thromboembolism *New England Journal of Medicine* 1995; **332(25)**: 1661–5.

34 • Palareti G, Cosmi B, Legnani C, *et al.*; PROLONG Investigators. D-dimer testing to determine the duration of anticoagulation therapy *New England Journal of Medicine* 2006; **355(17)**: 1780–9.

35 • Baglin TP, Rose PE, Walker ID, *et al.* Guidelines on oral anticoagulation: third edition *British Journal of Haematology* 1998; **101(2)**: 374–87.

36 • Wildberger JE, Mahnken AH, Das M, *et al.* CT imaging in acute pulmonary embolism: diagnostic strategies *European Radiology* 2005; **15(5)**: 919–29.

37 • Simonneau G, Sors H, Charbonnier B, *et al.* A comparison of low-molecular-weight heparin with unfractionated heparin for acute pulmonary embolism. The THESEE Study Group. Tinzaparine ou heparine standard: evaluations dans l'embolie pulmonaire *New England Journal of Medicine* 1997; **337(10)**: 663–9.

38 • Carson J, Kelley M, Duff A, *et al.* The clinical course of pulmonary embolism *New England Journal of Medicine* 1992; **326(19)**: 1240–5.

39 • Hull R, Hirsh J, Jay R. Different intensities of oral anticoagulation therapy in the treatment of proximal vein thrombosis *New England Journal of Medicine* 1982; **307(27)**: 1676–81.

40 • Fennerty T. The diagnosis of pulmonary embolism *British Medical Journal* 1997; **314(7078)**: 425–9.

41 • PIOPED Investigators. Value of ventilation/perfusion scan in acute pulmonary embolism *Journal of the American Medical Association* 1990; **263(20)**: 2753–9.

42 • Bradbury A, Evans C, Allan P, *et al.* What are the symptoms of varicose veins? Edinburgh vein study cross sectional population survey *British Medical Journal* 1999; **318(7180)**: 353–6.

43 • Kim J, Richards S, Kent PJ. Clinical examination of varicose veins: a validation study *Annals of the Royal College of Surgeons of England* 2000; **82(3)**: 171–5.

44 • London NJM, Nash R. ABC of arterial and venous disease: varicose veins *British Medical Journal* 2000; **320(7246)**: 1391–4.

45 • Ruckley CV. Caring for patients with chronic leg ulcer *British Medical Journal* 1998; **316(7129)**: 407–8.

Emergency care

11

Olaolu Erinfolami and Matthew Cooke

Aims

The aims of this chapter are to provide a guide to the management of patients with undifferentiated chest pain (and other common or potentially lethal cardiovascular conditions), signpost those patients that require immediate referral to specialist care and offer an appreciation of the seamless role of the GP in the prevention, treatment and rehabilitation of patients with cardiovascular disease. This chapter will specifically cover the emergency management of patients with:

▷ chest pain and/or shortness of breath of unclear cause
▷ acute coronary syndrome (ACS)
▷ pulmonary embolism (PE)
▷ structural heart disease (myocarditis and pericarditis)
▷ thoracic aortic dissection and aneurysms
▷ syncope
▷ palpitations
▷ cardiac arrest in primary care.

Key learning points

▶ Immediate life-threatening conditions must be ruled out.
▶ Some serious disorders, particularly coronary ischaemia and PE, often do not have a classic presentation.
▶ The degree of symptoms is a poor indicator of a patient's risk of having a serious condition.
▶ The type of chest discomfort (pain), pattern of radiation and concomitant symptoms – such as nausea, sweating and cold, pale skin – are valuable signs of a possible serious condition.
▶ A patient who is haemodynamically unstable (shock, low blood pressure) or who has a potentially malignant arrhythmia (severe bradycardia/tachycardia) needs immediate attention regardless of the underlying cause.

▶ If a serious, life-threatening condition is suspected, time should not be spent reaching a diagnosis unless there are therapeutic options such as fibrinolysis and a defibrillator available.

▶ Optimise the patient's condition by relieving pain, reducing anxiety and stabilising any haemodynamic disturbance.

▶ If an acute myocardial infarction (MI) is suspected, treatment should be initiated with aspirin, short-acting nitrate and morphine.

Chest pain and/or shortness of breath of unclear cause

Introduction

Patients presenting with an underlying cardiovascular disease often present with chest pain and/or shortness of breath.

Chest pain and shortness of breath are a common presentation to the GP, as discussed in Chapter 1. There is a broad differential diagnosis for these symptoms that includes several life-threatening diseases. Making an accurate diagnosis can be more difficult because of a frequent disassociation between intensity of signs and symptoms and seriousness of underlying pathology. Accurately discerning the correct diagnosis and treatment of the patient with chest pain and/or shortness of breath remains one of the most difficult tasks for the physician.

Many disorders produce chest pain or discomfort. These disorders may involve the cardiovascular, gastrointestinal (GI), pulmonary, neurologic, or musculoskeletal systems. Painful stimuli from thoracic organs can produce discomfort described as pressure, tearing, 'gas' with the urge to belch, indigestion, burning, aching, stabbing, and sometimes sharp needle-like pain. When the sensation is visceral in origin, many patients deny they are having pain and insist it is merely 'discomfort'. Acute coronary syndromes, pulmonary embolus, pericarditis with tamponade, dissecting aortic aneurysm, acute pulmonary oedema, pneumothorax, and oesophageal rupture are potentially catastrophic causes of chest pain.

Patients with chest pain may go to their GP surgery, call an ambulance or attend the emergency department (ED). They often 'self-stratify', and the severity of the underlying cause reflects where they choose to present.[1] Evidence shows that a paramedic sees a higher proportion of chest pain of cardiac origin compared with GPs who see chest pain more commonly due to musculoskeletal disorders.

Evaluation

A careful evaluation of each patient presenting with a suspected cardiovascular emergency in primary care must include a history and examination, as described in Chapter 1. The extent and precise components of the evaluation will depend on the urgency of the situation and will, in some cases, be limited to an 'Airway, Breathing, Circulation' type of appraisal prior to commencing resuscitation. In most circumstances there is time to do a more thorough evaluation but help (for instance an ambulance) may need to be summoned before the evaluation is complete.

The extent of subsequent testing will depend on the stability of the patient, the suspected underlying diagnosis and the setting in which the patient presents. For example, a patient presenting to a primary care setting with suspected acute MI should at the most have a 12-lead ECG and be transferred as soon as possible to a centre capable of providing thrombolysis or primary percutaneous coronary intervention. On the other hand, a patient with costo-chondritis does not require any further specialised test. Details of suggested tests for other suspected diagnoses will be discussed further in the relevant sections of this chapter.

Pre-hospital (primary care) evaluation

The key steps in the management are 1) initial evaluation, 2) diagnosis and risk assessment and 3) management within primary care setting or referral to hospital.

When confronted with a patient suffering from acute chest pain, the first priority is to decide whether the patient has a life-threatening disease or not. In primary care settings, this judgement is based on the patient's previous history, presenting symptoms, clinical signs and, if available, ECG findings. Laboratory tests such as troponin are not rapidly available to GPs and it would be inappropriate to delay definitive treatment while awaiting test results. If an ischaemic cause for chest pain is likely, the patient should be further investigated in a hospital setting. Troponin T (cTnT) and troponin I (cTnI) are found in cardiac muscle and rise 3 to 6 hours after MI, peak at about 20 hours and remain detectable for 4 to 10 days.[2-4]

Severe prolonged chest pain of acute onset is rarely a decision-making problem. If not caused by a trauma (fractured ribs or contusion) this symptom calls for immediate action whatever its cause. The differential diagnosis of potentially life-threatening conditions includes acute MI or unstable angina, aneurysm of the aorta, pulmonary embolism and pneumothorax. Immediate hospital care is required for all of these conditions. The physical examination contributes almost nothing in diagnosing acute MI (unless there is associated shock). General predictors for infarction are age, male gender, type of pain and pattern of radiation, nausea and sweating, and prior cardiovascular disease.[5]

When telephoned by a patient with a history of acute chest pain suggestive of acute MI, the GP should call for an ambulance. This is especially the case within 1 hour of onset of the symptoms, when the risk for ventricular fibrillation is greatest.[6] If an acute MI is suspected and the GP is with the patient, a short-acting nitrate (typically sublingual GTN) may be given if the patient does not have bradycardia or low blood pressure. Fast-acting aspirin (chewable or water soluble) should be given as soon as possible and opiates should be considered to relieve pain and anxiety. In a case like this, the GP should stay with the patient until the ambulance arrives.

Attacks of chest pain that are not very severe or prolonged, but distressing enough to make contact with a GP, present a more difficult problem in diagnosis and management. Musculoskeletal pain is the most prevalent diagnosis and most of the time a GP can make a diagnosis based on the medical history and physical examination.[1]

In the presence of a typical history of angina, the odds for coronary artery disease (CAD) are high. In patients without a previous history of CAD, the highest diagnostic information against the presence of angina is pain affected by palpation, breathing, turning, twisting, bending or from multiple sites.[7] In any event, if in doubt, it is best to assume an underlying CAD, in which case referral to a 'Rapid-Access Chest Pain Clinic' is appropriate.

Emergency department and hospital management

The key steps in hospital management are similar to that in a primary care setting, but ED management may involve treatment of a patient before ascertaining a comprehensive history or completing a detailed physical examination. The emergency management of an unstable patient is structured in the sequence of 1) primary survey and resuscitation, 2) secondary survey and ongoing treatment and 3) definitive management.

The initial primary assessment and resuscitation should include a 12-lead ECG and should be followed by measures to stabilise the patient, obtain a focused history and perform further immediate investigations as necessary, such as plain chest X-ray (CXR) to diagnose conditions such as pneumothorax and pneumonia, or a CT pulmonary angiogram (CTPA) to diagnose pulmonary embolism. Following this, a definitive management plan, such as primary percutaneous coronary intervention (PCI) or thrombolysis for acute MI or PE, is made. This will depend on the availability of PCI locally and the time period from onset of chest pain. Unless there are contraindica-

280

tions, reperfusion therapy is indicated in all patients with ST-segment elevation myocardial infarction (STEMI) (or presumed new left bundle branch
block [LBBB]) of less than 12 hours' duration.[8] In patients presenting early
(<2 hours after symptom onset), primary PCI is the preferred therapy, provided the time from first medical contact (FMC) to balloon inflation is <90
minutes.[8]

The approach to the stable patient is also based on an orderly approach,
but is more in line with the traditional mode of medical management:

▷ directed history
▷ physical examination
▷ investigations, such as 12-lead ECG, CXR, CTPA, echocardiogram, etc.
▷ therapeutic interventions.

In these patients, the overriding principle is to ensure that there are no
underlying life-threatening conditions such as acute coronary syndromes
(acute MI and unstable angina), thoracic aortic dissection and PE. Overall,
the most common causes are 'idiopathic', chest wall tenderness and GI disorders (e.g. oesophageal reflux). It is not uncommon for no cause to be found
even after full evaluation.

Follow-up care

The follow-up in the community by the GP depends on the diagnosis. While
it is important to consider the results of hospital tests and the discharge diagnosis, it is important to appreciate that some of the test results, especially
12-lead ECGs and cardiac enzymes, are 'snapshots' of the transient physiological status of the myocardium. Thus, in a patient with the right history
and the right profile, a recent negative 12-lead ECG or a negative cardiac
enzyme result does not rule out an acute MI if such a patient were to present
again to the GP with a similar history of chest pain.

Some of the required follow-up may be incidental to the hospital visit. For
example, as part of the investigation in a patient presenting with chest pain,
a previously unidentified hyperlipidaemia may be detected in hospital. Such
patients, especially if a non-cardiac diagnosis is made, may need further
advice regarding lifestyle or statin treatment, and follow-up by the GP.

Acute coronary syndrome

Introduction

Ischaemic heart disease (IHD) consists of angina pectoris and MI. Angina pectoris is a clinical syndrome of precordial discomfort or pressure due to transient myocardial ischemia without infarction. It is typically precipitated by exertion or psychological stress, and relieved by rest or sublingual nitrates. Diagnosis is by symptoms, ECG and myocardial imaging. Changes such as rest angina, new-onset angina and increasing angina are termed unstable angina and require prompt evaluation and treatment.

The spectrum of IHD can be further subdivided into stable angina, unstable angina, non-ST-segment elevation myocardial infarction (NSTEMI) and STEMI.

ACS refers to unstable angina, NSTEMI and STEMI. Unstable angina can be further stratified into low, moderate and high risks, using various clinical parameters such as ECG changes, severity and duration of pain, and associated systemic features such as heart failure. Alternatively, there are clinical tools such as Thrombolysis In Myocardial Infarction (TIMI) Risk Stratification scores to aid stratification (see Table 11.1), in conjunction with clinical assessment.[9]

Table 11.1 ○ *TIMI risk stratification score*

Risk factor	Points
1 Age 65 years or older	1
2 Three or more risk factors for coronary disease (family history, hypertension, diabetes, currently smoking, or hypercholesterolaemia)	1
3 Prior coronary stenosis of 50% or more	1
4 ST-segment deviation on electrocardiogram at presentation	1
5 At least two anginal events in prior 24 hours	1
6 Use of aspirin in prior 7 days	1
7 Elevated serum cardiac markers	1

Coronary heart disease (CHD) is the most common cause of death (and premature death) in the UK, with 1 in 5 men and 1 in 6 women dying from the disease; this translates to 101,000 deaths from CHD in the UK each year.[10] The average incidence of MI is 600 per 100,000 in men aged 30–69 and 200 per 100,000 in women.[10] Of note, overall mortality from

CHD is falling but morbidity in terms of numbers surviving a coronary event appears to be rising.

Evaluation

The history remains the cornerstone of the assessment of the patient with suspected myocardial ischemia. Many studies have shown that patients with classic features for ischemia, such as pressure-like discomfort, radiation of discomfort, diaphoresis, and male gender, have a high likelihood for ACS despite an initially normal or non-diagnostic 12-lead ECG.[11,12]

The initial evaluation provides information about the diagnosis and prognosis, and should attempt to simultaneously answer two questions:

▷ What is the likelihood that the signs and symptoms represent ACS are secondary to obstructive CAD?
▷ What is the likelihood of an adverse clinical outcome? Outcomes of concern include death, MI (or recurrent MI), stroke, heart failure, recurrent symptomatic ischaemia, and serious arrhythmia.

Pre-hospital (primary care) evaluation

Patients presenting with a history consistent with ACS should be assumed to have an acute MI until proven otherwise. Chest pain itself is a poor predictor of the pre-hospital diagnosis of acute MI; diaphoresis (sweating) in the patient with chest pain, however, is very suggestive of acute MI.[13]

Management in the primary care setting would depend on the differential diagnosis. In patients known to have stable angina who present with symptoms consistent with this, diagnosis may require an up-titration of their current medication and/or lifestyle advice.

By definition, any patient suspected of having a new onset of IHD (CAD) has unstable angina. If such a patient presents to the GP with ongoing chest pain, the best mode of management is to send to hospital in an ambulance following immediate vital signs, a brief history and physical examination, treatment with aspirin if there are no contraindications and administration of oxygen as appropriate [15 litres/min if SpO2 is <85 per cent; 5–10 L/min (via simple face mask) or 2–6 L/min (via nasal cannulae) if SpO2 >85–93 per cent].[14] The guiding principle for oxygen therapy in MI and acute coronary syndromes is to aim at an oxygen saturation of 94–98 per cent or 88–92 per cent if the patient is at risk of hypercapnoeic respiratory failure. However, for critically ill patients, high concentrations of oxygen should be administered immediately at $15 \, L/min^{-1}$ via a reservoir mask or bag-mask.[14]

The ambulance personnel would be expected to initiate cardiac monitoring and perform a 12-lead ECG and gain intravenous access *en route* to hospital. Persistent chest pain should be treated with sublingual nitrates (and intravenous morphine if not relieved by the nitrate).

Recognising the importance of rapid identification and treatment of acute MI and advances in technology has influenced pre-hospital emergency cardiac care. Pre-hospital 12-lead ECG is one important new development and paramedics can accurately identify thrombolytic candidates with a 12-lead ECG in an average of 3 to 5 additional minutes on the scene.[15] Other studies have shown that, when 12-lead ECGs are transmitted prior to arrival at the hospital, thrombolytic treatment is initiated up to 55 minutes earlier, highlighting the interaction of pre-hospital and ED care.[16]

Patients may however present with a history of new-onset chest pain symptoms that are intermittent and may not be present when they are seen in the surgery. These patients require urgent referral to A Rapid-Access Chest Pain Clinic; however, they should be advised to seek urgent medical attention if the chest pain recurred before they are seen in the clinic.

Emergency department and hospital management

The history remains the cornerstone of effective diagnosis and management, but the initial first few minutes are focused on reducing likelihood of an adverse clinical outcome. Patients have a quick, focused history, measurement of vital signs and a 12-lead ECG within 15 minutes of arrival, if not already done by the paramedic. This approach is aimed at quick identification of those whose physiological parameters are unstable and/or those who require immediate resolution of the coronary artery blockage by thrombolysis or primary PCI (depending on the local setting).

Once an acute STEMI has been excluded, the patient is assessed and stratified into ACS or stable angina. Those with stable angina are often discharged back to their GPs without further intervention. Those deemed to have ACS are stratified into low, moderate or high risk using various clinical parameters or clinical scoring tools such as TIMI Risk Stratification scores.[9] Depending on the local arrangements, those with low-risk ACS are managed within the 'Clinical Decision Unit' of the ED and undergo serial ECGs, cardiac enzyme testing and non-invasive cardiac stress testing. The cardiologist manages those with high-risk ACS, while general/acute physicians or cardiologists manage those with moderate risk. The procedures carried out depend on the persistence of the chest pain, results of cardiac enzyme tests and serial ECGs, and the outcome of a non-invasive stress test if indicated. If any of these suggest ongoing myocardial damage (positive enzymes) or significant IHD, the patient should have a coronary angiogram while in hospital, with coronary intervention appropriate to the findings (e.g. stenting).

Medical treatment should be individualised to the specific needs of each patient based on the in-hospital findings, and this includes aspirin, clopidogrel, beta-blockers, cholesterol-lowering agents, ACE inhibitors, nitrates, calcium antagonists and treatment of major risk factors such as hypertension and diabetes mellitus.

Follow-up care

The acute phase of unstable angina/NSTEMI is usually over within 1 to 3 months. The risk of progression to acute MI or the development of recurrent MI or death is highest during that period. At 1 to 3 months after the acute phase, most patients resume a clinical course similar to that in patients with chronic stable coronary disease. The broad goals during the hospital discharge phase are two-fold: 1) to prepare the patient for normal activities to the extent possible; and 2) to use the acute event as an opportunity to re-evaluate long-term care, particularly lifestyle and risk factor modification.

Risk factor modification is the mainstay of the long-term management of stable CAD. Low-risk patients requiring non-invasive stress testing are typically evaluated and discharged on the day of, or day after, testing. However, this depends on whether the patients were referred to the 'Rapid-Access Chest Pain Clinic' or admitted via the ED. Patients who have undergone successful PCI with an uncomplicated course are usually discharged the next day, and patients who undergo uncomplicated coronary artery bypass graft (CABG) are generally discharged 4 to 7 days after surgery.

In most cases, the in-patient anti-ischaemic medical regimen used in the non-intensive phase (other than intravenous nitrate) should be continued after discharge, and the antiplatelet/anticoagulant medications should be changed to an out-patient regimen.

The goals for continued medical therapy after discharge relate to potential prognostic benefits (aspirin, beta-blockers, cholesterol-lowering agents, and ACE inhibitors), control of ischaemic symptoms (nitrates, beta-blockers and calcium antagonists), and treatment of major risk factors such as hypertension, smoking, hyperlipidaemia and diabetes mellitus. The selection of a medical regimen is individualised to the specific needs of each patient based on the in-hospital findings and events, the risk factors for CAD, drug tolerance, or the type of recent procedure.

Pulmonary embolism

Introduction

PE and deep-vein thrombosis (DVT) are two clinical presentations of venous thromboembolism (VTE) and share the same predisposing factors. In most cases, PE is a consequence of DVT. Among patients with proximal DVT, about 50 per cent have an associated, usually clinically asymptomatic, PE on lung scan.[17] In about 70 per cent of patients with PE, DVT can be found in the lower limbs if sensitive diagnostic methods are used.[18] Venous thromboembolic disease (PE and DVT) is known as the 'silent killer' because patients and clinicians are often unaware of its presence until it is too late.

PE is uncommon in ambulatory patients in the community, but common in hospitalised patients, especially in elderly or medically complex patients.

Evaluation

An important aspect of making a diagnosis of PE is suspicion and awareness of the presence of risk factors in the individual patient; this includes immobilisation (e.g. post-operatively or after a long flight), pregnancy, oral contraceptives, heart disease, cancer and previous DVT or PE. The likelihood of PE increases with the number of predisposing factors present. However, in around 30 per cent of cases PE occurs in the absence of any predisposing factors (unprovoked or idiopathic PE).

While individual clinical signs and symptoms are not very helpful, as they are neither sensitive nor specific enough,[19] a combination of certain clinical symptoms raises the suspicion of PE; in several series, dyspnoea, tachypnoea or chest pain were present in more than 90 per cent of patients with PE.[20,21] Pain is more often lateral and pleuritic. It is usually abrupt in onset and maximal at the start, but it may be episodic or intermittent. Dyspnoea is a common symptom and is often more prominent than pain. Patients often have a respiratory rate over 16/minute and tachycardia is also common.

Apart from tachypnoea and tachycardia, patients often have no positive signs, unless the patient has significant PE with signs of right ventricular strain and/or signs of shock. Uncommonly, examination findings may include inspiratory râles, an increased pulmonary second heart sound or a low-grade fever. Patients with massive PE may have a raised jugular venous pressure (JVP), tachycardia, hypotension, diaphoresis or reduced conscious level.

While routine tests such as 12-lead ECG, arterial blood gases and plain CXR are helpful during the evaluation of patients suspected of having PE, none of these allows the exclusion or confirmation of acute PE. The main value of these tests lies in the exclusion of alternative diagnosis.

If PE is suspected, the key management strategy is to stratify the likelihood of significant morbidity and mortality. This can be done using clinical tools such as the British Thoracic Society (BTS) PE guidelines (see Box 11.1), Wells score or the Geneva Score.[22-25]

Box 11.1 ○ *British Thoracic Society's PE guidelines*

Criteria

1 Most patients with PE are breathless and/or tachypnoeic >20/min; in the absence of these, pleuritic chest pain or haemoptysis is usually due to another cause.

2 Clinical probability in patients with possible PE may be assessed by asking:

▶ is another diagnosis unlikely (chest radiograph and ECG are helpful)?

▶ is there a major risk factor (recent immobility/major surgery/lower-limb trauma or surgery, pregnancy/postpartum, major medical illness, previous proven VTE)?

Risk classification

Low = neither; intermediate = either; high = both.

Stable patients who are deemed low or intermediate risk should have D-dimer tests. Although all D-dimer tests are sufficiently sensitive to rule out a PE in low-risk patients, only VIDAS (ELISA) or MDA (latex) tests are sufficiently sensitive to rule out those with intermediate risk.[23] In those with a positive D-dimer or a high risk of having PE, CTPA or, less commonly, a ventilation/perfusion scan can be used to make a definitive diagnosis. Immediate echocardiogram is also useful in making a diagnosis of PE in unstable patients.[26]

In a pregnant patient suspected of having a PE, the recommended first line of investigation is ultrasound of both lower-limb veins. A positive test confirms the diagnosis of VTE without recourse to irradiation exposure. If negative, a CTPA should be carried out, as the current machines have exposure within safe limits and the irradiation dose is less than that for ventilation/perfusion scan and similar to isolated perfusion scan.[19]

Pre-hospital (primary care) evaluation

As described above, appreciation of the underlying risk factors is key to the suspicion of PE as the underlying diagnosis. Unstable patients are unlikely to present to the GP, and patients suspected of having PE should be assessed in hospital; it is unlikely that the patient will have any discriminatory symptoms or signs that could confidently rule out PE if the diagnosis is suspected.

Emergency department and hospital management

The key is taking a good history and having a high index of suspicion. In stable patients, the key management strategies are to rule out other differential diagnosis such as STEMI (with a 12-lead ECG) and risk-stratify the patient on the basis of history and simple tests such as D-dimer (when appropriate). The definitive diagnosis can be made using appropriate investigation such as CTPA, V/Q scan or lower-limb duplex (in suspected associated DVT or as a first-line test in pregnant patients).

Patients with a definitive diagnosis of VTE who are stable may be managed as out-patients, once anticoagulation with concomitant subcutaneous low molecular weight heparin (LMWH) and warfarin have been initiated. LMWH may be discontinued once the INR is in the therapeutic range (INR 2.5, range 2–3) and warfarin should be continued for 6 months.[27,28]

In patients presenting with suspected PE and who are in shock (with or without features of right heart failure), echocardiogram is useful as a diagnostic tool. Such patients may benefit from immediate thrombolysis. The potential benefits are improved survival, fewer recurrences of PE and long-term prevention of pulmonary hypertension, but these have to be balanced against the adverse effects associated with thrombolysis such as intracranial haemorrhage.

Follow-up care

Patients with VTE initiated on anticoagulation should be regularly followed up to ensure adequate anticoagulation. Patients with a first episode of VTE should receive anticoagulation for 6 months, but those with recurrent VTE should receive life-long therapy.[19,23]

Structural heart disease (myocarditis and pericarditis)

Introduction

Pericarditis is inflammation of the pericardium, with or without fluid accumulation. There are many possible causes of pericarditis (e.g. infection, MI, trauma, tumours and metabolic disorders) but it is often idiopathic. It is a rare presenting diagnosis in both primary care and hospital settings. Cardiac tamponade is an even more rare complication.

Myocarditis is associated with inflammatory changes in the heart muscle and is characterised by myocyte necrosis. The cause may be infectious, toxic or immunologic. Viral infection is the commonest cause, and idiopathic myocarditis is also likely to be due to an undiagnosed viral cause. Depending on the cause and severity, clinical presentation of myocarditis can range from no symptoms at all, to life-threatening heart failure and rarely sudden death. However, most people recover completely from myocarditis.

Evaluation

Patients with pericarditis may present with dyspnoea, diaphoresis and pain, which is often worse when supine, but improves when sitting up. Patients may give a history of a preceding viral illness or underlying disease such as SLE or uraemia. On examination of the patient's chest a friction rub may be heard, often fleeting and position dependent (in 50 per cent of patients). An essential diagnostic tool is a 12-lead ECG that may show a typical pattern of ST-segment elevation across the precordial leads. Erythrocyte sedimentation rate (ESR) may be elevated. A plain CXR or echocardiogram may show evidence of pericardial fluid accumulation.

Myocarditis is frequently a diagnosis of exclusion. Flu-like symptoms are common initial symptoms and approximately 12 per cent of patients have chest pain. On clinical examination, a tachycardia disproportionate to the temperature or apparent toxicity may be apparent but cardiac examination is often unremarkable.[29]

Most tests do not give a specific diagnosis of myocarditis. ECG changes include sinus tachycardia, but it can also show a prolonged corrected QT interval, atrioventricular (AV) block, or acute MI pattern. Cardiac enzymes, white blood cell count and ESR may all be elevated. The echocardiographic features of myocarditis are non-specific, but can show multi-chamber dysfunction.

While myocarditis can masquerade as acute MI, patients with myocarditis are usually young (usually <35 years of age) and have few risk factors for CAD. In myocarditis, chest pain continues with no further evolution of the ECG to indicate ischemia.

Pre-hospital (primary care) evaluation

The diagnosis of pericarditis is essentially made on the history and a 12-lead ECG. If there are no complications such as a pericardial effusion or tamponade, patients can be managed with non-steroidal anti-inflammatory drugs (NSAIDs) without the need for further investigation or referral to hospital. If a pericardial effusion or tamponade is suspected, the patient will require an echocardiogram, which should be carried out urgently if tamponade is likely.

All patients with suspected myocarditis should be admitted, and those with haemodynamic instability may require admission to the intensive care unit (ICU).

Emergency department and hospital management

Patients presenting to the ED with a history consistent with pericarditis should have a 12-lead ECG and a plain CXR. Patients with a suspected pericardial effusion or tamponade should have an echocardiogram. Treatment depends on the cause and the complications, but general measures include analgesics and anti-inflammatory drugs.

The key element in the evaluation of myocarditis is assessment of physiological instability and directed admission into the appropriate area: general ward, cardiology ward or ICU. The current treatment for myocarditis is supportive therapy, with bed rest accepted as being of benefit. Patients with a fulminant clinical course require cardiac transplantation.

Follow-up care

Young, previously healthy patients with uncomplicated idiopathic (or suspected viral) pericarditis do not require any specific follow-up and attempts at differentiating idiopathic from viral aetiology is often futile and of little practical importance. Others should be monitored for complications such as effusion, tamponade and constrictive pericarditis. Follow-up is usually dependent on the underlying cause, for example, those patients with pericarditis due to uraemia may require more frequent dialysis.

Thoracic aortic dissection

Introduction

This is a very rare presentation to primary care or hospital settings. The median age for presentation is 59 years. The patients often have a history of hypertension (in 70–90 per cent of patients) and the condition is commoner in males. There is an increased incidence in patients with Marfan's syndrome.

Evaluation

Most patients have rapid-onset severe chest pain that is maximal at the start. The pain radiates anteriorly from the chest to the back, the interscapular area or into the abdomen, and the pain often has a 'tearing' character.

The patient may present with neurological complications such as paresis or paraplegia. They may also present with abdominal or peripheral ischaemia. On examination, the patient often presents with elevated BP and poor peripheral perfusion. In most cases, there is an asymmetrical decrease or absence of peripheral pulses.

An initial plain CXR often shows an abnormal aortic silhouette, and may show widening of the mediastinum. While a transoesophageal echo is useful in screening, and aortic angiography is the gold standard investigation for dissection, in clinical practice the diagnosis is often made on CT chest (with contrast).

Pre-hospital (primary care) evaluation

If a diagnosis of dissecting thoracic aortic aneurysm is suspected in the primary care setting, the patient should be transferred to hospital urgently by ambulance.

Emergency department and hospital management

If aortic dissection is suspected, patients are managed in a high-risk area (usually resuscitation in the ED), and rapidly evaluated and resuscitated as appropriate with oxygenation and IV fluids prior to an emergency CT chest with contrast.

The definitive treatment is guided by the type (Stanford classification). Type A involves true ascending aorta and usually requires surgery, while Type B (descending aorta distal to left subclavian artery) is usually managed medically, with beta-blockers to control heart rate to target of 60–80 b.p.m. Beta-blockers, alone or in conjunction with other antihypertensives, are also used to reduce the rate of change of blood pressure (dP/dt) and to maintain a target blood pressure of 100–120 mmHg.

Follow-up care

Risk factor modification is the mainstay of long-term management after discharge from hospital. The goals for continued medical therapy relate to treatment of major risk factors such as hypertension, smoking, hyperlipidaemia, diabetes mellitus and strict blood pressure control.

Syncope

Introduction

Syncope is a transient loss of consciousness (T-LOC) due to transient global cerebral hypoperfusion characterised by rapid onset, short duration, and spontaneous complete recovery.[30]

This definition of syncope includes the cause of the unconsciousness, i.e. transient global cerebral hypoperfusion, thereby differentiating syncope from other causes of T-LOC, such as epileptic seizures and concussion.

Other conditions incorrectly diagnosed as syncope are:

▷ disorders with partial or complete loss of consciousness but without global cerebral hypoperfusion, e.g. hypoglycaemia, hypoxia, hyperventilation with hypocapnia, intoxication and vertebrobasilar transient ischaemic attack (TIA)
▷ disorders without impairment of consciousness, e.g. fall, TIA of carotid origin, cataplexy, drop attacks and psychogenic pseudosyncope.

The causes of syncope can be:

▷ reflex syncope (vasovagal; situational such as post-micturition; carotid sinus syncope and atypical or idiopathic)
▷ syncope due to orthostatic hypotension (primary autonomic failure such as Parkinson's disease; secondary autonomic failure such as uraemia; drug-induced such as due to alcohol, vasodilators and diuretics; volume depletion due to haemorrhage, vomiting, etc.)
▷ cardiovascular syncope (arrhythmia; structural cardiac disease such as aortic stenosis, hypertrophic cardiomyopathy; others such as PE and aortic dissection).

Reflex syncope is the commonest, and, while many cases never have a firm diagnosis or lead to any apparent harm, a small number of cases have a serious cause, usually cardiac. In the elderly, syncope often has more than one cause. For example, the combination of taking several heart and BP drugs and standing in a hot church during a long or emotional service may lead to syncope.

Evaluation

The diagnosis depends on a careful history and eyewitness account so an evaluation should be carried out as soon as possible after the event.

The history should ascertain events leading up to the syncope, including the patient's activity, position (e.g. lying down or standing) and, if standing, for how long. The history should also include important associated symptoms immediately before the event (warning symptoms such as dizziness, nausea and sweating) and after the event, such as the time to full recovery (prompt, a few minutes, up to an hour or over several hours).

The history should include system review, enquiring about symptoms such as episodes of palpitations, chest pain with/without exertion, bloody or tarry stools, heavy menses, vomiting and diarrhoea. Enquiries about previous syncopal events, known cardiovascular disease, current medications and a family history should note presence at a young age of heart disease or sudden death in any family member.

Measurement of the pulse rate and BP are essential; the BP should be measured with the patient supine and after 2 minutes of standing, and the pulse palpated for irregularity. Auscultation for the presence of heart murmurs is also important as well as checking for any signs of injury (e.g. bruising, swelling, tenderness, tongue bite).

Certain findings raise suspicion of a more serious aetiology of syncope. These include syncope during exertion, multiple recurrences within a short time, heart murmur or other findings suggesting structural heart disease (e.g. chest pain), older age, significant injury during syncope and a family history of sudden unexpected death.

The specific tests for each patient would depend on the differential diagnosis resulting from the history, including the age, medications and family history, and the examination findings.

Pre-hospital (primary care) evaluation

Syncope is a common presentation to primary care.[31] The diagnosis is based upon a carefully taken medical history and the context of the event. Most are due to a simple faint that can be diagnosed by the patient's GP and needs only reassurance.

An active searching for alarming symptoms is however necessary to rule out more significant pathology. These symptoms include syncope during exertion, syncope in the lying-down position, absence of external factors, family history of hypertrophic obstructive cardiomyopathy (HOCM), or slow recovery from syncope. An ECG can be helpful in identifying an underlying rhythm disorder. If the diagnosis remains uncertain then the patient should be referred to a cardiologist, neurologist or psychologist/psychiatrist as appropriate. If the syncope is due to medications, the GP should address this issue by adjusting dose or stopping the causative agent.

Emergency department and hospital management

A flexible, focused approach is required to diagnose syncope. The features of the initial history and physical examination help guide diagnostic testing.

The evaluation of syncope in the setting of ED is focused on risk stratification rather than attempting to make a definitive diagnosis of the cause of syncope. This aims to 1) recognise patients with life-threatening conditions and admit them to the hospital; 2) recognise patients with low-risk conditions to be discharged and referred later to the appropriate out-patient clinic; 3) recognise those who do not need any further evaluation and treatment; and 4) choose a time and setting where further diagnostic tests should be performed in patients with inconclusive initial evaluation.

For all patients with new-onset syncope of unknown cause, 12-lead ECG is recommended. The ECG may reveal arrhythmia, a conduction abnormality, ventricular hypertrophy, pre-excitation, QT prolongation, pacemaker malfunction, myocardial ischaemia or MI. Other specialised testing is suggested only in certain circumstances; in general, if syncope results in an injury or is recurrent (particularly within a brief period) more intensive evaluation is warranted.[32]

Pulse oximetry should be carried out during or immediately after an episode to identify hypoxaemia (which may indicate pulmonary embolism); if hypoxaemia is present, a CT scan or lung scan is indicated to rule out pulmonary embolism. Laboratory tests are done based on clinical suspicion; full blood count is measured if anaemia is suspected and electrolytes are measured if an abnormality is clinically suspected (e.g. by symptoms or drug use). Echocardiography is indicated for patients with exercise-induced syncope, cardiac murmurs, or suspected intracardiac tumours. Tilt-table testing can be carried out if history and physical examination indicate vasodepressor or other reflex-induced syncope. It can also be used to evaluate exercise-induced syncope if echocardiography or exercise stress testing is negative. Stress testing (exercise or pharmacological) is done when intermittent myocardial ischaemia is suspected. EEG can be helpful if a seizure disorder is suspected and a CT scan and/or an MRI of the head and brain are indicated only if signs and symptoms suggest a focal neurological disorder.

Patients with suspected arrhythmias, myocarditis, or ischaemia should be evaluated as in-patients, whereas others may be evaluated as out-patients.

Specific treatment depends on the cause and its pathophysiology: for example, severe bradycardia is treated with atropine; inadequate venous return can be improved by keeping the patient supine, raising the legs, and giving IV normal saline.

Follow-up care

This will depend on the underlying cause. For most patients with syncope, the cause is vasovagal or another benign reflex syncopal cause, and they do not require any further follow-up.

Syncope due to medications may require follow-up to monitor the adverse effect, any change in current medications or for monitoring electrolytes (if caused by electrolyte disturbance secondary to the medication). If syncope is due to HOCM, the first-degree relatives will require screening.

Palpitations

Introduction

Palpitations are common and they are the perception of cardiac activity. They may be described as a fluttering, racing or skipping sensation, but the mechanisms responsible for the sensation are unknown. They can occur in the absence of heart disease or can result from life-threatening heart disorders.

The key to diagnosis and treatment is to 'capture' the rhythm on ECG and make careful observations during the palpitations. Some patients simply have heightened awareness of normal cardiac activity, particularly when exercise, febrile illness or anxiety increase heart rate. However, in most cases, palpitations result from an arrhythmia or ectopic beats.

The most common and usually harmless arrhythmias include premature atrial contractions (PACs) and premature ventricular contractions (PVCs). Other common arrhythmias include paroxysmal supraventricular tachycardia (PSVT), atrioventricular nodal re-entrant tachycardia, atrial fibrillation or flutter, ventricular tachycardia, bradyarrhythmias and the heart blocks.

The cause of palpitations can be cardiac or non-cardiac. Cardiac causes include myocardial ischaemia, congenital heart disease, valvular heart disease and conduction system disturbances. Non-cardiac disorders include thyrotoxicosis, anxiety, drugs (e.g. digoxin, salbutamol), caffeine, cocaine, hypoxia, hypovolaemia, anaemia and electrolyte imbalances such as hypokalaemia.

Evaluation

A complete history and physical examination are essential. The history should include the frequency and duration of palpitations, the provoking or exacerbating factors, and should cover symptoms suggestive of the causative disorders (e.g. IHD, thyroid problem and current medication).

During the examination, asking the patient to tap out the rate and cadence of palpitations is better than a verbal description, and often allows a definitive diagnosis, as in the 'missed beat' of atrial or ventricular extrasystoles or the rapid total irregularity of atrial fibrillation. Vital signs should be measured to highlight fever, hypertension, hypotension, tachycardia, bradycardia, tachypnoea and low O_2 saturation. Examination directed to check for an underlying cause such as thyroid disease should be performed (thyroid enlargement or tenderness and exophthalmos).

Features suggestive of a serious underlying aetiology include associated chest pain, significant underlying heart disease, family history of sudden death and syncope.

The specific tests for each patient would depend largely on the nature of the pulse (rate, rhythm and volume), the underlying history and the age of the patient.

In patients with tachycardia and/or in whom features suggestive of a serious underlying aetiology are present, a 12-lead ECG is mandatory. Unless the recording is carried out while symptoms are occurring, it may not provide a diagnosis. Patients with intermittent (paroxysmal symptoms) will require Holter monitoring for 24 to 48 hours. If very infrequent, the patient can wear an event recorder for a longer period, which can be activated by the patient when he or she is aware of symptoms.

Laboratory testing is indicated for some patients. Measurement of FBC, serum electrolytes and cardiac markers (e.g. troponin) is appropriate in those with chest discomfort, or other symptoms suggesting active or recent coronary ischaemia, myocarditis or pericarditis. Thyroid function tests are indicated when atrial fibrillation is newly diagnosed or there are symptoms of hyperthyroidism. Patients with paroxysms of high BP should be evaluated for pheochromocytoma. Tilt-table testing can be helpful in patients with postural syncope, and patients with findings suggesting cardiac dysfunction or structural heart disease require echocardiography. Patients with symptoms on exertion require stress testing.

Pre-hospital (primary care) evaluation

Palpitations are a frequent but relatively non-specific symptom, and, while a thorough history and examination is mandatory, the timing and extent of investigations should be determined by the likelihood of a serious underlying cause.

Palpitations are not a reliable indicator of a significant arrhythmia, but palpitations in a patient with structural heart disease or an abnormal ECG may be a sign of a serious problem and warrant investigation. A normal ECG in a symptom-free interval does not rule out significant disease, therefore an ECG or other recording done during symptoms is essential.

Those with tachycardia, new-onset irregularity or with features suggestive of a serious underlying aetiology should be referred to hospital for further evaluation. Further details on common arrhythmias can be found in Chapter 6.

Emergency department and hospital management

In a patient presenting with palpitations and cardiovascular compromise due to arrhythmia, DC shock should quickly follow brief assessment and ECG analysis.

The approach to the patient with a stable arrhythmia should be based on a structured assessment designed to ascertain the nature and cause of the underlying rhythm. This consists of a directed history, physical examination, ECG recording of the rhythm, and diagnostic and therapeutic interventions. Diagnostic evaluation should be carried out as described above and management directed at the underlying cause.

Follow-up care

This depends on the underlying pathology. Precipitating drugs and substances should be stopped and, if a necessary therapeutic drug causes dangerous or debilitating arrhythmias, a different agent should be tried. For isolated PACs and PVCs in patients without structural heart disease, simple reassurance is appropriate. A beta-blocker can be helpful in an otherwise healthy patient if these phenomena are disabling. The anxious patient should be made fully aware of the cause of their symptoms and reassured that they do not have a serious disorder.

Cardiac arrest

Cardiac arrest is an infrequent event in primary care; however, all GPs should be able to give basic life support and operate an automated electronic defibrillator. All practices should offer annual basic life support training to all their staff. The Resuscitation Council *Adult Basic Life Support Guideline 2005*[33] gives a clear description of what to do in the event of cardiac arrest and is summarised overleaf.

Figure 11.1 ○ *Adult basic life support algorithm*

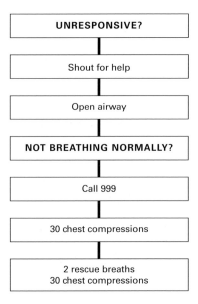

Source: Resuscitation Council. *Adult Basic Life Support Guideline 2005*. www.resus.org.uk/
pages/bls.pdf. Reproduced with permission.[33]

Summary

This chapter has focused on those cardiovascular conditions or complaints
that may present in a primary care setting, but require emergency or urgent
referral to hospital.

Chest pain of unknown cause and syncope are relatively common presentations to the GP. A directed history is key in diagnosing the underlying cause and often dictates if and what investigations are required. While
the majority of patients with chest pain may have a benign condition, it is
important to rule out serious pathology such as CAD. Further assessment
and tests may be required either by direct access or by referral to the ED or
hospital specialists; the timing and access are determined by the patient's
vital signs and/or the suspected underlying cause. If a serious, life-threatening condition is suspected, time should not be lost in reaching a definitive
diagnosis; the patient is better served by being transferred immediately to
the most appropriate hospital where definitive management is available.

References

1 • Bertrand ME, Simoons ML, Fox KA, *et al*. Management of acute coronary syndromes in patients presenting without persistent ST-segment elevation *European Heart Journal* 2002; **23(23)**: 1809–40.

2 • Tucker JF, Collins RA, Anderson AJ, *et al*. Early diagnostic efficiency of cardiac troponin I and troponin T for acute myocardial infarction *Academic Emergency Medicine* 1997; **4(1)**: 13–21.

3 • Bertinchant JP, Larue C, Pernel I, *et al*. Release kinetics of serum cardiac troponin I in ischemic myocardial injury *Clinical Biochemistry* 1996; **29(6)**: 587–94.

4 • Ebell MH, Flynn A. A systematic review of troponin T and I for diagnosing acute myocardial infarction *Journal of Family Practice* 2000; **49(6)**: 550–6.

5 • Grijseels EWM, Deckers JW, Hoes AW, *et al*. Implementations of a pre-hospital decision rule in general practice. Triage of patients with suspected myocardial infarction *European Heart Journal* 1996; **17(1)**: 89–95.

6 • Norris RM on behalf of the United Kingdom Heart Attack Study Collaborative Group. Fatality outside hospital from acute coronary events in three British health districts, 1994–5 *British Medical Journal* 1998; **316(7137)**: 1065–70.

7 • Short D. Diagnosis of slight and subacute coronary attacks in the community *British Heart Journal* 1981; **45(3)**: 299–310.

8 • Van de Werf F, Bax J, Betriu A, *et al*. Management of acute myocardial infarction in patients presenting with persistent ST-segment elevation *European Heart Journal* 2008; **29(23)**: 2909–45.

9 • Antman E, Cohen M, Bernick PJ, *et al*. The TIMI risk score for unstable angina/ non-ST elevation MI: a method for prognostication and therapeutic decision making *Journal of the American Medical Association* 2000; **284(7)**: 835–42.

10 • British Heart Foundation Statistics Database; *Coronary Heart Disease Statistics*. 2007 edition.

11 • Tierney WM, Roth BJ, Psaty B, *et al*. Predictors of myocardial infarction in emergency room patients *Critical Care Medicine* 1985; **13(7)**: 526–31.

12 • Jayes RL, Beshansky JR, D'Agostino R, *et al*. Do patients' coronary risk factor reports predict acute cardiac ischemia in the emergency department? A multicenter study *Journal of Clinical Epidemiology* 1992; **45(6)**: 621–6.

13 • Hargarten KM, Aprahamian C, Stueven H, *et al*. Limitations of prehospital predictors of acute myocardial infarction and unstable angina *Annals of Emergency Medicine* 1987; **16(12)**: 1325–9.

14 • O'Driscoll BR, Howard LS, Davidson AG (on behalf of BTS Emergency Oxygen Guideline Development Group). BTS guideline for emergency oxygen use in adult patients *Thorax* 2008; **63(Suppl 6)**: vi1–68.

15 • Aufderheide TP, Hendley GE, Thakur RK, *et al*. The diagnostic impact of prehospital 12-lead electrocardiography *Annals of Emergency Medicine* 1990; **19(11)**: 1280–7.

16 • Aufderheide TP, Hendley GE, Woo J, *et al*. A prospective evaluation of prehospital 12-lead ECG application in chest pain patients *Journal of Electrocardiology* 1992; **24(Suppl)**: 8–13.

17 • Moser KM, Fedullo PF, Littejohn JK, *et al*. Frequent asymptomatic pulmonary embolism in patients with deep venous thrombosis *Journal of the American Medical Association* 1994; **271(3)**: 223–5.

18 • Kearon C. Natural history of venous thromboembolism *Circulation* 2003; **107(23 Suppl 1)**: I22–I30.

19 • Torbicki A, Perrier A, Konstantinides S, *et al.*; Task Force for the Diagnosis and Management of Acute Pulmonary Embolism of the European Society of Cardiology (ESC). Guidelines on diagnosis and management of acute pulmonary embolism *European Heart Journal* 2008; **29(18)**: 2276–315.

20 • Wells PS, Ginsberg JS, Anderson DR, *et al.* Use of a clinical model for safe management of patients with suspected pulmonary embolism *Annals of Internal Medicine* 1998; **129(12)**: 997–1005.

21 • Miniati M, Prediletto R, Formichi B, *et al.* Accuracy of clinical assessment in the diagnosis of pulmonary embolism *American Journal of Respiratory and Critical Care Medicine* 1999; **159(3)**: 864–71.

22 • Value of the ventilation/perfusion scan in acute pulmonary embolism. Results of the Prospective Investigation of Pulmonary Embolism Diagnosis (PIOPED). The PIOPED Investigators *Journal of the American Medical Association* 1990; **263(20)**: 2753–9.

23 • British Thoracic Society Standards of Care Committee Pulmonary Embolism Guideline Development Group. British Thoracic Society guidelines for the management of suspected acute pulmonary embolism *Thorax* 2003; **58(6)**: 470–83.

24 • Wells PS, Anderson DR, Rodger M, *et al.* Derivation of a simple clinical model to categorize patients' probability of pulmonary embolism: increasing the model's utility with the SimpliRED D-dimer *Thrombosis and Haemostasis* 2000; **83(3)**: 416–20.

25 • Wicki J, Perneger TV, Junod AF, *et al.* Assessing clinical probability of pulmonary embolism in the emergency ward: a simple score *Archives of Internal Medicine* 2001; **161(1)**: 92–7.

26 • Breitkreutz R, Walcher F, Seeger F. ALS conformed use of echocardiography or ultrasound in resuscitation management *Resuscitation* 2008: **77(2)**: 270–2.

27 • Wells PS, Kovacs MJ, Bormanis J, *et al.* Expanding eligibility for outpatient treatment of deep venous thrombosis and pulmonary embolism with low-molecular-weight heparin: a comparison of patient self-injection with homecare injection *Archives of Internal Medicine* 1998; **158(16)**: 1809–12.

28 • Kovacs MJ, Anderson D, Morrow B, *et al.* Outpatient treatment of pulmonary embolism with dalteparin *Thrombosis and Haemostasis* 2000; **83(2)**: 209–11.

29 • Olinde KD, O'Connell JB. Inflammatory heart disease: pathogenesis, clinical manifestations, and treatment of myocarditis *Annual Review of Medicine* 1994; **45**: 481.

30 • The Task Force for the Diagnosis and Management of Syncope of the European Society of Cardiology (ESC). Guidelines for the diagnosis and management of syncope (version 2009) *European Heart Journal* 2009; **30(21)**: 2493–537.

31 • Olde Nordkamp LAR, van Dijk N, Ganzeboom KS, *et al.* Syncope prevalence in the ED compared to that in the general practice and population: a strong selection process *American Journal of Emergency Medicine* 2009; **27(3)**: 271–9.

32 • Linzer M, Yang EH, Estes NA, *et al.* Diagnosing syncope. Part 1: value of history, physical examination, and electrocardiography. Clinical Efficacy Assessment Project of the American College of Physicians *Annals of Internal Medicine* 1997; **126(12)**: 989–96.

33 • Resuscitation Council. *Adult Basic Life Support Guideline 2005.* www.resus.org.uk/pages/bls.pdf [accessed September 2010].

Appendix

Evidence-based indicators related to cardiovascular disease in the 2010/11 Quality and Outcomes Framework

The indicators detailed in this section have been extracted from the 2010/11 Quality and Outcomes Framework (QoF) guidance with the agreement of NHS Employers and the General Practitioners Committee of the BMA.

Please note that indicators are subject to change in subsequent years. The current, complete version of the guidance is available to download from the QoF section of the NHS Employers website (link below). These pages also outline the process by which changes are made to the QoF.

www.nhsemployers.org/PayAndContracts/GeneralMedicalServicescontract/qof/Pages/QualityOutcomesFramework.aspx

Secondary prevention of coronary heart disease

Indicator	Points	Payment stages
Records		
CHD 1 ▶ The practice can produce a register of patients with coronary heart disease (CHD)	4	
Diagnosis and initial management		
CHD 2 ▶ The percentage of patients with newly diagnosed angina (diagnosed after 1 April 2003) who are referred for exercise testing and/or specialist assessment	7	40–90%
Ongoing management		
CHD 5 ▶ The percentage of patients with CHD whose notes have a record of blood pressure in the previous 15 months	7	40–90%
CHD 6 ▶ The percentage of patients with CHD in whom the last blood pressure reading (measured in the previous 15 months) is 150/90 or less	17	40–70%

Indicator	Points	Payment stages
CHD 7 ▶ The percentage of patients with CHD whose notes have a record of total cholesterol in the previous 15 months	7	40–90%
CHD 8 ▶ The percentage of patients with CHD whose last measured total cholesterol (measured in the previous 15 months) is 5 mmol/L or less	17	40–70%
CHD 9 ▶ The percentage of patients with CHD with a record in the previous 15 months that aspirin, an alternative antiplatelet therapy, or an anticoagulant is being taken (unless a contraindication or side effects are recorded)	7	40–90%
CHD 10 ▶ The percentage of patients with CHD who are currently treated with a beta-blocker (unless a contraindication or side effects are recorded)	7	40–60%
CHD 11 ▶ The percentage of patients with a history of myocardial infarction (diagnosed after 1 April 2003) who are currently treated with an ACE inhibitor or angiotensin II antagonist	7	40–80%
CHD 12 ▶ The percentage of patients with CHD who have a record of influenza immunisation in the preceding 1 September to 31 March	7	40–90%

Cardiovascular disease – primary prevention

Indicator	Points	Payment stages
Initial diagnosis		
PP 1 ▶ In those patients with a new diagnosis of hypertension (excluding those with pre-existing CHD, diabetes, stroke and/or TIA) recorded between the preceding 1 April to 31 March: the percentage of patients who have had a face-to-face cardiovascular risk assessment at the outset of diagnosis (within 3 months of the initial diagnosis) using an agreed risk assessment tool	8	40–70%
Ongoing management		
PP 2 ▶ The percentage of people diagnosed with hypertension diagnosed after 1 April 2009 who are given lifestyle advice in the last 15 months for: increasing physical activity, smoking cessation, safe alcohol consumption and healthy diet	5	40–70%

Heart failure

Indicator	Points	Payment stages
Records		
HF 1 ▶ The practice can produce a register of patients with heart failure	4	
Initial diagnosis		
HF 2 ▶ The percentage of patients with a diagnosis of heart failure (diagnosed after 1 April 2006) that has been confirmed by an echocardiogram or by specialist assessment	6	40–90%
Ongoing management		
HF 3 ▶ The percentage of patients with a current diagnosis of heart failure due to left ventricular dysfunction (LVD) who are currently treated with an ACE inhibitor or angiotensin receptor blocker (ARB), who can tolerate therapy and for whom there is no contraindication	10	40–80%
HF 4 ▶ The percentage of patients with a current diagnosis of heart failure due to LVD who are currently treated with an ACE inhibitor or ARB, who are additionally treated with a beta-blocker licensed for heart failure, or recorded as intolerant to or having a contraindication to beta-blockers	9	40–60%

Stroke and transient ischaemic attack

Indicator	Points	Payment stages
Records		
STROKE 1 ▶ The practice can produce a register of patients with stroke or transient ischaemic attack (TIA)	2	
STROKE 13 ▶ The percentage of new patients with a stroke or TIA who have been referred for further investigation	2	40–80%
Ongoing management		
STROKE 5 ▶ The percentage of patients with TIA or stroke who have a record of blood pressure in the notes in the preceding 15 months	2	40–90%

303

Indicator	Points	Payment stages
STROKE 6 ▶ The percentage of patients with a history of TIA or stroke in whom the last blood pressure reading (measured in the previous 15 months) is 150/90 or less	5	40–70%
STROKE 7 ▶ The percentage of patients with TIA or stroke who have a record of total cholesterol in the last 15 months	2	40–90%
STROKE 8 ▶ The percentage of patients with TIA or stroke whose last measured total cholesterol (measured in the previous 15 months) is 5 mmol/L or less	5	40–60%
STROKE 12 ▶ The percentage of patients with a stroke shown to be non-haemorrhagic, or a history of TIA, who have a record that an antiplatelet agent (aspirin, clopidogrel, dipyridamole or a combination), or an anticoagulant is being taken (unless a contraindication or side effects are recorded)	4	40–90%
STROKE 10 ▶ The percentage of patients with TIA or stroke who have had influenza immunisation in the preceding 1 September to 31 March	2	40–85%

Hypertension

Indicator	Points	Payment stages
Records		
BP 1 ▶ The practice can produce a register of patients with established hypertension	6	
Ongoing management		
BP 4 ▶ The percentage of patients with hypertension in whom there is a record of the blood pressure in the previous 9 months	18	40–90%
BP 5 ▶ The percentage of patients with hypertension in whom the last blood pressure (measured in the previous 9 months) is 150/90 or less	57	40–70%

Diabetes mellitus

Indicator	Points	Payment stages
Records		
DM 19 ▶ The practice can produce a register of all patients aged 17 years and over with diabetes mellitus, which specifies whether the patient has Type 1 or Type 2 diabetes	6	
Ongoing management		
DM 2 ▶ The percentage of patients with diabetes whose notes record BMI in the previous 15 months	3	40–90%
DM 5 ▶ The percentage of patients with diabetes who have a record of HbA1c or equivalent in the previous 15 months	3	40–90%
DM 23 ▶ The percentage of patients with diabetes in whom the last HbA1c is 7 or less (or equivalent test/reference range depending on local laboratory) in the previous 15 months	17	40–50%
DM 24 ▶ The percentage of patients with diabetes in whom the last HbA1c is 8 or less (or equivalent test/reference range depending on local laboratory) in the previous 15 months	8	40–70%
DM 25 ▶ The percentage of patients with diabetes in whom the last HbA1c is 9 or less (or equivalent test/reference range depending on local laboratory) in the previous 15 months	10	40–90%
DM 21 ▶ The percentage of patients with diabetes who have a record of retinal screening in the previous 15 months	5	40–90%
DM 9 ▶ The percentage of patients with diabetes with a record of the presence or absence of peripheral pulses in the previous 15 months	3	40–90%
DM 10 ▶ The percentage of patients with diabetes with a record of neuropathy testing in the previous 15 months	3	40–90%
DM 11 ▶ The percentage of patients with diabetes who have a record of the blood pressure in the previous 15 months	3	40–90%
DM 12 ▶ The percentage of patients with diabetes in whom the last blood pressure is 145/85 or less	18	40–60%

Indicator	Points	Payment stages
DM 13 ▶ The percentage of patients with diabetes who have a record of micro-albuminuria testing in the previous 15 months (exception reporting for patients with proteinuria)	3	40–90%
DM 22 ▶ The percentage of patients with diabetes who have a record of estimated glomerular filtration rate (eGFR) or serum creatinine testing in the previous 15 months	3	40–90%
DM 15 ▶ The percentage of patients with diabetes with a diagnosis of proteinuria or micro-albuminuria who are treated with ACE inhibitors (or A2 antagonists)	3	40–80%
DM 16 ▶ The percentage of patients with diabetes who have a record of total cholesterol in the previous 15 months	3	40–90%
DM 17 ▶ The percentage of patients with diabetes whose last measured total cholesterol within the previous 15 months is 5 mmol/L or less	6	40–70%
DM 18 ▶ The percentage of patients with diabetes who have had influenza immunisation in the preceding 1 September to 31 March	3	40–85%

Chronic kidney disease

Indicator	Points	Payment stages
Records		
CKD 1 ▶ The practice can produce a register of patients aged 18 years and over with chronic kidney disease (CKD) (US National Kidney Foundation: Stage 3 to 5 CKD)	6	
Initial management		
CKD 2 ▶ The percentage of patients on the CKD register whose notes have a record of blood pressure in the previous 15 months	6	40–90%
Ongoing management		
CKD 3 ▶ The percentage of patients on the CKD register in whom the last blood pressure reading, measured in the previous 15 months, is 140/85 or less	11	40–70%

Indicator	Points	Payment stages
CKD 5 ▶ The percentage of patients on the CKD register with hypertension and proteinuria who are treated with an angiotensin-converting enzyme inhibitor (ACE-I) or angiotensin receptor blocker (ARB) (unless a contraindication or side effects are recorded)	9	40–80%
CKD 6 ▶ The percentage of patients on the CKD register whose notes have a record of a urine albumin: creatinine ratio (or protein: creatinine ratio) test in the previous 15 months	6	40–80%

Atrial fibrillation

Indicator	Points	Payment stages
Records		
AF 1 ▶ The practice can produce a register of patients with atrial fibrillation	5	
Initial diagnosis		
AF 4 ▶ The percentage of patients with atrial fibrillation diagnosed after 1 April 2008 with ECG or specialist confirmed diagnosis	10	40–90%
Ongoing management		
AF 3 ▶ The percentage of patients with atrial fibrillation who are currently treated with anticoagulation drug therapy or an antiplatelet therapy	12	40–90%

Obesity

Indicator	Points	Payment stages
Records		
OB 1 ▶ The practice can produce a register of patients aged 16 and over with a BMI greater than or equal to 30 in the previous 15 months	8	

Smoking

Indicator	Points	Payment stages
Ongoing management		
Smoking 3 ▶ The percentage of patients with any or any combination of the following conditions: coronary heart disease, stroke or TIA, hypertension, diabetes, COPD, CKD, asthma, schizophrenia, bipolar affective disorder or other psychoses whose notes record smoking status in the previous 15 months	30	40–90%
Smoking 4 ▶ The percentage of patients with any or any combination of the following conditions: coronary heart disease, stroke or TIA, hypertension, diabetes, COPD, CKD, asthma, schizophrenia, bipolar affective disorder or other psychoses who smoke whose notes contain a record that smoking cessation advice or referral to a specialist service, where available, has been offered within the previous 15 months	30	40–90%

Index

309